CHOLECYSTECTOMIES

PROCEDURES, PROGNOSIS AND POTENTIAL COMPLICATIONS

HEPATOLOGY RESEARCH AND CLINICAL DEVELOPMENTS

Additional books in this series can be found on Nova's website under the Series tab.

Additional E-books in this series can be found on Nova's website under the E-book tab.

SURGERY - PROCEDURES, COMPLICATIONS, AND RESULTS

Additional books in this series can be found on Nova's website under the Series tab.

Additional E-books in this series can be found on Nova's website under the E-book tab.

CHOLECYSTECTOMIES

PROCEDURES, PROGNOSIS AND POTENTIAL COMPLICATIONS

MIYU AKIYAMA

AND

SATOMI KUNOMASU

EDITORS

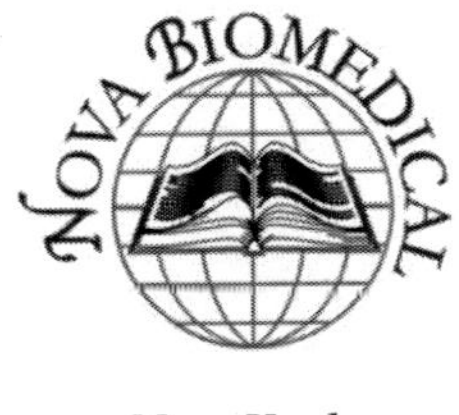

New York

For permission to use material from this book please contact us:
Telephone 631-231-7269; Fax 631-231-8175
Web Site: http://www.novapublishers.com

NOTICE TO THE READER

Additional color graphics may be available in the e-book version of this book.

Library of Congress Cataloging-in-Publication Data

ISBN: 978-1-62257-890-0
Library of Congress Control Number: 2012947881

Published by Nova Science Publishers, Inc. † New York

Contents

Preface

Cholecystecomy is the surgical removal of the gallbladder. It is the definitive treatment for symptomatic gallstones and non-neoplastic gallbladder disease. In this book, the authors present current research in the study of the procedures, prognosis and potential complications of cholecystectomies. Topics include the techniques and indications of cholecystectomy; traditional laparoscopic cholecystectomy; iatrogenic bile duct injuries after cholecystectomy; surgical strategy for gallbladder carcinoma; cholecystectomy in patients with suspected choledocholithiasis and cholecystitis in the elderly; and single-incision laparoscopic cholecystectomy.

Chapter I – Cholecystectomy is the procedure of choice to treat uncomplicated cholelithiasis. The classical open approach is increasingly being replaced by the less invasive laparoscopic approach, which minimizes postoperative discomfort and shortens in-hospital stay. More recently, single incision laparoscopic cholecystectomy (SILC) and natural orifice translumenal endoscopic surgery (NOTES) have been introduced, although their possible advantages and indications are currently under debate. In case of biliary acute pancreatitis, cholecystectomy is also necessary. Here the timing of surgery is important, since although the procedure must be performed with no delay, upon recovery, waiting until resolution is advisable if fluid collections are present.

Cholecystectomy is also the procedure of choice in case of acute cholecystitis. The timing of surgery has been controversial until recent years. Although the classical therapeutic scheme consisted of initial antibiotic treatment followed by cholecystectomy several months later, now there is enough evidence to support emergency cholecystectomy (usually in the first 72 hours). In addition to surgery, it is necessary to put patients on antibiotic treatment covering the expected microbes, including the extended-spectrum beta-lactamase-producing organisms in high-risk cases. A controversial issue, seldom analyzed in the literature, is antibiotic therapy duration in the postoperative period. In our own experience, there is no indication to prolong therapy in uncomplicated cases after four days.

An alternative procedure to surgery in high-risk cases is percutaneous cholecystostomy. This procedure, combined with antibiotics, can achieve resolution of the inflammatory bout, although when compared with emergency surgery offers little advantage. It ought to be used only in patients with surgical contraindications.

Major complications, either intraoperative or postoperative, are uncommon, although potentially severe. Bleeding is possible from the surgical bed or the port sites. Surgical site infection can develop, especially in cases of acute cholecystitis. Biliary leak can arise from the gallbladder bed or the cystic duct. However the most severe complications are those produced by direct lesion of the biliary tree. Even in experienced hands, the rate is higher in laparoscopic than in open cholecystectomy. If the lesion is intraoperatively recognized and treated, the prognosis is better than those unrecognized and, therefore, treated with delay. Some of them can be managed by endoscopic methods but others need major surgical procedures.

Chapter II – Removal of the gallbladder has been long recognized as the best treatment for symptomatic gallstones. Incisions have evolved from laparotomy and extended Kocher's incision to "minilap" cholecystectomy. The revolutionary era of multi-port laparoscopic surgery in the 1980's- 90's saw transformation in the approach with much improved outcomes to the patient especially in terms of recovery. This is currently accepted as the standard operation for gallbladder disease. The authors are now witnessing another change that is not yet accepted as standard. Single port laparoscopy is "in vogue" and is still trying to prove itself as a sustainable alternative to multi- port laparoscopy. The obvious benefit is cosmesis but the long-term issues with hernia and pain are still to be discerned. Natural orifice cholecystectomy is still investigational and the advantages unproven.

In open cholecystectomy, a right subcostal incision is preferred. The "dome down" technique is utilized with careful dissection performed from the gallbladder fundus towards the neck. Along this path, the cystic artery must be identified and ligated. The cystic duct must be identified with absolute certainty prior to ligation. The incision must be carefully closed to avoid future hernia.

Laparoscopic Cholecystectomy possesses more versatility. The multiple incision approach involves placing a 12mm port peri-umbilically, a 5mm port in the right abdomen for gallbladder retraction and 2 left abdominal operating ports (5-10mm). The single incision approach involves a larger umbilical incision and specialized port that allows for 3 instruments. In either technique the gallbladder can be approached from a "dome down" perspective, similar to open surgery, or by exposing the "critical view". The latter entails retracting the gallbladder cranio-laterally to expose Calot's triangle and identifying the cystic duct and artery carefully before ligation. Various energy sources can then be utilized to dissect the gallbladder off of its bed and gain hemostasis. Specialized retrieval devices aid extraction of the organ from the umbilical incision.

Injury to the common bile duct (CBD) remains the most feared pitfall of gallbladder surgery. The 1990's saw a wave of high laparoscopic CBD injuries but with time, this has settled to be on par with open cholecystectomy. Proponents of intra-op cholangiography argue that it reduces the incidence, but this is unproven. Minor injuries may be repaired primarily with the support of a T-tube but larger injuries usually require hepaticojejunostomy for definitive repair. Additionally, repair should only be attempted by experienced surgeons. The morbidity associated with CBD injuries is significant. Other potential complications include retention of calculi within the biliary system, bleeding, hernias and infection. As with all procedures, complication rates decrease with as the surgeon gains experience.

Chapter III – Iatrogenic Bile duct injuries (IBDI) are complex clinical situations usually caused by surgeons in healthy patients, and are associated with significant morbidity and low, but no negligible, mortality. IBDI can result from surgery (cholecystectomy, liver transplants and other procedures) or non-surgical procedures (tumour ablative therapies [RF], liver biopsies, TIPS or external radiation therapy). Most of IBDI occurs performing a cholecystectomy. Since Carl Langebuch performed the first open cholecystectomy in 1882 until now, IBDI has been an inherent complication of this surgery due to the surgeon's perceptive error. Laparoscopic cholecystectomy (LC) has led to a decrease in postoperative pain and hospital stay, but unfortunately has increased some complications such as IBDI. In a meta-analysis of more than 78 747 LCs, the IBDI incidence ranged from 0.36%-0.47%. For treating IBDI correctly, high level of scrutiny in the intraoperative and immediate postoperative phases is required, and also a multidisciplinary approach between surgeons, radiologists and gastroenterologists to offer the patient the best initial diagnosis, the best treatment options and better management of complications and follow-up is needed.

This chapter is intended to describe the current status of the literature on this type of injury and its therapeutic management.

Chapter IV – Background: Bile duct injury (BDI) following cholecystectomy is a severe and potentially life-threatening complication associated with significant morbidity and mortality and high rates of medical malpractice litigation. With the small number of patients having BDI recognized in each center, a prospective comparative study is difficult to perform.

Methods: A review of the English language literature listed on Medline database, concerning BDI following cholecystectomy, was performed.

Results: Although a rate of BDI following cholecystectomy is recently stabilized at 0.1-0.7% in the literature, higher incidence of BDI is reported to be occurred in the setting of laparoscopic approach. In addition, BDI following laparoscopic cholecystectomy often involves complete disruption and excision of bile ducts, and may be associated with hepatic artery injuries. Factors which have been associated with BDI include surgeon experience, patient age, male sex, and acute cholecystitis. The safety of cholecystectomy requires careful dissection and correct identification of the relevant anatomy to ensure the "critical view of safety" prior to dividing any structures. Increasing evidence suggests that prompt recognition and diagnosis of BDI directly affect outcome, and that it should be managed by an experienced hepatobiliary surgeon. Since patients with BDI may require long-term follow-up due to possible delayed biliary stricture, the outcome and quality of life after BDI remains poor.

Conclusion: Although it can and should be regarded as preventable, bile duct injury following cholecystectomy is still one of the most severe and complicated events especially in the era of laparoscopic cholecystectomy. A great effort must continue to be taken to highlight seriousness of this catastrophic complication and to reduce its incidence.

Chapter V – In the treatment of patients with symptomatic cholelithiasis and possible choledocholithiasis (CBDS) there is not an algorithm that is fully accepted. Therefore the management of these patients depends upon the availability, capability and skill of the surgical and endoscopic teams involved in the process. There is consensus to perform preoperative ERCP if the patient can be classified as a high risk for CBDS following the ASGE guideline 2010. There is also complete agreement to not perform any other diagnostic or therapeutic radiologic or endoscopic studies if the patient has a low risk of CBDS. However when the patient has an intermediate risk of CBDS, and in order to avoid risky and unnecessary procedures (such as preoperative ERCP) there are a range of therapeutic options available to use (Intraoperative ERCP, Postoperative ERCP, Laparoscopic management of CBDS) whenever an intraoperative cholangiography (IOC) shows the CBDS. Magnetic resonance cholangiopancreatography (MRC) for imaging the biliary tract and endoscopic ultrasound (EUS) are very helpful to diagnose CBDS in this setting. However not every hospital in the world has these facilities available and nor have they easy or timely access to them. It is important to know that in spite of the fact of their availability there are patients with contradictory radiological and clinical results (normal MRCP with persistently pathologic liver tests not justifiable by other reasons). In these cases the authors can use IOC during Laparoscopic Cholecistectomy as a definitive radiological test to determine whether or not it will be necessary to use Intraoperative or postoperative ERCP or laparoscopic management of CBDS. Postoperative ECP is a good choice with some drawbacks such as it is a two-stage treatment that in case of failure can be followed by another surgical operation. The laparoscopic management of CBDS is a single–stage treatment which needs a very good and experienced surgical team, and in order to reach this skill it requires a long learning curve. Intraoperative ERCP has the advantage of being a single-stage treatment that can be used all over the world, that has a significant success rate, an easy learning curve, low morbidity involving a shorter hospital stay and lower costs than the two-stage treatments (postoperative and preoperative ERCP). Intraoperative ERCP is also a good salvage treatment when preoperative ERCP fails or when total laparoscopic management is not successful thereby avoiding open cholecystectomies. It also has some drawbacks such as the need for good coordination between surgical and endoscopic teams and that cholecistectomy must be practically completed before the ERCP is performed.

Chapter VI – *Background.* Complications from gallstone disease continue to cause patient morbidity and mortality, although less frequently now. Complications of gallstone disease are more likely to result in difficult cholecystectomies. A difficult cholecystectomy refers to a case in which exposure of the critical anatomy necessary to conduct a safe procedure is challenging as a result of acute inflammation, dense scarring, gallstone impaction, bleeding, liver pathology or hepatobiliary anatomy. These difficult laparoscopic cholecystectomies demand advanced strategies to ensure safe operative approaches.

Aim. To review the evidence-based advanced operative procedures for difficult laparoscopic cholecystectomies, and outcomes of these approaches for difficult gall bladder problems.

Methods. A review of literature databases of PubMed, MEDLINE, EMBASE, and SCOPUS was performed. Advanced operative approaches for difficult laparoscopic cholecystectomy and their outcomes in patients with gangrenous cholecystitis, inflamed mega-gall bladder, perforated gall bladder, a short or large cystic duct, Mirizzi syndrome and cholecystectomy in liver cirrhosis and portal hypertension are reviewed. Factors influencing the decision to convert to open cholecystectomy are discussed.

Results. From a review of 100 studies including 2 meta-analyses, 12 randomized controlled trials (RCTs), and 86 prospective and retrospective studies, several different operative approaches for a difficult cholecystectomy were identified. They include fundus-first/dome down approach, ultrasonic dissection with or without fundus first or half-dome approach and subtotal/partial cholecystectomy. Another approach, the half dome down approach, is also discussed.

From the existing literature, the fundus-first approach, ultrasonic dissection and subtotal cholecystectomy have been found to reduce the rate of conversion of a laparoscopic to open cholecystectomy with no associated increase in the risk of injury to the liver, duodenum, colon or the biliary tree. They have been found to lower the complication rates. Ultrasonic dissection has been demonstrated to be safe and very valuable for bloodless dissection especially in acute cholecystitis, but a learning curve exists. There is also a risk of thermal injury from instrument misuse. With these techniques, outcomes similar to standard retrograde cholecystectomy for uncomplicated and acute cholecystitis can be reached.

Conclusion. Advanced operative approaches for difficult laparoscopic cholecystectomy should be considered prior to converting to open cholecystectomy. In situation where it is still difficult to perform a safe laparoscopic cholecystectomy or the surgeon is inexperienced, conversion to open cholecystectomy should be considered or the patient referred to an experienced center.

Chapter VII – *Background.* Acute cholecystitis in the elderly is a serious condition with high operative mortality and morbidity. Both acute cholecystitis and high age are significant risk factors for mortality and prolonged hospital stay after cholecystectomy.

Methods. A review of the English language literature listed on Medline database, concerning cholecystectomy for acute cholecystitis in the elderly, was performed.

Results. It is generally accepted that early cholecystectomy is the preferred approach for most patients with acute cholecystitis, and laparoscopic cholecystectomy is increasingly advocated for experienced surgeons. Several randomized controlled trials that compared early surgery with delayed one found that early surgery had the advantages of shorter operation time, less blood loss, and less length of hospital stay. Results of randomized controlled trials comparing early and delayed laparoscopic cholecystectomy have also shown that early laparoscopic surgery is superior to delayed surgery in terms of the conversion rate to open surgery, complication rate, and total hospital stay. On the other hand, recent reports still showed that acute cholecystitis in the elderly may be associated with higher morbidity and mortality. Some encouraging papers demonstrated early laparoscopic cholecystectomy in the elderly patients suffering from acute cholecystitis is feasible and effective if an appropriate surgery candidate is selected.

Conclusion. The elderly patients with acute cholecystitis still represent a challenging group and need to be carefully managed. Early laparoscopic cholecystectomy is a safe, effective treatment option for acute cholecystitis if an appropriate selection for candidate is secured.

Chapter VIII – The surgical strategy for gallbladder carcinoma (GBC) depends on the extent of disease, especially the T-stage in TNM classification. Our institution has developed an original surgical strategy for GBC based on the accumulation of clinical and pathological studies. The previous study about the efficacy of extended surgical resection, such as hepatectomy, extrahepatic bile duct resection (BDR) or pancreatoduodenectomy (PD) in T2 and T3 GBC revealed that S4a+5 hepatectomy combined with BDR and regional lymphadenectomy is recommendable for the treatment of T2 or T3 GBC. An original scoring system, the "subserosal cancer invasion score (ss score)" was developed to discriminate favorable cases in T2 GBC. The score divides the lesion into three categories: ss minimum (ss min), ss medium (ss med), and ss massive (ss mas) and our previous study indicated the survival of an ss min GBC patient would be satisfactory with simple cholecystectomy. The authors focused on the phenomena of dedifferentiation (DD) and tumor budding (BD), which have been reported as markers predictive of poor prognosis in other malignancies, particularly in colorectal cancer and analyzed 80 consecutive patients with GBC exceeding stage T1b. This study revealed both BD and DD correlated significantly with survival in patients with T2 tumor whereas no prognostic impact was evident in patients with other T-stage of tumor. Our accumulated experience and studies enable us to select meticulous surgical strategies for individual patients. However, practical use of these strategies in clinical settings requires close cooperation between surgeons and pathologists.

Chapter IX – Laparoscopic cholecystectomy is the gold standard for the treatment of gallbladder stone disease. The advantages of this procedure compared with the open approach include less postoperative pain, shorter recovery time and better cosmetic results. In recent years, many surgeons have attempted to reduce the number and size of ports to decrease parietal trauma and improve cosmetic results. The first step was to remove the fourth trocar that is used to grasp the fundus of the gallbladder, pulling upward and outward to expose Calot's triangle or to retract the liver. A recent meta-analysis of randomized clinical trials confirms that three port technique has similar operating time, success rate, analgesia requirement and postoperative hospital stay.

In the past three years laparoendoscopic single-site surgery (LESS) has also gained greater interest and diffusion as a less invasive laparoscopic cholecystectomy. The cosmetic outcomes of LESS are expected to be better when the operation is performed through the umbilicus because the surgical wound is hidden within the umbilicus, leaving no visible abdominal scars, virtually "scarless" surgery. The best procedure to evaluate a new technology and/or an innovative surgical technique is a prospective trial comparing the new technique with the gold standard. Otherwise a literature review of the best available evidence is necessary to make the best choice. This critical review aims to evaluate the feasibility and safety of LESS cholecystectomy versus the three-port technique through a comparative analysis of five parameters: mean operative time, intraoperative and postoperative complications, conversion to open, conversion to the four-trocar technique and postoperative hospital stay. Although LESS cholecystectomy is a fashionable technique there are few data available for an evidence-based determination as to the real benefits of this technique. Well-designed comparative studies are suggested to validate the clinical benefits, missing the cosmetic outcome, and ensure that there are no new complications or added costs associated with the new technique. Laparoscopic cholecystectomy (LC) is the gold standard for the treatment of gallbladder stone disease. The advantages of this procedure compared with the open approach include less postoperative pain, shorter recovery time and better cosmetic results.

Chapter X – *Introduction:* In general, the term of single-incision laparoscopic cholecystectomy (SILC) has become familiar with the introduction of natural orifice transluminal endoscopic surgery (NOTES) technique. NOTES needs the special surgical instruments, however, SILC can perform by ordinary laparoscopic instruments without any limitations. Therefore, SILC became an attractive surgical procedure from 2007. In fact, the authors had already started SILC using an abdominal wall-lift method from 1997. However, its outcomes were not acceptable compared with conventional laparoscopic techniques regarding a long operation time, insufficient operative devices and more surgical stress for surgeons. After several novel surgical instruments were introduced into the laparoscopic surgery, SILC was rapidly progressed in many surgical fields. At this time, the authors are performing SILC using the several new devices consisting of Endo-Grab[TM], MIT port[TM] and pre-bent instruments for the purpose of the elimination of port or instruments, the reduction of clashing between the instruments and laparoscope. The authors report our technique of SILC and a review of the literature.

Patients and Surgical technique: SILC was performed in 74 patients (40 males, 34 females). The median age was 57 years (range, 30-86 years).The indications for surgery included gallbladder stones in 65 patients (87.7%) and polyps in 9 (12.3%). Under general anesthesia, the authors made a 2.5-cm skin incision at umbilicus. In pneumoperitoneum method, the incision was applied a wound retractor and a surgical glove or another devices. The authors used three 5-mm ports technique. In an abdominal wall-lift method, the authors created using the original abdominal-wall lift with a rigid bar.

Two or three 5-mm ports were placed through the same umbilical incision. After retracting the gallbladder upward using an Endo-Grab^{TM}, the cystic duct and artery were divided and identified using pre-bend forceps through the MIT port^{TM} and a laparoscopic coagulating shears (LCS). The cystic artery was dissected by LCS and the cystic duct was also dissected by shears after clipping. The gallbladder was free from the liver bed using LCS. The specimen was retrieved from the umbilical wound.

Results: All procedures were completed without a conversion to open laparotomy. There were no intraoperative complications. The additional ports were required in 3 (4%) cases. The abdominal wall-lift method was changed to pneumoperitoneum in 2 cases (16.7%) out of 10 due to the difficulty of procedure. The Endo-Grab^{TM} eliminated the retraction of the gallbladder by grasping forceps. The mean operative time was 67 min (range, 34-95 min) in the last 20 cases. The MIT port ^{TM} and pre-bend forceps reduced the clashing between the instruments and laparoscope at the intra- and extra-peritoneal cavities. The authors have to be careful to injure the viscera by the hook locating at the both sides of Endo-Grab^{TM}.

Conclusion: SILC is a feasible and safe procedure under the pneumoperitoneum by experienced surgeons. The Endo-Grab^{TM}, MIT port^{TM} and pre-bend forceps were very useful in the performance of SILC with the elimination of abdominal instruments and the reduction of clashing between the instruments and laparoscope.

Chapter XI – Laparoscopic cholecystectomy has been accepted by the surgical community as the "standard of care" for the treatment of biliary disease. When compared to open cholecystectomy, laparoscopic approaches do carry a higher complication rate for biliary injury but offer many beneficial advantages in reduced postoperative pain and shorter recovery times. With the introduction of single incision approaches to cholecystectomy, it is important that the surgical community maintain similar operative standards as these new techniques are introduced into clinical practice. This article will focus on the outcomes and complications of laparoscopic cholecystectomy as well as ways to reduce these potential injuries. The role for intraoperative cholangiography will also be addressed. It will also analyze the available data regarding single incision cholecystectomy with regards to advantages and potential complications from this new and evolving operative technique.

Chapter XII – Several case series have been published demonstrating the feasibility of single site laparoscopic cholecystectomy in both the adult and pediatric population with satisfactory results. The advantage of the procedure, as compared to traditional multi-port laparoscopic cholecystectomy, is to achieve better cosmesis and decrease post-operative pain. Several reports have addressed the outcomes and complication rates, reporting the safety and feasibility of the procedure. This chapter describes preoperative preparation, instrumentation and details of the procedure. Also, it discusses the outcomes and complication rates of laparoscopic single site cholecystectomy as compared to multi-port laparoscopic cholecystectomy. Being cosmetically superior with comparable outcomes to multi-port laparoscopic cholecystectomy, the single site approach can be easily performed with standard laparoscopic instruments and techniques.

In: Cholecystectomies
Editors: Miyu Akiyama and Satomi Kunomasu

ISBN: 978-1-62257-890-0
© 2013 Nova Science Publishers, Inc.

Chapter I

Cholecystectomies: Procedures, Prognosis and Potential Complications

Juan C. Rodríguez-Sanjuán, Roberto Fernández-Santiago, Federico Castillo, Luis A. Herrera and Manuel Gómez-Fleitas
Hepato-biliary Unit, Department of General Surgery
University Hospital Marqués de Valdecilla
University of Cantabria, Santander, Spain

Abstract

Cholecystectomy is the procedure of choice to treat uncomplicated cholelithiasis. The classical open approach is increasingly being replaced by the less invasive laparoscopic approach, which minimizes postoperative discomfort and shortens in-hospital stay. More recently, single incision laparoscopic cholecystectomy (SILC) and natural orifice translumenal endoscopic surgery (NOTES) have been introduced, although their possible advantages and indications are currently under debate. In case of biliary acute pancreatitis, cholecystectomy is also necessary. Here the timing of surgery is important, since although the procedure must be performed with no delay, upon recovery, waiting until resolution is advisable if fluid collections are present.

Cholecystectomy is also the procedure of choice in case of acute cholecystitis. The timing of surgery has been controversial until recent years. Although the classical therapeutic scheme consisted of initial antibiotic treatment followed by cholecystectomy several months later, now there is enough evidence to support emergency cholecystectomy (usually in the first 72 hours).

In addition to surgery, it is necessary to put patients on antibiotic treatment covering the expected microbes, including the extended-spectrum beta-lactamase-producing organisms in high-risk cases A controversial issue, seldom analyzed in the literature, is antibiotic therapy duration in the postoperative period. In our own experience, there is no indication to prolong therapy in uncomplicated cases after four days.

An alternative procedure to surgery in high-risk cases is percutaneous cholecystostomy. This procedure, combined with antibiotics, can achieve resolution of the inflammatory bout, although when compared with emergency surgery offers little advantage. It ought to be used only in patients with surgical contraindications.

Major complications, either intraoperative or postoperative, are uncommon, although potentially severe. Bleeding is possible from the surgical bed or the port sites. Surgical site infection can develop, especially in cases of acute cholecystitis. Biliary leak can arise from the gallbladder bed or the cystic duct. However the most severe complications are those produced by direct lesion of the biliary tree. Even in experienced hands, the rate is higher in laparoscopic than in open cholecystectomy. If the lesion is intraoperatively recognized and treated, the prognosis is better than those unrecognized and, therefore, treated with delay. Some of them can be managed by endoscopic methods but others need major surgical procedures.

Abbreviations

OC: open cholecystectomy
LC: laparoscopic cholecystectomy
AC: acute cholecystitis
SILC: single incision laparoscopic cholecystectomy
IOC: intraoperative cholangiography
NOTES: natural orifice translumenal surgery
BDI: bile duct injury
ERCP: Endoscopic retrograde cholangiopancreatography
PTC: percutaneous transhepatic cholangiography
MRCP: Magnetic resonance cholangiopancreatography

1. Cholecystectomy in Uncomplicated Gallstone Disease

A. Epidemiology

Gallstone disease is one of the most common of all digestive diseases. In 1999 it was estimated that 6.3 million men and 14.2 million women aged 20 to 74 in the United States had gallbladder disease (Everhart et al, 1999).

There are no known etiological factors of gallstone disease, but it appears related to hormonal factors and Western diet, there being an increased incidence in women over 40 years, multiparous and overweight. Age is also considered as a factor favoring the incidence of cholelithiasis since it is greater than 30% in those over 70 years (Attili et al, 1995).

Many studies have revealed a marked variation in overall gallstone prevalence between different ethnic populations. As a general rule, there appears to be higher rates of cholelithiasis in western Caucasian, Hispanic, and Native American populations and lower rates in eastern European, African American, and Japanese populations (Velo Bellver et al, 1996).

B. Clinical Picture and Diagnosis

Although cholelithiasis is highly prevalent in the general population, and increases with longevity, only a small proportion develops symptoms. The most common clinical manifestation (80%) of gallstones is biliary colic and appears annually in the 1 to 4% of patients with asymptomatic cholelithiasis (McSherry et al, 1985). The clinical picture consists of right upper quadrant pain, sometimes radiating to the back, with nausea and vomiting, but with normal abdominal examination. At other times it may present as epigastric pain or biliary dyspepsia. Laboratory studies are usually normal in patients with cholelithiasis both during asymptomatic periods and during biliary colic. However, some laboratory studies such as liver biochemical tests, serum amylase and lipase, complete blood count and urine analysis can be helpful for excluding other diagnoses. The most useful imaging study to detect the presence of gallstones is ultrasonography because it is non-invasive, readily available, inexpensive, does not expose the patient to ionizing radiation and sensitivity and specificity were estimated at 84% and 99% respectively (Shea et al, 1994).

In patients with cholelithiasis and biliary symptoms, surgical treatment is recommended (Schmidt et al, 2011) because the risk of more severe symptoms and complications occurs in 70% of cases in the first two years after the onset of symptoms (Thistle et al, 1984). This treatment consists of cholecystectomy, which has become one of the abdominal surgical procedures most commonly performed and in the last 25 years has undergone a revolution in terms of its approach.

C. Surgical Treatment

The first cholecystectomy was successfully performed by the German Karl Langenbuch on July 15, 1882 (Praderi, 1982). Previously, in 1474 in Paris, there was the first surgical examination of the gallbladder in a man with biliary colic and amazingly he survived the operation, earning him the pardon of his death sentence (Trinchet Hernandez et al, 1996). Open cholecystectomy (OC) was the technique of choice until the 1988 publication of the new technique of laparoscopic cholecystectomy (LC), first performed in Lyon in 1987 by Mouret and perfected and reported upon by Dubois in 1988 (Dubois et al, 1989) and that meant one of the best innovations of modern surgery. In recent years the laparoscopic technique has become the gold standard but it is evolving into other minimally invasive techniques such as single-incision laparoscopic cholecystectomy (SILC) and natural orifice translumenal endoscopic surgery (NOTES), in order to further minimize postoperative sequelae.

Open Cholecystectomy

OC was the commonest performed surgery for the treatment of cholelithiasis from 1882 until the 1980s. Today the most frequent indication for OC is the inability to safely complete a LC. Currently the overall rate of conversion to open surgery is between 8.9% and 11% (Kaafarani et al, 2010; Ingraham et al, 2010; Navez et al, 2012) although in uncomplicated cholelithiasis this rate is lower. Predictors of conversion to OC include age, male gender, emergency status, serum albumin (<1g/dL) and previous abdominal surgery (Kaafarani et al, 2010). The causes of conversion from laparoscopic to open surgery include the inability to access the surgical site due to adhesions, surgical failure to identify with certainty the cystic duct and cystic artery after 20-30 minutes, presence of anatomical variants – which may involve vascular or biliary injury- suspected gallbladder cancer and uncontrollable intraoperative complications by laparoscopy (Keus et al, 2006).

In some cases, the operation should not be started laparoscopically and OC should be planned in patients who are unable to tolerate pneumoperitoneum, patients who are suspected to have gallbladder cancer, critically ill patients who require open surgery for other intraabdominal pathology, patients with a history of a cholecystoenteric fistula and patients with cirrhosis or portal hypertension.

Before performing OC, the patient should be given antibiotic prophylaxis. In most centers a single dose of intravenous cefazolin 2 g. in the hour prior to surgical incision is recommended (Bratzler et al, 2004). Prophylaxis of thromboembolic disease with low molecular weight heparin must also be performed.

The incision used is the right subcostal –Kocher incision-, 3 cm. under the costal margin (García Valdecasas et al, 1988). After exposure of the surgical field, it is necessary to identify the cystic duct and cystic artery at Calot's triangle -the region in the liver bed bounded by the cystic artery, cystic duct, and common hepatic duct (Calot 1890). Unequivocal identification of the cystic duct and cystic artery is critical in order to avoid injury to the common duct, right hepatic artery, and aberrant right hepatic branch duct. Identification of the cystic duct and artery begins with proper retraction and careful dissection. The fundus of the gallbladder is grasped with a clamp and retracted superiorly. This helps to expose the infundibulum of the gallbladder. The area above the infundibulum is grasped and retracted inferiorly and to the right. The peritoneum over the infundibulum of the gallbladder is incised and stripped down along with the fat toward the common duct. The "critical view of safety" must be achieved prior to the clipping or ligation of the cystic duct and artery (Avgerinos et al, 2009). The critical view of safety is achieved by dissecting Calot's triangle free of all tissue except for the cystic duct and cystic artery and by exposing the base of the liver bed by freeing the lower part of the gallbladder from the liver. When this view is achieved, the only structures entering the gallbladder can be the cystic duct and artery, and injury to major structures is avoided. It is not necessary to visualize the common duct to obtain the critical view of safety. The cystic duct should not be clipped or divided until the surgeon is certain that the cystic duct goes directly into the gallbladder, and that there are no other ductal structures coursing between the base of the gallbladder and the liver bed. It is not necessary to routinely open the peritoneum over the common duct. If a top down approach is planned, the cystic duct is left looped until it is ready for ligation at the completion of the dissection. Often, the cystic artery can be unequivocally identified going onto the gallbladder and this can be doubly looped or ligated prior to freeing the gallbladder from the liver bed. An unusually wide cystic duct should prompt the surgeon to recheck the anatomy. If the structure is unequivocally identified as the cystic duct, it may be opened and "milked" if it is suspected to harbor substantial stone debris. It should then be sutured or ligated. If possible, a long or large cystic duct remnant, possibly harboring stone debris and sludge, should be avoided since it may predispose to postcholecystectomy complications or choledocholithiasis.

After the cystic duct is identified, the cystic artery is located. The cystic artery usually has an anterior and posterior branch, and can typically be found in Calot's triangle with its anterior branch going up onto the gallbladder. The anterior branch is ligated on the gallbladder. The cystic artery is ligated in Calot's triangle if it is small. Otherwise, it is secured with a double loop of silk suture and temporarily occluded. If there is concern that the structure could be a diminutive right hepatic artery, a vessel loop can be used for temporary occlusion. Then, the vessel must be dissected to the entrance into the gallbladder wall or, otherwise, to the entrance in the liver.

For the dissection of the gallbladder from the liver, there are two options: While most surgeons perform LC "from the bottom of the gallbladder (infundibulum) up", (bottom up) many surgeons perform OC from the "top of the gallbladder (fundus or dome) down" (top down) in order to avoid injury to major structures. The top down approach should be used if there is uncertainty about the location of the cystic duct and artery in relation to other named structures in the hilum of the liver. If the surgeon has identified the cystic duct and artery with certainty, it should be equally safe to remove the gallbladder from the top down or from the bottom up (Salembier, 1988).

Abdominal drains are not routinely recommended since there is risk of increasing surgical site infections (Gurusamy et al, 2007). Two plane closure of the abdominal incision is recommended.

Laparoscopic Cholecystectomy

Cholecystectomy is probably the laparoscopic procedure most often performed, and is today considered the "gold standard" surgical treatment of uncomplicated cholelithiasis. Approximately 90% of these are performed laparoscopically (Csikesz et al, 2010). It is a safe and effective procedure, of low technical complexity, fast and with a low rate of conversion to open surgery. In addition, patients undergoing LC exhibit less postoperative pain, lower rate of surgical wound infection, shorter hospital stay and faster postoperative return to their work (Soper et al, 1992, Schirmer et al, 1991; Gurusamy et al, 2008). Its drawback is a slightly higher complication rate than open surgery, especially injury of the bile duct (Vollmer et al, 2007).

The only absolute contraindication to performing LC in uncomplicated cholelithiasis is the inability of the patient to tolerate general anesthesia and or pneumoperitoneum (Keus et al, 2006). Other conditions such as morbid obesity, pregnancy, previous abdominal surgery and severe associated comorbidities are considered relative contraindications as they will depend on the anesthesia team and the surgeon's experience.

Preoperative preparation with regard to thromboembolic and antibiotic prophylaxis is the same as that used in open surgery (Bratzler et al, 2004). The necessary laparoscopic instruments consist of four trocars or working ports (2 of 10 mm and 2 of 5 mm), an optical sight that can be angled 0° or 30°, two atraumatic graspers, curved dissector, curved scissors, a suction-irrigator with a blunt end, an automatic clip applier and isolated hook connected to monopolar coagulation.

In the art for performing LC there are two variants that differ in the position of the surgeon and trocar placement. In the U.S. position the surgeon stands on the patient's left side and puts a 10 mm trocar at umbilicus for the camera, a 10 mm trocar in the subxyphoid midline to introduce the working instruments, a 5 mm trocar in the right midclavicular line for grasping Hartmann's pouch and another of 5 mm in the right anterior axillary line for cranial traction of the gallbladder. In the French technique the patient is placed in a modified lithotomy position with legs apart while at the same level as the operating table. The surgeon stands between the patient's legs and the assistant on the left. A 10 mm umbilical trocar is inserted for the camera, another 10 mm trocar for the working instruments on the left flank, at the umbilicus level, outside the rectus sheath, a 5-mm trocar symmetric to the previous position on the right side for traction and gallbladder infundibulum and another one of 5 mm for the separation of the liver and gallbladder cranial traction (Paredes et al, 2003; Targarona Soler et al, 2010). Neither position has shown advantages over the other and the choice will depend on the training and preferences of each surgeon (Overby et al, 2010).

The first step after the initial preparation is the creation of pneumoperitoneum aimed at creating space for operative laparoscopy. The gas used is CO_2 as it has high diffusion, is not flammable and the risk of embolism is very low. The initial CO_2 insufflation can be performed in several ways. The first is using a Veress needle percutaneously inserted through the supraumbilical linea alba or, alternatively, at the left upper quadrant level. With a syringe with saline solution the placement in the abdominal cavity is confirmed. Then a 10 mm trocar is blindly inserted. The second way is the open technique with a Hasson trocar. This is done through a small minilaparotomy at umbilicus (Hasson, 1971) under direct vision, and is preferred in patients with previous abdominal surgery. There are no demonstrable differences in the safety of open versus closed techniques for establishing access (Ahmad et al, 2008); as a result SAGES guidelines recommend that decisions regarding choice of technique are left to the surgeon and should be based on individual training, skill, and case assessment (Overby et al, 2010). Other techniques are direct trocar placement without prior pneumoperitoneum, and the optical view technique, in which laparoscope placement within the trocar allows direct visualization of the layers of the abdominal wall as they are being traversed (Overby et al, 2010). Some surgeons have combined pneumoperitoneum with abdominal wall lift by using special devices, which leads to lower pressure. This decreases cardiopulmonary changes and thus, can help in high-risk patients, although it cannot be recommended routinely (Gurusamy et al, 2012).

The second step is exposure of the gallbladder and release of adhesions. Perivesicular adhesions are common but most may be freed with a gentle pull. If adhesions are fibrous they are sectioned with scissors or with a hook, progressing to fully release of the bladder neck. Then, the assistant pushes the gallbladder upward while the surgeon moves the infundibulum to the right and down.

The next step is cystic pedicle dissection. The most important consideration in a cholecystectomy is clear identification of the cystic artery and duct prior to division. A thorough dissection of Calot's triangle, bounded by the gallbladder wall, cystic duct, and common hepatic duct, to obtain the "critical view of safety", is a key step. The surgeon grasps the infundibulum with the left hand forceps and retracts it inferiorly and laterally to open the angle between the cystic duct and common duct. This instrument is used to provide retraction in various angles to give anterior and posterior exposure of the triangle. The dissection of the junction of the gallbladder and cystic duct is initiated by the surgeon gently stripping the peritoneum beginning high on the gallbladder. Keeping the dissection on a known safe structure (the gallbladder) to develop visualization of the unknown structures is an important principle.

The postero-lateral aspect of the gallbladder is the safest area for initial dissection and can be exposed by retracting the infundibulum medially and superiorly. The surgeon can use minimal cautery or blunt dissection to incise the superficial layer of peritoneum attaching the gallbladder neck to the liver in order to allow further retraction of the infundibulum. Anterior and posterior dissection continues with alternating infero-lateral and supero-medial retraction of the neck until the gallbladder is dissected away from the liver, creating a "window" crossed by two structures: the cystic duct and artery. This is the "critical view of safety" that should be achieved prior to clipping or dividing any tubular structure (Avgerinos et al, 2009). There is no need to dissect down to the cystic duct-common bile duct junction unless the cystic duct is very short. The cystic artery should be dissected in a similar fashion. Calot's node or cystic duct lymph node is usually encountered adjacent and anterior to the artery and can be a useful landmark. Electrocautery may be needed for hemostasis before the node can be bluntly swept down.

The surgeon should be aware of certain anatomic variations in order to avoid misidentification of structures. A common anomaly is the right hepatic artery looping onto the infundibulum and being mistaken for the cystic artery. A short cystic duct is also seen quite frequently and could drain into the right hepatic duct, the common duct, or a low-lying aberrant right sectoral duct. If there is a large stone in the neck of the gallbladder, the infundibulum may be "tethered" to the hepatic duct, which may lead the surgeon to misidentify the common bile duct for the cystic duct.

Sometimes the biliary anatomy is unclear or there is a high suspicion of choledocholithiasis, making it necessary to perform intraoperative cholangiography (IOC). A catheter is directly introduced in the abdominal cavity through the abdominal wall. Once clipped, the cystic duct is partially opened and the catheter is inserted (or in the gallbladder if the cystic duct is doubtful) and the dye is introduced under direct vision by fluoroscopy. This test should allow visualizing the cystic duct, the junction with the main bile duct, the presence of stones in the common bile duct or intrahepatic ducts and the passage of contrast into the duodenum as well as integrity of the entire biliary tree (Mellinger et al, 2008). There is no agreement among surgeons concerning the need of routinely performing IOC in the absence of suspicion of choledocholithiasis or bile duct injury (Overby et al, 2010). Some studies have suggested that routine use may decrease the risk of injury and improve lesion recognition (Waage et al, 2006), while other papers have suggested that IOC does not prevent them, although it helped in early identification (Debru et al, 2005). Intraoperative ultrasonography is also useful for identifying possible stones in bile duct but it requires much more experience (Perry et al, 2008). If common bile duct stones are found, they can be managed intraoperatively or postoperatively, through ERCP (Overby et al, 2010). This issue is beyond the scope of this chapter.

Next follows section of the duct and cystic artery. Once both structures are fully individualized, two clips are placed across the pedicle of the cystic duct and one on the gallbladder, cutting it with scissors. Cystic artery was clipped and sectioned in the same way. Once the two structures have been cut, the infundibulum is pulled up and out away from the biliary tree.

Retrograde gallbladder dissection is carried out from the bladder neck to the bottom. The vesicular peritoneum leaves are cut with the hook coagulator or scissors. The dissection plane is that closest to the gallbladder to minimize injury to the liver parenchyma and therefore, the risk of bleeding. The traction exerted by the counter assistant to lift up the gallbladder bed greatly facilitates dissection. During this dissection, much attention must be paid to the possible presence of accessory bile ducts that drain directly into the gallbladder.

Finally the gallbladder is extracted after it has been completely freed. It is introduced into a bag which enables extraction without risk of bile or stone leakage. The bag is left in the right subdiaphragmatic space and checks for hemostasis and biliostasis are carried out. Usually gallbladder extraction is performed through the umbilical trocar. Some surgeons feel that the subxyphoid site may be better for specimen extraction since it has a lower likelihood of hernia formation, although no formal study has ever been undertaken (Tonouchi et al, 2004). The fascial opening of 10 mm is closed with absorbable stitches and skin staples. Injection with local anesthetics of the trocar path reduces postoperative pain (Paredes et al, 2010; Borie et al, 2003).

Some surgeons perform the same technique but using only three trocars; at present there is no difference between surgical time, postoperative analgesia requirement and hospital stay (Sun et al, 2009), but with this technique the exposure of Calot's triangle is more difficult so there may be a higher risk of biliary or vascular injury.

Single-incision Laparoscopic Cholecystectomy (SILC)

Cholecystectomy through a single incision is an emerging technique that has been developed to improve outcomes of classical LC (Bresadola et al, 1999; Navarra et al, 1997). In this procedure, a special port with several orifices is inserted at the umbilicus –through a 1.5-2 cm incision-, to introduce a 5 mm camera and two articulating instruments which allow for triangulation on the target by crossing them. The theoretical advantages include reduced risk of wound infection, less postoperative pain, faster recovery and no cosmetic sequelae (Cuesta et al, 2008). Potential disadvantages of this technique include increased surgical time, long surgeon's learning curve and poorer exposure and vesicular mobilization (Edwards et al, 2010, Elsey et al, 2010; Ma et al, 2011) because it requires a modification to the conventional operative procedures, such as the level of triangulation of instruments and less room for retraction and manipulation of the gallbladder. All this implies a possible increase in iatrogenic injuries. At this moment, SILC offers no advantage over traditional LC with respect to patient satisfaction, postoperative pain or quality of life of patients (Ma et al, 2011). Large randomized studies are still needed in the long term to see if there are real advantages over traditional laparoscopy.

Cholecystectomy by Natural Orifice Translumenal Endoscopic Surgery (NOTES)

To maximize the potential benefits of minimally invasive surgery, a new concept in surgery, natural orifice translumenal endoscopic surgery, has been developed (Kalloo et al, 2004). NOTES is an emerging field within gastrointestinal surgery and interventional gastroenterology in which the surgeon accesses the peritoneal cavity via a hollow viscus and performs diagnostic and therapeutic procedures. The initial approach was transgastric, but more recently NOTES has been performed through other orifices, resulting in transcolonic, transvaginal, and transurethral/transcystic approaches. The approach has also been extended from the peritoneum to other compartments in the body, such as transesophageal approaches to the mediastinum and heart, transgastric intrauterine interventions in pregnant animals, and novel approaches to the vertebral column (Kantsevoy et al, 2006; Fritscher-Ravens et al, 2007; Giday et al, 2008; Magno et al, 2008).

At present, intervention most commonly performed by NOTES is cholecystectomy (85% in the German registration) (Lehmann et al, 2010) and the most widely used approach has been transvaginal, although most procedures have been hybrid, with laparoscopic assistance, and not pure NOTES (Zornig et al, 2009). Complications have been reported in 3% of patients and the rate of conversion to open or laparoscopic surgery is approximately 5%. One problem is that transvaginal access can lead to complications not directly related to cholecystectomy such as dyspareunia, infertility and urinary tract infections secondary to urinary catheterization (Varadarajulu et al, 2008; Strickland et al, 2010). Transgastric access is more complex as it requires further technological development, especially for safe gastric closure. Up to now, laparoscopic assistance has been needed to achieve this end (Chukwumah et al, 2010). Furthermore, the NOTES approach prevents control of serious intraoperative complications which always lead to conversion to open surgery or laparoscopy.

These intraoperative limitations, added to the financial costs of technical development and training requirements, mean that NOTES should be currently considered an experimental procedure.

2. Cholecystectomy in Gallstone Acute Pancreatitis

After a bout of acute pancreatitis in a patient having cholelithiasis, additional episodes may be expected over the following weeks. As a result, cholecystectomy is recommended upon clinical and laboratory recovery, preferably by laparoscopic approach (Overby et al, 2010; Van Baal et al, 2012). Some authors have reported good results in the first 48 hours after admission even before full clinical improvement in the case of mild pancreatitis (Aboulian et al, 2010). On the contrary, cholecystectomy should be delayed if peripancreatic fluid collections or pseudocysts develop, until either resolution or persistence beyond 6 weeks (Nealon et al, 2004).

Table 1. Diagnostic criteria for acute cholecystitis (Hirota et al, 2007)

A. Local signs of inflammation etc.:
(1) Murphy's sign, (2) RUQ mass/pain/tenderness
B. Systemic signs of inflammation etc.:
(1) Fever, (2) elevated CRP, (3) elevated WBC count
C. Imaging findings: imaging findings characteristic of acute cholecystitis

Definite diagnosis
(1) One item in A and one item in B are positive
(2) C confirms the diagnosis when acute cholecystitis is suspected clinically
Note: acute hepatitis, other acute abdominal diseases, and chronic
cholecystitis should be excluded

3. Cholecystectomy in Cholecystitis

A. Epidemiology of Cholecystitis

Acute cholecystitis (AC) can develop in about 20% of symptomatic patients having untreated cholelithiasis (Strasberg et al, 2008). These patients are somewhat older than those with uncomplicated symptomatic cholelithiasis. Most patients with AC have had attacks of biliary colic, but in some cases it is the first manifestation of the biliary disease. After an initial attack of AC, new episodes of pain or inflammation are common, so cholecystectomy, either emergent or scheduled, is recommended. AC is more frequent in women, although the relative frequency in men is higher, considering the lower prevalence of cholelithiasis.

Acalculous AC is less common - accounting for approximately 10 % of cases of AC- and usually associated to very ill patients, frequently those in intensive care units, after trauma, burns or surgery (Chrichlow et al, 2012). Its pathogeny is obscure although believed to be related with ischemic changes and bile stasis. Occasional reports of acalculous AC caused by treatment with sorafenib (Ajhara et al, 2012), or hepatic arterial embolization (Shah et al, 2011) have been published. This entity has a higher tendency to progress to gangrenous cholecystitis and is associated with greater mortality, as high as 21% (Chrichlow et al, 2012).

B. Diagnosis and Grading

The diagnostic suspicion is usually based on a clinical picture of pain in the upper right abdominal quadrant for several hours –usually more than 4 to 6- without any relief, either spontaneously or after NSAID treatment, accompanied by fever and leukocytosis. Physical examination usually shows pain, tenderness or a palpable mass in the right abdominal upper quadrant as well as Murphy's sign.

Diagnosis is usually confirmed by ultrasonography. Cholescintigraphy can also be used. Since there may be wide clinical variations, the Tokyo consensus conference defined diagnostic criteria as shown in table 1 (Hirota et al, 2007).

Cholecystitis severity is variable, depending upon several factors such as time from onset to diagnosis, immunodepression settings or diabetes. Other factors such as a body mass index lower than 25 kg/m^2, advanced age, or male sex have been related to the development of complicated AC (Lee et al, 2009). The Tokyo consensus conference also developed a grading system of severity which classifies cholecystitis cases into mild, moderate and severe according to the criteria shown in table 2 (Hirota et al, 2007).

C. Rationale for Treatment

If the disease is left untreated, the symptoms can spontaneously disappear after 7-10 days. In many patients however, complications such as gallbladder gangrene and subsequent perforation may occur. Other possible adverse consequences are cholecystoenteric fistula and gallstone ileus. As a result, current practice recommends treatment in every case. The options used are cholecystectomy –as the main component, either emergent or delayed-, antibiotic treatment, and percutaneous drainage of the gallbladder.

D. Timing for Surgery

The classical approach, even currently performed in many centers worldwide, has been initial medical treatment (with antibiotics, nothing by mouth and supportive therapy) to induce bacterial eradication and inflammation control, followed by cholecystectomy after 6-8 weeks. This strategy has several drawbacks. First, on some occasions control of the septic source cannot be achieved in up to 41% of patients (Casillas et al, 2008) and emergent surgical treatment becomes necessary at the worst moment, due to local conditions, with higher risks, especially biliary tract injury. Second, in the interval between infection control and cholecystectomy, new bouts of cholecystitis may happen as well as pancreatitis, choledocholithiasis and biliary colics (Wilson et al, 2010). Third, although these events do not happen, overall hospital stay – including the initial episode plus the operation admission-increases as do costs (Wilson et al, 2010).

On the other hand, there is a strategy in which cholecystectomy is performed in the first episode, thus avoiding the above mentioned drawbacks.

The argument against this approach has been a supposed higher risk of intraoperative morbidity, especially biliary tract injury. The rationale for this supposition has been the inflammatory changes that occur in the acute episode of cholecystitis. This is true several days after the clinical onset, but in the first 48-72 hours, edema predominates, making surgical dissection even easier.

Evidence from meta-analysis, systematic reviews and large case series is currently available, showing similar morbidity and mortality rates for emergent and delayed cholecystectomy. As a result, the emergent approach seems to be associated with both clinical and financial benefits (Papi et al, 2004; Gurusamy et al, 2006; Wamashita et al, 2007; Overby et al, 2010; Banz et al, 2011; Skouras et al, 2012).

Table 2. Grading criteria of severity (Hirota et al, 2007)

---

1. Criteria for mild (grade I) acute cholecystitis:

It does not meet the criteria of "severe (grade III)" or "moderate (grade II)" acute cholecystitis. Grade I can also be defined as acute cholecystitis in a healthy patient with no organ dysfunction and only mild inflammatory changes in the gallbladder, making cholecystectomy a safe and low-risk operative procedure.

2. Criteria for moderate (grade II) acute cholecystitis

It is accompanied by any one of the following conditions:

1. Elevated WBC count ($>$18 000/mm^3)
2. Palpable tender mass in the right upper abdominal quadrant
3. Duration of complaints $>$72 h
4. Marked local inflammation (biliary peritonitis, pericholecystic abscess, hepatic abscess, gangrenous cholecystitis, emphysematous cholecystitis)

3. Criteria for severe (grade III) acute cholecystitis:

It is accompanied by dysfunctions in any one of the following organs/systems:

1. Cardiovascular dysfunction (hypotension requiring treatment with inotropic agents)
2. Neurological dysfunction (decreased level of consciousness)
3. Respiratory dysfunction (PaO2/FiO2 ratio $>$300)
4. Renal dysfunction (oliguria, creatinine $>$2.0 mg/dl)
5. Hepatic dysfunction (PT-INR $>$1.5)
6. Hematological dysfunction (platelet count $>$100 000/mm^3)

E. Open Cholecystectomy

Classically, the surgical approach (historically, after cholecystostomy) has been OC, until recently. Even today, it is performed in many centers worldwide since it is less technically demanding than the laparoscopic approach. Data from the National Hospital Discharge Survey (NHDS) of the United States show that as many as 15% of the cases were upfront operated through an open approach between 2000 and 2005, with no trend to decrease (Csikesz et al, 2008).

Their clinical results concerning morbidity, mortality and healing rates (the main aims of treatment) are acceptable enough to justify its use (Navez et al, 2012). However, the data from the NHDS suggest that OC is associated with higher morbidity - 37% vs. 25% - and higher unadjusted mortality - 3.4% vs. 0.4% - than LC (Csikesz et al, 2008).

The open approach can be a good upfront option in case of previous upper abdominal surgery or cases with a long interval between symptom onset and admission and also when the attendant surgeon has less experience in laparoscopic surgery.

F. Laparoscopic Cholecystectomy

Although the laparoscopic approach in case of AC is currently considered the standard treatment (Yamashita et al, 2007; Csikesz et al, 2008; Kim et al, 2008; Navez et al, 2012), it is not generalized worldwide. It needs a higher degree of expertise than cholecystectomy in non-inflammatory cases.

It is possible that surgeons dealing with these patients are younger and less skilled than those who usually perform most laparoscopic and complex procedures. However, in our experience and that of others, LC can be accomplished in most cases without higher morbidity or mortality rates; of 539 patients emergently operated on for AC in our department, treatment was laparoscopic in 71.8% with a conversion rate of 22% with an overall morbidity rate of 19.9% and mortality of 1% (data not published). Others have reported conversion rates of 10-11% (Csikesz et al, 2008; Navez et al, 2012).

As mentioned above, in the first 48-72 hours, edema predominates, making the surgical dissection relatively easy. In our experience, even 72 hours after onset, a large proportion of cases - 73% - could be successfully and safely managed by laparoscopy. However, we found a higher conversion rate in those operated on in the first 72 hours - 20.5% - than in those operated on later - 32.6%.

Others have reported both higher conversion and morbidity rates as well as longer operation time with longer intervals between admission and surgery (Banz et al, 2011).

Some have claimed lower morbidity and mortality rates for LC (even when converted) than for OC (Csikesz et al, 2008). The laparoscopic approach offers the advantages of more patient comfort and shorter in-hospital stay (Csikesz et al, 2008; Skouras et al, 2012).

The main reported complications are intraabdominal bleeding (0.7-5.7%), surgical site infection (0.1-0.3%) and extrahepatic bile duct injury (0.01-0.2%) (Csikesz et al, 2008; Banz et al, 2011). Less common complications are injury of vessels or organs by trocar or Veress needle. Detailed discussion of complications is made below.

In some especially difficult cases, subtotal or anterior cholecystectomy can be performed.

G. Subtotal Cholecystectomy

In complex cases as well as in cirrhotic patients, coagulopathy, or anticoagulant treatment, the posterior gallbladder wall can be left in situ, thus avoiding difficult and bloody separation from the liver bed (Ji at al, 2006). The remnant mucosa can be optionally destroyed by electrocoagulation. The spilled stones must be carefully removed with forceps and irrigation to avoid further abdominal abscesses. In these difficult cases, a suction drain seems reasonable.

H. Anterior Cholecystectomy

In cases with high degree of local inflammation or firm adhesions in Calot's triangle, making further dissection difficult and dangerous, anterior cholecystectomy can be used (Sinha et al, 2006).

In some papers it is also called "subtotal" cholecystectomy (Philips et al, 2008). It can be employed in both laparoscopic and open surgery and consists of excision of the anterior wall of the gallbladder, leaving in situ the posterior wall and Hartmann's pouch (figure 1). No attempt at cystic duct ligation (or dissection) is necessary. The spilled stones must be carefully removed as in the case of subtotal cholecystectomy.

A drain must be left for any eventual biliary fistula. If fistula is finally established, many are transient. In case the biliary drainage persists, ERCP and sphincterotomy should be performed, which allows most fistulas to heal. In some of these cases, a common bile duct stone is found (facilitating fistula) and removed. Occasionally, a retained stone makes it necessary to perform a delayed excision of the gallbladder remnant (Philips et al, 2008).

This strategy was originally applied to LC, with the aim of reducing conversion rates. However it increases safety since if Calot's triangle dissection is difficult and dangerous by laparoscopy it is also difficult by open surgery. As a result, in our opinion anterior cholecystectomy is a technical maneuver useful in any difficult cholecystectomy, irrespective of the approach.

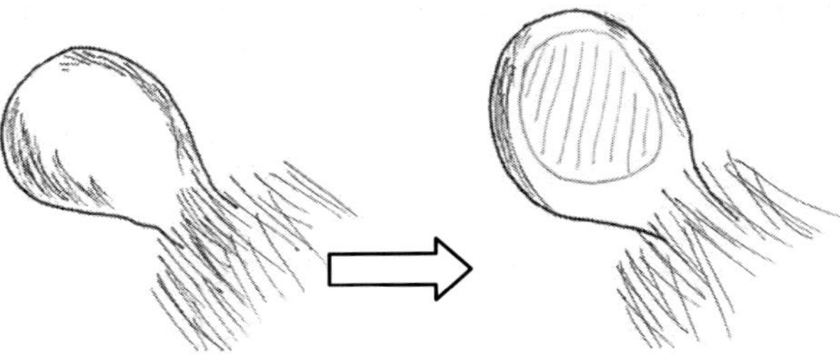

Figure 1. Anterior cholecystectomy.

I. Single-incision Laparoscopic Cholecystectomy (SILC)

SILC has also been used in treating AC, with reports of conversion (7.7%) and complication (3.8%) rates not significantly different than in uncomplicated cholelithiasis, although the performed technique included the use of a couple of 2-mm wire loop retractors

(Sasaki et al, 2012). Of note, in this report additional trocars were required frequently and surgery was delayed after antibiotic treatment, with no case of emergent cholecystectomy.

More results are needed before acceptance in clinical practice. In our opinion, the SILC approach ought to be considered under evaluation.

J. Cholecystectomy in Case of Cholecystitis in the Elderly

Significant comorbidity and limited functional reserve is frequently associated with advanced age, which could complicate a postoperative course, especially in the case of a septic process such AC. LC in patients aged over 75 years is feasible and effective but is associated with a higher morbidity rate -frequently unrelated to the surgical site- as well as a higher mortality rate compared with younger patients. Also, their in-hospital stay tends to be longer (Kirshtein et al, 2008).

Studies comparing the safety of both open and LC in patients over 75 have been done. Both approaches appear safe with no significant difference in mortality although with lower morbidity in the case of laparoscopy (Chau et al, 2002).

K. Antibiotic Treatment

Normal bile in the absence of lithiasis is sterile. When cholelithiasis is present, bacteria are expected, as well as in clinical cholecystitis. However, not all patients with cholecystitis have infected bile as shown in several studies where the proportion of positive cultures ranged 47-54% (Yoshida et al, 2007). In our own experience, only 95 (52.5%) out of 181 cultures from bile or peritoneal exudates taken at surgery were positive. Despite all, current agreement in the indication of antibiotic coverage exists, with the exception of mild cases (Yoshida et al, 2007, Solomkin et al, 2010). In case of community-acquired cholecystitis, the expected species are enteric gram-negative aerobic and facultative bacilli as well as anaerobes. As a result, antibiotic treatment aiming at these germs is usually initiated upon diagnosis. Activity against enterococci is not required in community-acquired cases except in those of high risk (Solomkin et al, 2010). The main recommended empirical regimes are shown in table 3. Of note, carbapenems ought to be used in case of risk factors of harboring extended-spectrum beta-lactamase-producing bacteria (Guirao et al, 2010). Nevertheless, these regimes have to be adapted to local patterns of bacterial resistance.

Antibiotics can be used in several circumstances. In high surgical risk cases, they can be used as the sole treatment. In other cases they are used until the inflammatory process becomes controlled and then scheduled cholecystectomy is performed. Interestingly, a recent paper has challenged the need of antibiotics to overcome the acute phase, at least in mild cases, since they did not find any clinical difference (percutaneous cholecystostomy tube placement, readmissions or perioperative course after delayed cholecystectomy) between patients receiving intravenous antibiotics or not (Mazeh et al, 2012). However, the main practice guidelines currently recommend the use of intravenous antibiotics (Yoshida et al, 2007; Solomkin et al, 2010). These should be given until symptomatic relief occurs as well as laboratory normalization of the leukocyte counts, and probably, the C-reactive protein.

Finally, antibiotics can be used as adjuvant therapy to emergent cholecystectomy. They have to be initiated preoperatively, upon diagnosis. Duration after cholecystectomy is controversial, mainly because of the scanty literature available concerning this issue. Long courses of antibiotics, lasting 7-10 days or even more, have often been used. Only a few papers have addressed the duration of antibiotic therapy. One article gives only a description of clinical practices concerning duration of antibiotics and surgeons' preferences, without any definitive conclusion or recommendation (Kanafani et al, 2003). In a randomized trial of cefamandole use in patients with AC who underwent OC, a short course (three doses) was as effective as a 7-day course (Lau et al, 1990). In another old study (Kune et al, 1975), longer treatment did not show any reduction in septic complications. The scanty recommendations available come from clinical guidelines.

The Spanish Consensus on antibiotic therapy of intraabdominal infections (Guirao et al, 2010) gives only generic recommendations of limiting the antibiotics to 3 days, provided the septic source has been removed and there are no risk factors of bad evolution, although there is no specific reference to the case of AC.

The Infectious Diseases Society of America guidelines (Solomkin et al, 2010) give the recommendation of discontinuing antibiotics 24 hours after cholecystectomy, unless evidence of infection outside the gallbladder wall exists. The Tokyo guidelines recommend that antimicrobial agents should be administered to patients diagnosed with AC, except in mild cases (Yoshida et al, 2007). However treatment duration is not stated nor is it in the literature. Our own investigations revealed that there is no benefit, in terms of reduction of surgical site infections, in case of prolonging antibiotic treatment over 4 days after cholecystectomy in the absence of clinical or laboratory data suggesting active or persistent infection (data not published).

L. Alternatives to Cholecystectomy: Percutaneous Cholecystostomy and Endoscopic Transpapillary Gallbladder Drainage

The first surgical approach to cholecystitis was surgical cholecystostomy. After the development and success of cholecystectomy, cholecystostomy was abandoned. In recent years, when more elderly patients with more co-morbidity present with AC, cholecystostomy regained interest. However surgical cholecystostomy was no longer performed since currently cholecystostomy can be safely performed by means of percutaneous ultrasound-guided catheter drainage.

The tube is placed transhepatically to avoid bile leakage into the peritoneal cavity. High risk patients are increasingly being managed with this procedure. In some cases this is used as the sole treatment. In others, it allows patient improvement and is followed by delayed cholecystectomy. Also, patients having severe gallbladder inflammation can benefit from this procedure until resolution of local inflammatory changes, thus allowing a safer delayed cholecystectomy (Yamashita et al, 2007)

In our experience, cholecystectomy is safe enough and with similar mortality to cholecystostomy in most cases. Cholecystectomy warrants definite treatment and cholecystostomy does not. As a result, we advise cholecystectomy unless absolute surgical contraindication exists (Rodríguez-Sanjuán et al, 2012), as do others (Kim et al 2008, Abi-Haidar et al, 2012).

Table 3. Antibiotics recommended in acute cholecystitis

Mild
Yoshida et al, 2007
    Oral fluoroquinolones (Levofloxacin, ciprofloxacin)
    Oral cephalosporins Cefotiam, cefcapene
    First-generation cephalosporins: cefazolin
    Wide-spectrum penicillin/ Ampicillin/sulbactam
Guirao et al, 2010
    amoxycilline-clavulanate, ampicilline/sulbactam or Ertapenem
Solomkin et al, 2010
    cefazolin, cefuroxime, or ceftriaxone
Moderate
Yoshida et al, 2007
    Wide-spectrum penicillin/β-lactamase Piperacillin/tazobactam, ampicillin/sulbactam
    Second-generation cephalosporins Cefmetazole, cefotiam, oxacephem, flomoxef
Guirao et al, 2010
    amoxycilline-clavulanate, ampicilline/sulbactam or Ertapenem
Solomkin et al, 2010
    cefazolin, cefuroxime, or ceftriaxone
Severe cases or immunocompromised patients
Yoshida et al, 2007
    Third- and fourth-generation cephalosporins Cefoperazon/sulbactam, ceftriaxone, ceftazidime, cefepime, cefozopran
    Monobactams: Aztreonam
    One of above + metronidazole (when anaerobic bacteria are detected or are expected to co-exist)
Guirao et al, 2010
    piperacilline/tazobactam, imipenem or meropenem
Solomkin et al, 2010
    Imipenem-cilastatin, meropenem, doripenem, piperacillin-tazobactam, ciprofloxacin, levofloxacin, or cefepime, each in combination with metronidazole

After resolution of the acute phase and subsequent improvement of physiological status, the patient can be either discharged or scheduled to delayed cholecystectomy. Removal of the cholecystostomy tube without cholecystectomy is associated with a high incidence of recurrent cholecystitis and bad prognosis (Morse et al, 2010).

Occasionally percutaneous cholecystostomy cannot be performed for several reasons (anatomic, coagulopathy). In these patients gallbladder drainage can be placed transpapillary using an endoscopic approach, with a high rate of clinical response (Itoi et al, 2008).

4. Complications of Cholecystectomy

LC offers many benefits for patients compared to the open approach but unfortunately with an overall serious complication rate that remains higher than that seen in OC, despite increasing experience with the procedure (Vollmer et al, 2007; Khan et al, 2007). LC has been associated with significant increase in bleeding, bowel lesions, bile leaks and bile duct injury (BDI) ranging from 0.5 to 0.8% (Flum et al, 2003; Karvonen et al, 2007; Nordin et al,

2011). By comparison, in a large analysis conducted in the 1990s, the incidence rate of BDI in OC was approximately 0.2 % (Roslyn et al, 1993).

The complication rate of OC has increased as well, due to overall declining experience of younger surgeons in open surgery in the use of this approach, now reserved for the most complicated and challenging cases (Visser et al, 2008).

A. Laparoscopic Access Injuries

Establishing access and the creation of the initial pneumoperitoneum necessary to perform laparoscopic procedures of the biliary tract may lead to significant complications. Reviews of data regarding device-related injury and death reported vascular and visceral injuries as the major causes of morbidity and mortality related to abdominal access (Fuller et al, 2005; Larobina et al, 2005). As mentioned before, there are no demonstrable differences in the safety of open and closed techniques for establishing access and initial creation of the pneumoperitoneum (Ahmad et al, 2008) and, therefore, decisions regarding the choice of technique are left to the surgeon's preference and based on individual training, skill assessment and case (Larobina et al, 2005; Overby et al, 2010). Trocar injury to blood vessels or bowel can be more dangerous than Veress needle injury to the same structure. Bowel injuries can result from percutaneous or open insertion of the first trocar. With the open technique, the bowel injury could be immediately obvious and repaired through the umbilical incision. If bleeding occurs after removal of a trocar, the hole can be occluded with finger pressure to maintain pneumoperitoneum allowing hemorrhage control by cauterization or suture repair.

B. Intraoperative Complications

These problems have been related to three main causes: Dangerous surgery, dangerous anatomy, and dangerous pathology (Johnston. 1986). Dangerous surgery and anatomy derive from inadequate adhesion to the technical principles of cholecystectomy, poor experience, and lack of exposure or inadequate assistance leading to unclear anatomy. Dangerous pathology includes portal hypertension, severe inflammation or fibrosis, adhesions and infection. The situation can even worsen in case of hemorrhage (Smith et al, 1979; Gertsch et al, 2007).

In a review that combined the data from seven large studies with a total of 8856 LC, severe complications occurred in 2.6% (Strasberg et al, 1995). A combined analysis of eight large studies of LC reported the following types and frequencies of major complications: bleeding (0.11-1.97%), abscess (0.14-0.3%), bile leak (0.3-0.9%), biliary injury (0.26-0.6%), and bowel injury (0.1-0.35%) (Thurley et al, 2008). The rate of wound infections and surgical site infections is lower with the laparoscopic approach than with the open approach, but there is no advantage in terms of intra-abdominal abscess formation (Biscione et al, 2007).

The overall incidence of laparoscopic complications is also related to the experience of the surgeon. A report of over 8800 procedures performed by 55 surgeons estimated that 90% of BDI occurred in the first 30 cases for each surgeon, with the incidence falling from 1.7% in the first case to 0.17 % at the 50th case (Moore et al, 1995).

BDI is the most common severe complication of cholecystectomy (Strasberg et al, 2011). Laparoscopic BDI stems principally from misperception, not errors of skill, knowledge, or judgment. The most frequent cause of BDI is misidentification of the common bile duct (CBD), the right or common hepatic duct, or an aberrant duct (Way et al, 2003; Nordin et al, 2011). Biliary injuries are often associated with vascular injuries, especially arterial injuries (Davidoff et al, 1992).

A vasculobiliary injury is a lesion of both a bile duct and a hepatic artery or portal vein; the BDI may be caused by operative trauma, be ischemic in origin or both, and may or may not be accompanied by various degrees of hepatic ischemia (Strasberg et al, 2011).

Intraoperative Diagnosis

If BDI is suspected during LC, intraoperative cholangiography (IOC) should be performed to establish the diagnosis and to find out the type of the injury. If this is confirmed or suspected, conversion to open surgery is usually mandatory (Nordin et al, 2011). The negative effects of conversion or even aborting the procedure in case of suspicion are minor compared with the negative effect of BDI (Strasberg, 2005).

As mentioned before, recognition of biliary injury may be more likely if routine IOC is performed (Waage et al, 2006). Some studies found no overall benefit of routine IOC which, it was suggested, should be limited to patients suspected of having a common bile duct stone or if biliary anatomy is unclear or lesion suspected (Overby et al, 2010).

Classification of Lesions

Several classification systems have been proposed based on the anatomical level of injury or on the mechanism, with the aim to standardize the description, to guide the treatment and to compare the outcomes of BDI. The initial system, designed to categorize biliary strictures, was developed by Bismuth (Bismuth, 1982; Bismuth et al, 2001). Strasberg modified Bismuth classification into a new classification for BDI of LC that describes strictures, leaks, complete transections and occlusions (Strasberg et al, 1995).

Other proposed classifications give more subcategories including concomitant vascular injuries, but these systems become more complex, leaving the Strasberg-Bismuth classification as the most useful in giving sufficient description and being the most relevant to management (Wu et al, 2010; Lau et al, 2007).

The Strasberg classification establishes several types of lesions (figure 2):

Type A. These are injuries that involve leakage into the gallbladder bed from either the minor hepatic ducts or the cystic duct, with no loss in continuity of the biliary tree.

Types B and C. These are occlusion (Type B) and transection (Type C) injuries of aberrant right hepatic ducts. They are associated with cystic duct drainage into an aberrant right hepatic duct, an abnormality seen in as many as 2% of patients. In this setting, the right hepatic duct can be mistaken for the cystic duct at the point of insertion into either the main hepatic duct or common bile duct.

When the injury to the duct is an occlusion (Type B), the patient may remain asymptomatic for years and then present with upper right quadrant pain and fever due to recurrent cholangitis. As a result segmental fibrosis and/or atrophy may occur. By comparison, a biliary leak happens when the duct is transected but not occluded (Type C). Concomitant injuries to the right hepatic artery are frequently associated with this particular problem.

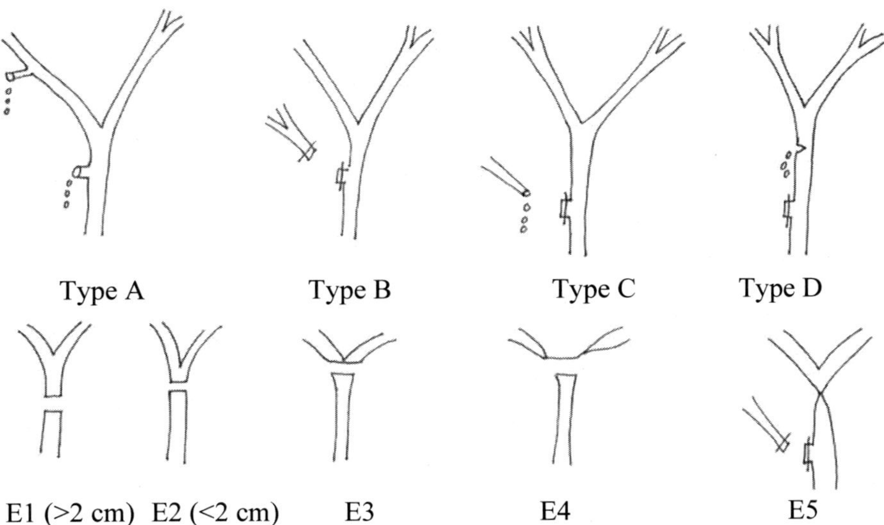

Figure 2. Strasberg Classification.

Type D. These are injuries with lateral damage to the common bile duct resulting in a biliary leak; they can usually be managed endoscopically but may progress to the more serious Type E injury.

Type E. These involve the main duct and are classified according to the level of injury in the biliary tree (Bismuth classification).

E1 (Bismuth Type I) - Transection >2 cm far from the confluence
E2 (Bismuth Type II) - Transection <2 cm far from the confluence
E3 (Bismuth Type III) - Transection in the hilum
E4 (Bismuth Type IV) - Separation of major ducts in the hilum
E5 (Bismuth Type V) - Type C injury plus injury in the hilum.

C. Early Postcholecystectomy Problems

Most patients have an uncomplicated course following cholecystectomy. Bile leakage after cholecystectomy does not cause pain initially and the elevation of liver enzymes may be slight. Vague symptoms, such as abdominal fullness, swelling, nausea, vomiting, fever and chills and finally, abdominal pain, should alert the surgeon.

If unrecognized, biliary leak may lead to bilomas, fistulas, cholangitis, sepsis, or even to multiorgan failure (Sicklick et al, 2005). Bile duct obstruction without significant leak may cause initially only mild symptoms, which may even subside and return later as cholangitis, obstructive jaundice, and later secondary biliary cirrhosis.

Following a careful history and physical examination, laboratory testing should include liver function tests and imaging test.

D. Primary Diagnostic Methods

The primary investigation methods are ultrasound and contrast enhanced computerized tomography scan (CT) to detect intra-abdominal fluid collections and biliary dilatation. CT reveals possible vascular or liver parenchymal lesions. Intra-abdominal collections should be drained immediately.

ERCP can delineate bile duct anatomy and help diagnose leaks and retained common bile duct stones. It also acts as a therapeutic modality to allow interventional procedures such as sphincterotomy, nasobiliary drainage, stent placement or stone removal (Karvonen et al, 2007). If major injury is suspected, ERCP should be performed as an emergency procedure to evaluate the injury. In delayed suspicion of BDI, laparotomy should be avoided before further diagnosis, classification and possible therapy at ERCP.

In case of complete obstruction, the proximal parts of the biliary tree may be visualized by percutaneous transhepatic cholangiography (PTC), which can aid to plan the corrective operation. Magnetic resonance cholangiopancreatography (MRCP) may give valuable information of intrahepatic biliary tree not visible by ERCP or PTC, such as obstruction of segmental or sectoral ductal systems.

Scintigraphy hepatobiliary imaging (technetium-99m iminodiacetic acid) assesses hepatocellular function, flow of bile into the duodenum, and collections of extrabiliary radionuclide.

Following LC, the cystic duct stump can be the source of the bile leak, and endoscopic sphincterotomy and stent placement usually provides adequate therapy. The goal of endoscopic therapy is to eliminate the transpapillary pressure gradient.

E. Late Postcholecystectomy Problems

The effect of cholecystectomy on bowel function is controversial. Following cholecystectomy, approximately 20% of patients have abdominal complaints, which may include pain, indigestion, bloating, and flatulence. In addition, chronic diarrhea is a known postcholecystectomy complication and may result from bile acid malabsorption. A small group of patients experience recurrent symptoms secondary to an impacted stone in a long cystic duct or gallbladder remnant following a partial/subtotal cholecystectomy. This late sequela is likely to occur more often with LC than with OC.

In these patients, ERCP or MRCP is usually performed to exclude common duct stones; however, surgeons should bear in mind that a cystic duct stone or remnant gallbladder may be present. Stones in the cystic duct that are difficult to extract may benefit from fragmentation techniques. Completion cholecystectomy with removal of cystic duct stones also represents definitive treatment and can often be performed laparoscopically (Desai et al, 2004).

F. Late Complications of BDI

Late stenosis is related to inflammatory phenomena and fibrosis or bile leaks secondary to vascular injury associated with ischemia. Usually the treatment is initiated by ERCP and or transhepatic drainage to solve cholangitis. In some cases, biliary reconstruction or liver resection may be required.

Portal hypertension may be due to prolonged biliary obstruction, portal damage during cholecystectomy, portal thrombosis or coexistence with previous liver disease such as cirrhosis (Agarwal et al, 2008). The incidence of portal hypertension and secondary biliary cirrhosis (SBC) in case of BDI is about 8% (Braasch et al, 1981). The presence of cirrhosis during repair predicts an increase in morbidity and mortality (Röthlin et al, 1998).

G. Postcholecystectomy Syndrome

Postcholecystectomy syndrome (PCS) comprises a heterogeneous group of symptoms and disorders including persistent abdominal pain and dyspepsia that recur and persist after cholecystectomy (Schofer, 2010; Jaunoo et al, 2010; Girometti et al, 2010). PCS is divided as "early" if it occurs in the postoperative period and "late" if it occurs months or years after cholecystectomy. The symptoms of pain and dyspepsia referred to as PCS can be caused by a wide spectrum of conditions, both biliary and extrabiliary. About half of the patients with PCS are found to have biliary, pancreatic, or gastrointestinal disorders, while the remaining patients have extraintestinal disease (Girometti et al, 2010).

Biliary causes of PCS include biliary injury, retained cystic duct, or common bile duct stones for the early PCS. Late PCS can be due to recurrent CBD stones, bile duct strictures, an inflamed cystic duct or gallbladder remnant, papillary stenosis or inflammation, or biliary dyskinesia. (Schofer 2010, Girometti et al 2010).

Extrabiliary causes of PCS include gastrointestinal causes such as irritable bowel syndrome, pancreatitis, pancreatic tumors, pancreas divisum, hepatitis, peptic ulcer disease, mesenteric ischemia, diverticulitis, or esophageal diseases. Extraintestinal causes are intercostal neuritis, wound neuroma, coronary artery disease, or Psychiatric and/or neurological disorders (Schofer 2010; Girometti et al, 2010).

Treatment for PCS is adapted to the specific cause of the symptoms. Diagnosis of the problem causing PCS usually requires imaging to exclude retained or recurrent stones or identify a bile duct leak, stricture, or transection. This can be accomplished in most cases with ultrasound or CT followed by direct cholangiography or MRCP. This provides a noninvasive alternative to direct cholangiography for evaluation of the biliary tract.

References

Abi-Haidar Y, Sanchez V, Willimans SA, Itani KMF. Revisiting Percutaneous Cholecystostomy for Acute Cholecystitis Based on a 10-Year Experience. *Arch Surg.* 2012; 147: 416-22.

Aboulian A, Chan T, Yaghoubian A et al. Early Cholecystectomy Safely Decreases Hospital Stay in Patients With Mild Gallstone Pancreatitis A Randomized Prospective Study. *Ann Surg* 2010; 251: 615-9.

Agarwal AK, Gupta V, Singh S, et al. Management of patients of postcholecystectomy benign biliary stricture complicated by portal hypertension. *Am J Surg* 2008; 195: 421-6.

Ahmad G, Duffy JM, Phillips K, Watson A. Laparoscopic entry techniques. *Cochrane Database Syst Rev* 2008 Feb 15; (2) CD006583.

Attili AF, Carulli N, Roda E, et al. Epidemiology of gallstone disease in Italy: prevalence data of the Multicenter Italian Study on Cholelithiasis (M.I.COL.). *Am J Epidemiol* 1995; 141: 158-65.

Avgerinos C, Kelgiorgi D, Touloumis Z, et al. One thousand laparoscopic cholecystectomies in a single surgical unit using the "critical view of safety" technique. *J Gastrointest Surg* 2009; 13: 498-503.

Banz V, Gsponer T, Candinas D, Güller U. Population-based analysis of 4113 patients with acute cholecystitis: defining the optimal time-point for laparoscopic cholecystectomy. *Ann Surg* 2011; 254: 964-70.

Braasch JW, Bolton JS, Rossi RL. A technique of biliary tract reconstruction with complete follow-up in 44 consecutive cases. *Ann Surg* 1981; 194: 635-8.

Biscione FM, Couto RC, Pedrosa TM, Neto MC. Comparison of the risk of surgical site infection after laparoscopic cholecystectomy and open cholecystectomy. *Infect Control Hosp Epidemiol* 2007; 55: 317-23.

Bismuth H. Postoperative strictures of the bile ducts. In: Blumgart LH, editor. *The Biliary Tract*. Vol. V. New York, NY: Churchill-Livingstone; 1982. p. 209–8.

Bismuth H, Majno PE. Biliary strictures: Classification based on the principles of surgical treatment. *World J Surg* 2001; 25: 1241-4.

Borie F, Millat B. Colecistectomía mediante laparoscopia. In: *Enciclopedia Médico-Quirúrgica-40-950*. Ed. Elsevier, Paris 2003.

Bratzker DW, Houck PM, Surgical Infection Prevention Guidelines Writers Workgroup, et al. Antimicrobial prophylaxis for surgery: an advisory statement from the National Surgical Infection Prevention Project. *Clin Infect Dis* 2004; 38: 1706-15.

Calot. De la cholecystectomie (ablation de la vesicule biliaire). *Thèse, Paris* 1890; 52 p.

Casillas RA, Yegiyants S, Collins JC. Early laparoscopic cholecystectomy is the preferred management of acute cholecystitis. *Arch Surg* 2008; 143: 533-7.

Chau CH, Tang CN, Siu WT et al. Laparoscopic cholecystectomy versus open cholecystectomy in elderly patients with acute cholecystitis: retrospective study. *Hong Kong Med J* 2002; 8: 394-9.

Chrichlow L, Walcott-Sapp S, Moajor J et al. Acute acalculous cholecystitis after gastrointestinal surgery. *Am Surg* 2012; 78: 220-4.

Chukwumah C, Zorron R, Marks JM, Ponsky JL. Current status of natural orifice translumenal endoscopic surgery (NOTES). *Curr Probl Surg* 2010; 47: 630-68.

Csikesz N, Ricciardi R, Tseng JF, Shah SA. Current status of surgical management of acute cholecystitis in the United States. *World J Surg* 2008; 32: 2230-6.

Csikesz NG, Singla A, Murphy MM, et al. Surgeon volume metrics in laparoscopic cholecystectomy. *Dig Dis Sci* 2010; 55: 2398-405.

Cuesta MA, Berends F, Veenhof AA. The "invisible cholecystectomy": a transumbilical laparoscopic operation without a scar. *Surg Endosc* 2008; 22: 1211–3.

Davidoff AM, Pappas TN, Murray EA, et al. Mechanisms of major biliary injury during laparoscopic cholecystectomy. *Ann Surg* 1992; 215: 196-202.

Debru E, Dawson A, Leibman S et al. Does routine intraoperative cholangiography prevent bile duct transection? *Surg Endosc* 2005; 19: 589–93.

Desai KM, Strasberg SM, Soper NJ. in: *Current Surgical Therapy. 8th edition* (Eds), *Cameron* JL. Mosby Inc, 2004. pages 416-19.

Dubois F, Berthelot G, Levard H. Cholecystectomie par coelioscopie. *Presse Med* 1989; 18: 980-2.

Edwards C, Bradshaw A, Ahearne P, et al. Single-incision laparoscopic cholecystectomy is feasible: initial experience with 80 cases. *Surg Endosc* 2010; 24: 2241–7.

Elsey JK, Feliciano DV. Initial experience with single-incision laparoscopic cholecystectomy. *J Am Coll Surg* 2010; 210: 620–4.

Everhart JE, Khare M, Hill M, Maurer KR. Prevalence and ethnic differences in gallbladder disease in the United States. *Gastroenterology* 1999; 117: 632-9.

Flum DR, Cheadle A, Prela C et al. Bile duct injury during cholecystectomy and survival in medicare beneficiaries. *JAMA* 2003; 290: 2168-73.

Fritscher-Ravens A, Patel K, Ghanbari A, et al. Natural orifice transluminal endoscopic surgery (NOTES) in the mediastinum: long-term survival animal experiments in transesophageal access, including minor surgical procedures. *Endoscopy* 2007; 39: 870-5.

Fuller J, Ashar BS, Carey-Corrado J. Trocar-associated injuries and fatalities: an analysis of 1399 reports to the FDA. *J Minim Invasive Gynecol* 2005; 12: 302-7.

García Valdecasas JC, Almenara R, Cabrer C, et al. Subcostal incisión versus midline laparotomy in gallstone surgery: a prospective and randomized trial. *Br J Surg* 1988; 75: 473-5.

Gertsch P. The technique of cholecystectomy. In: Blumgart LH, Belghiti J, Jarnagin WR, et al Eds. *Surgery of the Liver and Biliary Tract,* 4rd ed. WB Saunders. 2007: p. 496-505.

Giday SA, Buscaglia JM, Althaus J, et al. Successful diagnostic and therapeutic intrauterine fetal interventions by NOTES (abstract). *Gastrointest Endosc* 2008; 67: AB 104.

Girometti R, Brondani G, Cereser L, Como G, Del Pin M, Bazzocchi M, Zuiani C. Post-cholecystectomy syndrome: spectrum of biliary findings at magnetic resonance cholangiopancreatography. *Br J Radiol* 2010; 83: 351-61.

Guirao X, Arias J, Badía JM et al. Recomendaciones en el tratamiento antibiótico empírico de la infección intraabdominal. *Cir Esp* 2010; 87: 63-81.

Gurusamy KS, Samraj K. Early versus delayed laparoscopic cholecystectomy for acute cholecystitis. *Cochrane Database Syst Rev* 2006 Oct 18; (4): CD005440.

Gurusamy KS, Koti R, Samraj K, Davidson BR. Abdominal lift for laparoscopic cholecystectomy. *Cochrane Database Syst Rev* 2012 May 16; (2): CD006574.

Gurusamy KS, Samraj K, Farouk M, Davidson BR. Meta-analysis of randomized controlled trials on the safety and effectiveness of day-case laparoscopic cholecystectomy. *Br J Surg* 2008; 95: 161-8.

Gurusamy KS, Samraj K, Mullerat P, Davidson BR. Routine abdominal drainage for uncomplicated laparoscopic cholecystectomy. *Cochrane Database Syst Rev* 2007 Oct 17; (4): CD006004.

Hasson HM. A modified instrument and method for laparoscopy. Am J Obstet Gynecol 1971; 110: 886-887.

Hirota M, Takada T, Kawarada Y et al. Diagnostic criteria and severity assessment of acute cholecystitis: Tokyo Guidelines. *J Hepatobiliary Pancreat Surg* 2007; 14:78–82.

Ingraham AM, Cohen ME, Ko CY, Hall BL. A current profile and assessment of north american cholecystectomy: results from the american college of surgeons national surgical quality improvement program. *J Am Coll Surg* 2010; 211: 176-86.

Itoi T, Sofuni A, Itokawa F et al. Endoscopic transpapillary gallbladder drainage in patients with acute cholecystitis in whom percutaneous transhepatic approach is contraindicated or anatomically impossible (with video). *Gastrointest Endosc* 2008; 68: 455-60.

Jaunoo SS, Mohandas S, Almond LM. Postcholecystectomy syndrome (PCS). *Int J Surg* 2010; 8: 15-7.

Ji W, Li LT, Li JS. Role of laparoscopic subtotal cholecystectomy in the treatment of complicated cholecystitis. *Hepatobiliary Pancreat Dis Int* 2006; 5: 584-9.

Johnston GW. Iatrogenic bile duct stricture: an avoidable surgical hazard? *Br J Surg* 1986; 73: 245-7.

Kaafarani HM, Smith TS, Neumayer L, et al. Trends, outcomes, and predictors of open and conversion to open cholecystectomy in Veterans Health Administration hospitals. *Am J Surg* 2010; 200: 32-40.

Kanafani ZA, Khalifé N, Kanj SS et al. Antibiotic use in acute cholecystitis: practice patterns in the absence of evidence-based guidelines. *J Infect* 2005; 51: 128–134.

Kallo AN, Singh VK, Jagannath SB, et al. Flexible transgastric peritoneoscopy: a novel approach to diagnostic and therapeutic interventions in the peritoneal cavity. *Gastrointest Endosc* 2004; 60: 114-7.

Kantsevoy SV, Hu B, Jagannath SB, et al. Transgastric endoscopic splenectomy: is it possible? *Surg Endosc* 2006; 20: 522-5.

Karvonen J, Gullichsen R, Laine S, et al. Bile duct injury during laparoscopic cholecystectomy: primary and long-term results from a single institution. *Surg Endosc* 2007; 21: 1069–73.

Keus F, de Jong JAF, Gooszen HG, van Laarhoven CJHM. Laparoscopic versus small-incision cholecystectomy for patients with symptomatic cholecystolithiasis. *Cochrane Database of Systematic Reviews.* 2006 Oct 18; (4): CD006229.

Keus F, Broeders IA, van Laarhoven CJ. Gallstone disease: Surgical aspects of symptomatic cholecystolithiasis and acute cholecystitis. *Best Pract Res Clin Gastroenterol* 2006; 20: 1031-51.

Khan MH, Howard TJ, Fogel EL et al. Frequency of biliary complications after laparoscopic cholecystectomy detected by ERCP: experience at a large tertiary referral center. *Gastrointest Endosc* 2007; 65: 247-52.

Kim JH, Kim JW, Jeong IH et al. Surgical outcomes of laparoscopic cholecystectomy for severe acute cholecystitis. *J Gastrointest Surg* 2008; 12: 829-35.

Kirshtein B, Bayme M, Bolotin A et al. Laparoscopic Cholecystectomy for Acute Cholecystitis in the Elderly Is it Safe? *Surg Laparosc Endosc Percutan Tech* 2008; 18: 334–9.

Kune GA, Burdon JG. Are antibiotics necessary in acute cholecystitis? *Med J Aust* 1975; 2: 627-30.

Larobina M, Nottle P. Complete evidence regarding major vascular injuries during laparoscopic access. *Surg Laparosc Endosc Percutan Tech* 2005; 15:119-23.

Lau WY, Lai EC. Classification of iatrogenic bile duct injury. *Hepatobiliary Pancreat Dis Int* 2007; 6: 457–63.

Lau WY, Yuen WK, Chu KW, et al. Systemic antibiotic regimens for acute cholecystitis treated by early cholecystectomy. *Aust N Z J Surg* 1990; 60: 539-43.

Lee HK, Han HS, Min SK. The association between body mass index and the severity of cholecystitis. *Am J Surg* 2009; 197: 455–458.

McSherry CK, Ferstenberg H, Calhoun WF, et al. The natural history of diagnosed gallstone disease in symptomatic and asymptomatic patients. *Ann Surg* 1985; 202: 59-63.

Ma J, Cassera MA, Spaun GO et al. Randomized controlled trial comparing single-port laparoscopic cholecystectomy and four-port laparoscopic cholecystectomy. *Ann Surg* 2011; 254: 22-7.

Magno P, Mas MA, Rivera Y, et al. NOTES Is Successful for vertebral spinal interventions with significant advantages for anterior spinal procedures (abstract). *Gastrointest Endosc* 2008; 67: AB114 .

Mazeh H, Mizrahi I, Dior U, et al. Role of Antibiotic Therapy in Mild Acute Calculus Cholecystitis: A Prospective Randomized Controlled Trial. *World J Surg* 2012 Mar 29. [Epub ahead of print].

Mercado MA, Chan C, Orozco H, et al. Acute bile duct injury. The need for a high repair. *Surg Endosc* 2003; 17: 1351–5.

Moore MJ, Bennett CL. The learning curve for laparoscopic cholecystectomy. The Southern Surgeons Club. *Am J Surg* 1995; 170: 55-9.

Morse BC, Smith JB, Lawdahl RB, Roettger RH. Management of acute cholecystitis in critically ill patients: contemporary role for cholecystostomy and subsequent cholecystectomy. *Am Surg* 2010; 76: 708-12.

Navarra G, Pozza E, Occhionorelli S, et al. One-wound laparoscopic cholecystectomy. *Br J Surg* 1997; 84: 695.

Navez B, Ungureanu F, Michiels M, et al. The Belgian Group for Endoscopic Surgery (BGES) and the Hepatobiliary and Pancreatic Section (HBPS) of the Royal Belgian Society of Surgery. Surgical management of acute cholecystitis: results of a 2-year prospective multicenter survey in Belgium. *Surg Endosc* 2012 Mar 10. [Epub ahead of print].

Nealon WH, Bawduniak J, Walser EM. Appropriate Timing of Cholecystectomy in Patients Who Present With Moderate to Severe Gallstone-Associated Acute Pancreatitis With Peripancreatic Fluid Collections. *Ann Surg* 2004; 239: 741–51.

Nordin A, Grönroos JM, Mäkisalo H. Treatment of biliary complications after laparoscopic cholecystectomy. *Scand J Surg* 2011; 100: 42-8.

Overby W, Apelgren KN, Richardson W, Fanelli R. SAGES guidelines for the clinical application of laparoscopic biliary tract surgery. *Surg Endosc* 2010; 24: 2368-86.

Papi C, Catarci M, D'Ambrosio L, et al. Timing of cholecystectomy for acute calculous cholecystitis: A meta-analysis. *Am J Gastroenterol* 2004; 99: 147-55.

Paredes JP, Puñal JA. Colecistectomía laparoscópica. In: *Cirugía Endoscópica, Guías Clínicas de la AEC*, Vol 6. Ed. Targarona EM. Ed. Arán, Madrid 2003; 239.

Perry KA, Myers JA, Deziel DJ. Laparoscopic ultrasound as the primary method for bile duct imaging during cholecystectomy. *Surg Endosc* 2008; 22: 208–13.

Philips JA, Lawes DA, Cook AJ et al. The use of laparoscopic subtotal cholecystectomy for complicated cholelithiasis. *Surg Endosc* 2008; 22: 1697-700.

Praderi RC. One hundred years of biliary surgery. *Surg Gastroenterol* 1982; 1: 269-87.

Rodríguez-Sanjuán JC, Arruabarrena A, Sánchez-Moreno L et al. Acute cholecystitis in high surgical risk patients: percutaneous cholecystostomy or emergency cholecystectomy. *Am J Surg* 2012; 204: 54-9.

Roslyn JJ, Binns GS, Hughes EF, et al. Open cholecystectomy. A contemporary analysis of 42,474 patients. *Ann Surg* 1993; 218: 129-37.

Röthlin MA, Löpfe M, Schlumpf R, Largiadèr F. Long-term results of hepaticojejunostomy for benign lesions of the bile ducts. *Am J Surg* 1998; 175: 22-6.

Ruiz Gómez F, Ramia Ángel JM, García-Parreño Jofré J, Figueras J. Lesiones iatrogénicas de la vía biliar. *Cir Esp* 2010; 88: 211-21.

Sasaki K, Watanabe G, Matsuda M, Hashimoto M. Original single-incision laparoscopic cholecystectomy for acute inflammation of the gallbladder. *World J Gastroenterol* 2012; 18: 944-51.

Salembier Y. *La lithiase biliaire. Traitement chirurgical.* Medsi/McGraw-Hill. New York. 1988; pp 45-84.

Schirmer BD, Edge SB, Dix J, et al. Laparoscopic cholecystectomy. Treatment of choice for symptomatic cholelithiasis. *Ann Surg* 1991; 213: 665-76.

Schmidt M, Søndenaa K, Vetrhus M, et al. A Randomized Controlled Study of Uncomplicated Gallstone Disease with a 14-Year Follow-Up Showed that Operation Was the Preferred Treatment. *Dig Surg* 2011; 28: 270-6.

Schofer JM. Biliary causes of postcholecystectomy syndrome. *J Emerg Med* 2010; 39: 406-10.

Shea JA, Berlin JA, Escarce JJ, et al. Revised estimates of diagnostic test sensitivity and specificity in suspected biliary tract disease. *Arch Intern Med* 1994; 154: 2573-81.

Sicklick JK, Camp MS, Lillemoe KD, et al. Surgical management of bile duct injuries sustained during laparoscopic cholecystectomy: perioperative results in 200 patients. *Ann Surg* 2005; 241: 786–92.

Smith L. Obstructions of the bile duct. *Br J Surg* 1979; 66: 69-79.

Solomkin JS, Mazuski JE, Bradley JS et al. Diagnosis and management of complicated intra-abdominal infection in adults and children: guidelines by the surgical infection society and the infectious diseases society of America. *Surg Infect (Larchmt)* 2010; 11: 79–109.

Soper NJ, Stockmann PT, Dunnegan DL, Ashley SW. Laparoscopic cholecystectomy. The new 'gold standard'? *Arch Surg* 1992; 127: 917-21.

Strickland AD, Norwood MG, Behnia-Willison F, et al. Transvaginal natural orifice translumenal endoscopic surgery (NOTES): a survey of women's views on a new technique. *Surg Endosc* 2010; 24: 2424-31.

Shah RP, Brown KT. Hepatic arterial embolization complicated by acute cholecystitis. *Semin Intervent Radiol* 2011; 28: 252-7.

Sinha I, Lawson Smith M, Safranek P, et al. Laparoscopic subtotal cholecystectomy without cystic duct ligation. *Br J Surg* 2007; 94: 1527–29.

Skouras C, Jarral O, Deshpande R, Zografos G, Habib N, Zacharakis E. Is early laparoscopic cholecystectomy for acute cholecystitis preferable to delayed surgery?: Best evidence topic (BET). *Int J Surg* 2012 Apr 21. [Epub ahead of print].

Strasberg SM. Biliary injury in laparoscopic surgery: Part 2. Changing the culture of cholecystectomy. *J Am Coll Surg* 2005; 201: 604–11.

Strasberg SM. Acute Calculous Cholecystitis. *N Eng J Med* 2008: 358: 2804-11.

Strasberg SM, Helton WS. An analytical review of vasculobiliary injury in laparoscopic and open cholecystectomy. *HPB (Oxford)* 2011; 13: 1-14.

Strasberg M, Hertl M, Soper NJ. An analysis of the problem of biliary injury during laparoscopic cholecystectomy. J Am Coll Surg 1995; 180: 101–25 .

Targarona Soler EM, Trías Folch M. Patología de la vesícula biliar. In: Cirugía AEC, *Manual de la Asociación Española de Cirujanos*. Ed. Médica Panamericana, Madrid 2010; 705.

Thistle JL, Cleary PA, Lachin JM, et al. The natural history of cholelithiasis: the National Cooperative Gallstone Study. *Ann Intern Med* 1984; 101: 171-5.

Thurley PD, Dhingsa R. Laparoscopic cholecystectomy: postoperative imaging. *AJR Am J Roentgenol* 2008; 191: 794-801.

Tonouchi H, Ohmori Y, Kobayashi M, Kusunoki M. Trocar site hernia. *Arch Surg* 2004; 139: 1248-56.

Trinchet Hernández M, Muñoz Calero A, Escat JL, Louredo A, de Tomás J, Lago J. Papel de la colecistectomía convencional en la actualidad. In: *Litiasis biliar*, Ed. Ergon, Madrid, 1996; 327.

Van Baal MC, Besselink MG, Bakker OJ et al. Timing of Cholecystectomy after Mild Biliary Pancreatitis: A Systematic Review. *Ann Surg* 2012; 255: 860-6.

Varadarajulu S, Tamhane A, Drelichman ER. Patient perception of natural orifice transluminal endoscopic surgery as a technique for cholecystectomy. *Gastrointest Endosc* 2008; 67: 854-60.

Velo Bellver JL, Gell Gómez E, Casariego García J, et al. *Epidemiología de la litiasis biliar. In: Litiasis biliar*, Ed. Ergon, Madrid, 1996; 15. .

Visser BC, Parks RW, Garden OJ. Open cholecystectomy in the laparoendoscopic era. *Am J Surg* 2008; 195: 108-14.

Vollmer CM Jr, Callery MP. Biliary injury following laparoscopic cholecystectomy: why still a problem? *Gastroenterology* 2007; 133: 1039-41.

Waage A, Nilsson M. Iatrogenic bile duct injury: a population-based study of 152 776 cholecystectomies in the Swedish Inpatient Registry. *Arch Surg* 2006; 141:1207–13.

Wilson E, Gurusamy K, Gluud C, et al. Cost–utility and value-of-information analysis of early versus delayed laparoscopic choleystectomy for acute cholecystitis. *Br J Surg* 2010; 97: 210-9.

Way LW, Stewart L, Gantert W, et al. Causes and prevention of laparoscopic bile duct injuries: analysis of 252 cases from a human factors and cognitive psychology perspective. *Ann Surg* 2003; 237: 460-9.

Wu YV, Linehan DC. Bile duct injuries in the era of laparoscopic cholecystectomies. *Surg Clin North Am* 2010; 90: 787– 802.

Yamashita Y, Takada T, Kawarada Y et al. Surgical treatment of patients with acute cholecystitis: Tokyo Guidelines. *Hepatobiliary Pancreat Surg* 2007; 14: 91–7.

Yoshida M, Takada T, Kawarada Y et al. Antimicrobial therapy for acute cholecystitis: Tokyo Guidelines. *J Hepatobiliary Pancreat Surg* 2007; 14: 83–90.

In: Cholecystectomies
Editors: Miyu Akiyama and Satomi Kunomasu

ISBN: 978-1-62257-890-0
© 2013 Nova Science Publishers, Inc.

Chapter II

Cholecystectomy: Traditional Laparoscopic and Open Techniques

Shiva Seetahal[1], Dilip Dan[2] and Vijay Naraynsingh[2]
[1]Howard University Hospital, Washington, DC, US
[2]University of the West Indies, St Augustine campus, Trinidad, West Indies

Abstract

Removal of the gallbladder has been long recognized as the best treatment for symptomatic gallstones. Incisions have evolved from laparotomy and extended Kocher's incision to "minilap" cholecystectomy. The revolutionary era of multi-port laparoscopic surgery in the 1980's- 90's saw transformation in the approach with much improved outcomes to the patient especially in terms of recovery. This is currently accepted as the standard operation for gallbladder disease. We are now witnessing another change that is not yet accepted as standard. Single port laparoscopy is "in vogue" and is still trying to prove itself as a sustainable alternative to multi- port laparoscopy. The obvious benefit is cosmesis but the long-term issues with hernia and pain are still to be discerned. Natural orifice cholecystectomy is still investigational and the advantages unproven.

In open cholecystectomy, a right subcostal incision is preferred. The "dome down" technique is utilized with careful dissection performed from the gallbladder fundus towards the neck. Along this path, the cystic artery must be identified and ligated. The cystic duct must be identified with absolute certainty prior to ligation. The incision must be carefully closed to avoid future hernia.

Laparoscopic Cholecystectomy possesses more versatility. The multiple incision approach involves placing a 12mm port peri-umbilically, a 5mm port in the right abdomen for gallbladder retraction and 2 left abdominal operating ports (5-10mm). The single incision approach involves a larger umbilical incision and specialized port that allows for 3 instruments. In either technique the gallbladder can be approached from a "dome down" perspective, similar to open surgery, or by exposing the "critical view". The latter entails retracting the gallbladder cranio-laterally to expose Calot's triangle and identifying the cystic duct and artery carefully before ligation. Various energy sources can then be utilized to dissect the gallbladder off of its bed and gain hemostasis. Specialized retrieval devices aid extraction of the organ from the umbilical incision.

Injury to the common bile duct (CBD) remains the most feared pitfall of gallbladder surgery. The 1990's saw a wave of high laparoscopic CBD injuries but with time, this has settled to be on par with open cholecystectomy. Proponents of intra-op cholangiography argue that it reduces the incidence, but this is unproven. Minor injuries may be repaired primarily with the support of a T-tube but larger injuries usually require hepaticojejunostomy for definitive repair. Additionally, repair should only be attempted by experienced surgeons. The morbidity associated with CBD injuries is significant.

Other potential complications include retention of calculi within the biliary system, bleeding, hernias and infection. As with all procedures, complication rates decrease with as the surgeon gains experience.

Introduction

Cholecystectomy is the term describing surgical removal of the gallbladder. It is the definitive treatment for symptomatic gallstones and non-neoplastic gallbladder disease. The operation has evolved significantly with time. The first documented cholecystectomy was performed by Carl Langenbuch in Germany in 1882 [1]. Prior to this, cholecystitis was treated with cholecystostomy and stone removal. Langenbuch recognized that removal of the source of calculi was the superior treatment approach, although his view on the dispensability of the gallbladder was met with controversy at that time [2]. Cholecystectomy would evolve from a laparotomy approach to smaller and more strategic incisions over the course of the twentieth century [3]. A major milestone came with the advent of laparoscopic surgery. The first laparoscopic cholecystectomy was performed by Eric Muhe in 1985. Remarkably, this surgery was also performed in Germany and was a source of significant controversy, much like that of his predecessor Dr Langenbuch. This technique would be adopted and modified over the subsequent years by several surgeons, but in 1999 Professor Muhe was officially recognized by the American Society of Gastrointestinal Surgeons (SAGES) as having performed the first laparoscopic cholecystectomy [4].

Today, laparoscopic cholecystectomy is the "gold-standard" treatment for symptomatic cholelithiasis. Advances in technology and technique have improved the efficiency of the procedure and reduced the complication rate. However, it remains imperative that the skills for performing open cholecystectomy are not lost; the open approach is still required for cases where laparoscopy is contra-indicated or inadequate. Minilaparotomy may also be used. With this in mind, we describe our approaches to laparoscopic, open and minilaparotomy cholecystectomy.

Laparoscopic Cholecystectomy

Preoperative Evaluation

Planning surgery for patients with gallbladder disease should begin in the same manner as that of any other surgical patient – with a detailed history and physical. Specifically related to this procedure however, the surgeon must also determine the extent of gallbladder disease and the suitability of the patient for laparoscopy. The spectrum of benign gallbladder disease can essentially be divided into two broad categories – inflammatory and non-inflammatory. Inflammatory disease encompasses relatively common afflictions such as acute cholecystitis to the rarer but potentially catastrophic empyema of the gallbladder. Patients with complications of acute cholecystitis may sometimes be better served with an open approach from the beginning, so careful history and exam, and accurate diagnosis is essential. Non-inflammatory disease usually describes cholelithiasis. However, choledocholithiasis can be a troublesome complication and alters the algorithms of management. The surgeon must be aware of the potential complications of gallstones during the initial assessment and tailor the evaluation to confirm or exclude these possibilities.

An often overlooked aspect of the history is an estimation of the number of previous episodes of acute cholecystitis. Prior episodes of inflammation produce scarring, making identification of structures and dissection more difficult [5, 6]. This itself is not a contra-indication to laparoscopy, but is useful for the surgeon to anticipate possible difficulties and plan accordingly. Additional factors to be considered include previous surgeries, patient body habitus and the presence of any co-morbidities that may complicate laparoscopy or surgery in general.

Laboratory investigations should include basic blood tests that are appropriate for the age and medical history of the patient. Additionally, all patients should have coagulation studies and liver function tests. Imaging of the gallbladder is best performed by ultrasonography. Despite its limitation of being operator dependent, it has a higher sensitivity and specificity than CT for detecting gallstone disease [7]. Ultrasound can identify abnormal dilatation of the common bile duct (CBD) which necessitates further imaging of the duct and/or intra-operative exploration. Appropriate imaging modalities include magnetic resonance cholangiopancreatography (MRCP), endoscopic ultrasound (EUS) and endoscopic retro-grade cholangiopancreatography (ERCP) [8, 9]. The latter has the advantage of being potentially therapeutic as well as diagnostic, and can be employed to explore and clear the CBD prior to surgery and avoid having to perform an intra-op exploration. Other imaging modalities that may be encountered include oral cholecystography – now largely of historical interest only, and intraductal ultrasonaography (IDUS) which is gaining in popularity [10, 11].

The goal of per-operative evaluation should be the acquisition of information that allows for correct diagnosis, selection of appropriate surgical procedure, patient counseling regarding potential risks and benefits and trouble-shooting potential dangers peri-operatively. From this perspective, the evaluation process demands a dynamic approach and relies on the clinical acumen of the surgical team involved.

Contra-Indications

Expertise and technology advancements in the field of minimally-invasive surgery have shortened the list of contra-indications to laparoscopy. However, certain conditions cannot be ignored. An absolute contra-indication to laparoscopic cholecystectomy is the potential of gallbladder carcinoma; suspicion of cancer warrants an open approach [13]. Additionally, any patient with co-morbidities that place them at excessive risk of cardio respiratory complications during pneumo-peritoneum should be considered for open approach.

Liver disease with portal hypertension is a tricky proposition. The benefits of the laparoscopic approach over the open is substantial, however even laparoscopic dissection in these patients can be hazardous. Such patients should be operated upon by experienced surgeons following multi-disciplinary pre-operative management [13,14]. Coagulopathy is a relative contra-indication since most abnormalities can be reversed with transfusion of blood products. Ventral hernias may be considered to be complicating factors, but are no longer considered contra-indications. Umbilical hernias can be repaired during closure of the abdominal wall and variation in the placement of trocars can avoid larger abdominal wall defects [15, 16]. Large hernias may well require excess insufflation but external buttressing can minimize these complications. Obesity is a common and potentially challenging obstacle, especially for the inexperienced surgeon. Voluminous abdominal cavity, excessive omental fat and large steatotic liver make for difficult identification of anatomy and dissection. Finally, in pregnancy the second trimester is considered the "safe" period for laparoscopic cholecystectomy as organogenesis in the fetus is mostly complete and the uterus is not yet large enough to obscure the operative field [17]. However, it is prudent to work at reduced insufflation pressure to minimize potential complications. Sickle-cell patients represent another patient population who benefit from lower pneumo-peritoneum pressures [18].

Operative Technique

Appropriate antibiotics should be given no more than 1 hour prior to incision. Thrombo-prophylactic measures should also be instituted before administration of general anesthesia as is appropriate. The pneumo-peritoneum creates an additional risk-factor for deep-vein thrombosis (DVT) [19].

The patient should be placed in a supine position with both arms tucked at the sides to allow easy access for both the surgeon and assistant. Alternatively the Lloyd Davies or lithotomy position may be used, with the surgeon standing between the legs of the patient. A urinary catheter is usually unnecessary as the bladder does not fall into the surgical field. However, if the surgeon anticipates a prolonged operating time a catheter may be useful to accurately measure urinary output. Clippers should be used to remove hair from the abdominal wall. An oro- or nasogastric tube should be inserted for decompression of the stomach; this facilitates visualization and also reduces the risk of injury to the stomach. Following induction of anesthesia, the operative field should be cleansed using iodine or alcohol solution. The entire abdomen should be prepared, including extension cranially above the lower margins of the costal cartilages. This ensures a sterile field even if conversion to open procedure is necessary. The patient is then draped.

The traditional approaches to laparoscopic cholecystectomy entail the surgeon standing to the left of the patient with the assistant on the opposite side. Monitors should be positioned so as to be within clear view and at eye-level of the operators to preserve ergonomic integrity. Access to the abdominal cavity can be attained by various methods. We prefer to use the open technique as it is associated with lower incidences of bowel injury [20]. Port placement using a bladeless trocar under direct vision has been gaining popularity; it reduces port-placement time but carries a higher risk of visceral injury [21]. As such, it is perhaps better suited to the more experienced surgeon. The first port should be placed peri-umbilically. A 12mm trocar is necessary as this port will provide the extraction point for the gallbladder. In a patient with an umbilical hernia, the port can be placed through the defect once it has been established that the hernia sac has been reduced into the abdomen. In a patient with previous abdominal surgery, scar tissue and bowel adhesion to the abdominal wall complicates access. The initial trocar should be placed in an area that is removed from scarring to avoid inadvertent bowel injury.

Following entry into the abdominal cavity, pneumoperitoneum is established. Typically, an average pressure of 14-18 mmHg is sufficient with carbon dioxide being the preferred gas. A 10mm laparoscope is used to first inspect the abdominal cavity and then to assist in placement of accessory trocars. The positioning of accessory trocars often varies according to the prerogative of the surgeon. We utilize a 5mm port in the epigastrum and another in the mid-clavicular to anterior-axillary line on the left side, approximately 5 cm below the costal margin. These represent the primary operating ports. Another 5 mm port is placed in the right abdomen 5cm below the costal margin for the purposes of gallbladder retraction. A common pitfall in laparoscopic surgery is improper placement of operating ports. It has been our experience that allocating a few extra minutes to ensure that all ports are strategically positioned for optimal access and maneuverability ultimately shortens overall operating time and greatly enhances the ease of the procedure.

Once all ports have been placed, the patient should be placed in "reverse-Trendelenburg" position and rotated to the left to optimize the visual field. A three port technique has also been described. A locking, atraumatic grasper is inserted into the right-sided port and used to grasp the fundus of the gallbladder.

This may be difficult in a distended gallbladder, in which case the organ should be decompressed first. This can be performed either with an aspiration instrument via the trocar or percutaneously with a needle and syringe under direct vision. Care is taken not to spill any bile into the abdominal cavity. The gallbladder fundus is then retracted cranially and laterally. This maneuver exposes the touted "critical view" [22].

The left hand of the operating surgeon then uses an atraumatic grasper to retract the lateral wall of the gallbladder at Hartmann's pouch (Figure 1). This completes the exposure of the vital structures within Calot's triangle (Figure 2). A dissecting forceps can be used to initiate exploration around the cystic duct. Care should be taken to stay close to the gallbladder during this dissection. The surgeon retracting the left-handed grasper antero-laterally assists greatly in this process.

Once a portal has been made into the peritoneum, the anatomy should be re-evaluated before continuing dissection to avoid irreparable injuries. The junction of the gallbladder neck and cystic duct should be exposed and identifiable without ambiguity. To gain circumferential control of the cystic duct, the proximal gallbladder can be maneuvered postero-medially giving access to the posterior aspect of the duct. When the cystic duct has been cleared circumferentially, with Calot's triangle exposed, the duct can be clipped and divided.

Attention can then turn to the cystic artery. In recent years, evidence has shown that ultrasonic shears are adequate for ligating and transecting the cystic artery [23]. However, many surgeons still prefer to carefully identify this vessel before ligation with hemostatic clips and transection.

For the young surgeon, dissecting and identifying the cystic artery provides valuable experience and frequently peace-of-mind. We recommend this approach as well because significant bleeding can occur from an enlarged, improperly cauterized cystic vessel. The cystic artery should be delineated and divided in a manner similar to the cystic duct; it usually resides posterior and medially to the duct. Once it has been successfully divided, dissection of the gallbladder off of its bed can proceed.

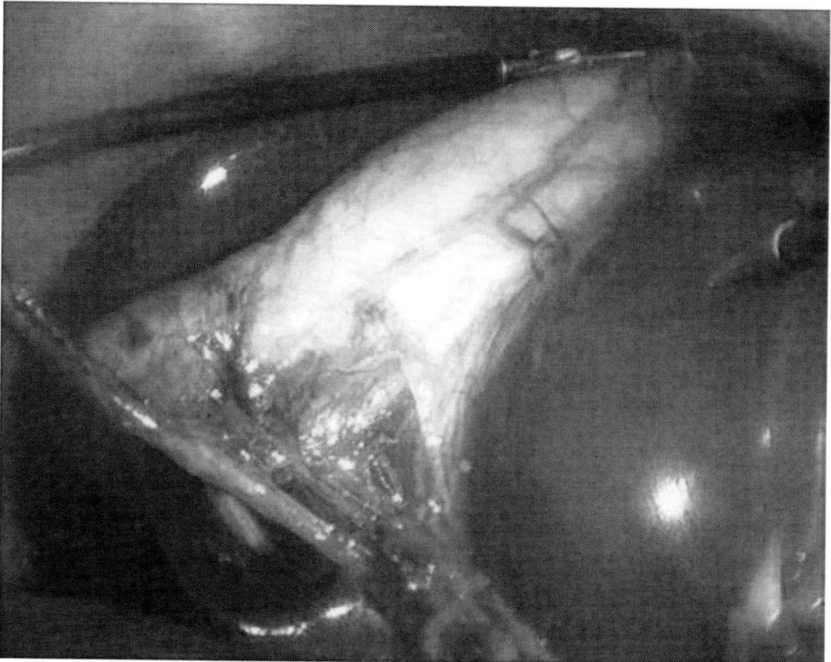

Figure 1. Retraction of the gallbladder to obtain the "critical view". Notice the fundus is retracted cranially and Hartman`s pouch antero-laterally.

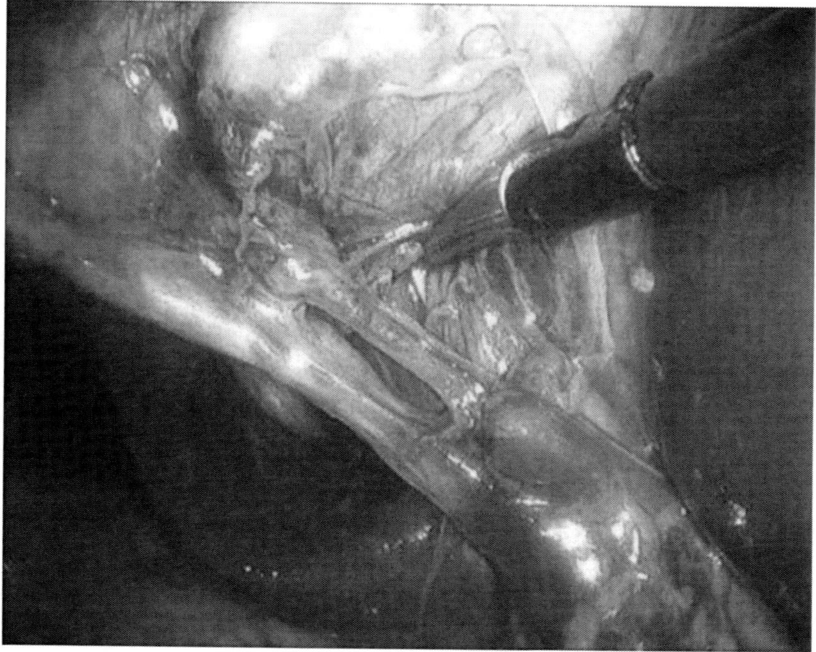

Figure 2. Close-up of the "critical view". The cystic duct (laterally), cystic artery (medial to the duct) and Calot`s node are shown.

We utilize harmonic shears to separate the gallbladder from the gallbladder fossa. Monopolar cautery is also appropriate with the advantage of being less costly. The mesentery of the gallbladder can vary in length, with shorter mesentery increasing the difficulty of the dissection. In such cases, caution should be exercised to avoid excessive injury to the hepatic parenchyma and troublesome bleeding. When this does occur, coagulation with the ultrasonic shears or cautery, topical hemostatic agents or even direct pressure with the aid of a gauze sponge are appropriate for hemostasis. Before the gallbladder is completely taken off of the bed, a final inspection should be performed to exclude the presence of any bleeding or bile leak (Figure 3).

Perforation of the gallbladder during dissection is not ideal as the bile spillage can cause peritoneal irritation. In instances of perforation, the gallbladder can be grasped at the defect with the non-traumatic grasper to stem the egress of bile. Alternatively, clips can be applied to the defect. Gallstones that escaped into the abdominal cavity should ideally be retrieved if easily identifiable; meticulous exploration for very small stones is not necessary however.

The gallbladder should be "bagged" within the abdominal cavity before removal from the abdomen. Commercially available plastic laparoscopic retrieval bags are popular, but improvisation using other materials can often accomplish the same results [24, 25, 26]. The 12mm periumbilical port is appropriate for specimen removal; the 12 mm laparoscope should be exchanged for a 5mm scope for the extraction. Specimens containing large gallstones may be difficult to extract. A Kelly forceps can be used to widen the fascial orifice or the fascial incision may need to be widened. Special caution must be taken to avoid perforating the retrieval bag and spilling bile into the abdominal cavity. Following extraction of the specimen, a final inspection of the abdomen is performed before removing the ports and beginning closure. Irrigation of the gallbladder bed and surrounding area should be performed following removal of the gallbladder and prior to closure in cases of bile spillage. The umbilical incision is the only one that requires fascial closure.

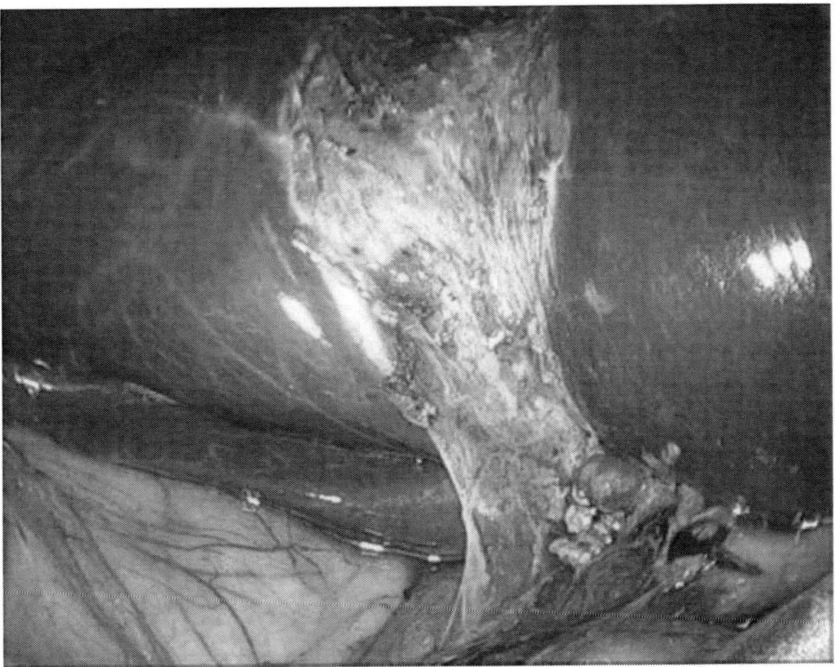

Figure 3. The gallbladder fossa and ligated cystic duct and artery following removal of the gallbladder.

Improper repair of these defects can spawn incisional hernias [27, 28]. We use a 0-Vicryl or 1-Prolene suture in a "figure-of- eight" configuration to bring the cut edges of the fascia together. Manual palpation of the repair will detect any weaknesses in the repair and additional interrupted sutures can be applied. The skin incisions are closed with 4/0 absorbable suture in the subcuticular layer. Dry dressings are then applied and the patient can be woken.

We do not practice routine intra-operative cholangiography although there are arguments for its inclusion; its place in standard laparoscopic cholecystectomy remains controversial [29]. The techniques involved are outside the scope of this chapter. Single-port laparoscopic cholecystectomy has emerged as a modification of the original technique that utilizes a single umbilical incision as opposed to 3- 4 separate, smaller ones. An umbilical incision is made to gain entry to the peritoneal cavity and a specialized access port is placed through this orifice. These ports vary according to manufacturer, but the general principle is that each allows for 3 instruments – the laparoscope and 2 additional instruments. Via this approach, the gallbladder is removed in similar fashion to that described. The challenges posed by this technique include the need for specialized ports and instruments, and a less ergonomic working space for the surgeons that usually requires specific practice and training. The purported advantage is the presence of only one incision thereby reducing peri-operative pain as well as post-operative scarring (the umbilical incision can be "hidden" within the recess of the umbilicus). We remain unconvinced as to the virtues of single-incision laparoscopy and prefer the more traditional method in our practice [30, 31, 32].

Complications

Peri-operative bleeding is uncommon but may occur. Intra-operatively, potential bleeding sources include the cystic artery, aberrant right hepatic artery and hepatic parenchyma in the gallbladder fossa. These can be addressed with combinations of hemostatic clips, cautery, ultrasonic shears and topical hemostatic agents or simple gauze pressure (see *Operative Technique*). Bleeding from the hepatic parenchyma can appear severe but will usually be self-limiting in patients with normal coagulation profiles. In such cases of persistent oozing, post-operative monitoring of the patient and measurement of hematocrit would be beneficial. Post-operatively, patients who present with persistent tachycardia, hypotension, severe abdominal pain, acidosis or dropping hematocrit levels should be suspected of suffering from post-operative hemorrhage. In the unstable patient, immediate re-exploration is warranted to identify and address the bleeding source. The hemodynamically stable with patient with declining hematocrit may be monitored with serial blood draws, and either CT scan or abdominal ultrasound should be performed. Imaging can offer insight into the severity and site of the bleeding. Persistent bleeding despite supportive care and transfusion demands re-exploration. Less commonly, angiography and embolization can be considered [33].

Biliary leakage occurs in approximately 1% of laparoscopic cholecytectomies [34, 35]. Cystic duct leaks constitute the majority of these complications. Patients present with persistent abdominal pain, tachycardia, fever and leucocytosis post-operatively. In severe cases, sepsis can occur. Suspicion of biliary leakage warrants imaging – CT, ultrasound or Hepatobiliary iminodiacetic (HIDA) scan. Fluid collections seen on imaging should be aspirated to determine etiology (blood versus bile). Aspiration of bilious fluid is also therapeutic as the inflammatory reaction and septic response is mitigated with removal of the offending fluid. Cystic duct leakage is treated by endoscopic decompression of the biliary tree via endoscopic retrograde cholangiopancreatography (ERCP) and stenting at the Ampulla of Vater. Leakage of bile from the ducts of Lushka is rarely clinically significant and often self-limiting. In cases of persistent bile leakage, aberrant ductal anatomy is usually the culprit and re-exploration may be required.

Injury to the common bile duct (CBD) is perhaps the most notorious complication of minimally-invasive cholecystectomy. The laparoscopic approach has been described as having a 2-3 fold increase in the incidence of these injuries [36, 37]. Pitfalls that predispose to CBD injuries include inexperience (a relative term that is married to the concept of the "learning curve"), difficult gallbladder anatomy and improper surgical technique [38]. The "critical view" technique has gained acceptance and popularity for its easy application and impressive results [22, 39]. Nevertheless, CBD injuries do occur and early detection remains an essential aspect of management. Intra-operative recognition of CBD injury allows the surgeon the option of immediate repair or temporization. In general, partial transections can be repaired with monofilamentous absorbable sutures over a T-tube. Larger or complete transections are best treated by choledocho- or hepato-jejunostomy. Both of these approaches require considerable skill and experience on the part of the surgeon.

If the surgeon harbors any doubt regarding their ability to perform CBD repair or salvage successfully, temporizing measures should be instituted and preparations made for transfer of the patient to an appropriate facility with better capabilities for repair.

Temporizing measures include placement of a closed suction drain to create a controlled biliary-cutaneous fistula. If the CBD has been accidentally clipped, drainage of the biliary tree is warranted with either a choledochotomy and T-tube intra-operatively, or a percutaneous tranhepatic cholangiographic (PTC) drain post-operatively. Proponents of intra-operative cholangiogram argue that bile duct injuries are less common and more likely to be detected on-table with the use of routine cholangiography [40] (Figure 4).

Post operatively, CBD injuries manifest with pain and jaundice. The main differential is the presence of retained bile duct stones. ERCP or HIDA scan are required to confirm diagnosis. With ERCP, PTC may also be required to delineate anatomy of the biliary tree as well as to decompress the proximal ducts.

When the diagnosis of CBD injury is delayed, there is some debate as to the optimal timing of repair. Arguments have been made for and against both early (within days of injury) and late (more than 6 weeks after injury) repair, with some consensus that "intermediate" repairs are the least efficient [41, 42].

Injury to right, left or common hepatic ducts should be treated using the same principles – hepatojejunostomy (in Roux-n-Y configuration).

Retained calculi within the CBD can manifest with post-operative pain and jaundice. Direct hyperbilirubinemia following surgery should arouse suspicion of retained stones. Intra-operative cholangiography can be a valuable adjunct to cholecystectomy in patients who are suspected of having choledocholithiasis and who have not had ERCP pre-operatively. Although the latter option is preferred in most centers for stones in the CBD pre-operatively, it is also a feasible option for obstructing stones discovered after surgery [43]. During cholecystectomy, if stones are discovered (via cholangiography or choledochoscopy) or suspected, intravenous glucagon should be administered and the CBD irrigated.

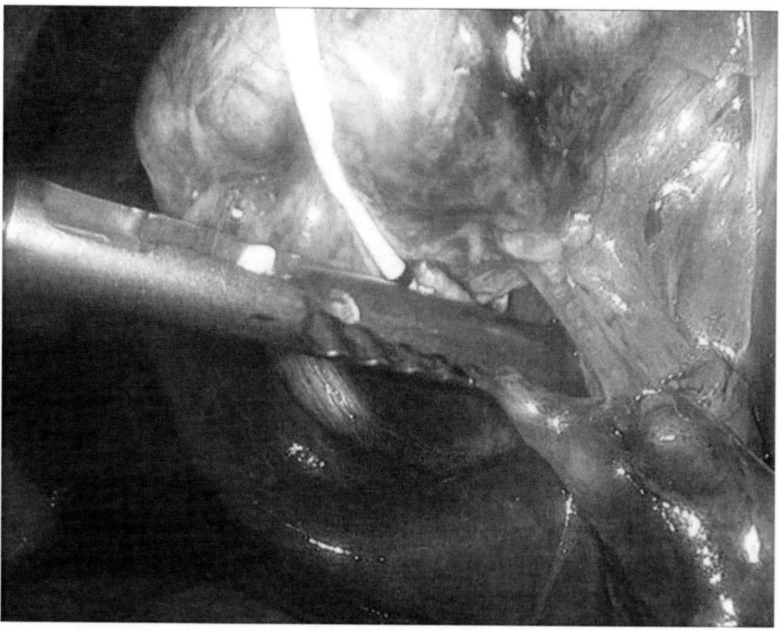

Figure 4. Insertion of a catheter into the cystic duct for an intra-operative cholangiogram.

Glucagon can cause relaxation in the Sphincter of Oddi and facilitate evacuation of calculi from the duct. Stones that cannot be flushed can be extracted by various techniques – "milking" toward the Sphincter of Oddi or cystic duct stump; choledochoscopic retrieval; choledochotomy and direct retrieval or fragmentation and flushing/extraction.

When there is concern for persistent debris with the duct, impacted stones or fears of subsequent cholangitis from duct manipulation, a T-tube can be secured within the duct and a controlled bilary-cutaneous fistula constructed. The advantage of this technique is that it allows for repeat cholangiography and access to the CBD while decompressing it.

The T-tube is generally kept for 4-7 weeks to allow maturation of the fistula before removal. Critics of this technique consider the potential complications and inconvenience of the T-tube to outweigh its possible benefits [44, 45].

Finally, incisional hernias are a rare complication given the increased attention paid to proper fascial closure. Special consideration must be afforded to fascial closure especially when difficult specimen extraction necessitates widening of the umbilical incision.

Open Cholecystectomy

Pre-Operative Evaluation

Pre-operative work-up for open cholecystectomy is essentially identical to that of laparoscopy. History, physical exam, routine laboratory investigations including liver function and coagulations tests, as well as appropriate adjunctive studies (EKG, chest radiograph, etc.) are required. Imaging of the gallbladder is also prudent, for the purposes of documenting underlying pathology as well as evaluation of the CBD for evidence of possible choledocholithiasis. In such instances, the algorithm is the same as for laparoscopic cases described earlier.

The decision to proceed with the open approach as opposed to the minimally-invasive approach is mitigated by several factors. Apart from the absolute and relative contra-indications to laparoscopy already discussed - previous upper abdominal surgery, the presence of a gangrenous gallbladder and to a lesser extent patient age are all indications to consider open approach [46]. Adhesions from prior surgeries increase the risk of bowel injury during port placement and increase the difficulty of maneuvering, and ultimately operating effectively [47]. Although these difficulties are surmountable, the experience level of the surgeon will often dictate the extent to which this challenge is accepted. Gangrenous gallbladders pose another set of difficulties, as sub-optimal control of the gangrenous tissue risks spreading of infected material throughout the peritoneal cavity. In these circumstances, where there is certainty or reasonable suspicion of gangrene or empyema, the open approach is considered safer [48, 49].

Gallbladder carcinoma is a unique entity that requires open cholecystectomy. Unfortunately, it is not always diagnosed prior to the removal of the organ and is commonly detected during routine pathological analysis following (usually laparoscopic) cholecystectomy. However, in the instances where it is suspected, the open approach is mandated [50, 51, 52]. These procedures may entail intra-operative "frozen-section" analysis and hepatic segmentectomy for invasive disease. A full discussion on gallbladder carcinoma is outside the scope of this chapter.

A significant number of open cholecystectomies begin as laparoscopic procedures. In the modern era, it has been lamented by some surgeons that the art of open surgery is being lost [53]. We offer no opinions on the veracity of this statement, but rather emphasize the point that conversion of a laparoscopic procedure to an open one is not a failure on the part of the surgeon, nor should it be considered a complication. Pre-operatively, the patient should be well aware of the potential risks that may require conversion and should be counseled appropriately. The surgeon should likewise have little compunction in converting if the safety and efficacy of the operation is in compromise. The decision to open may follow initial access and inspection of the abdomen and gallbladder. Organs discovered to be gangrenous, severely scarred or adherent to surrounding structures are all acceptable reasons for conversion. Additionally, during the procedure if there is difficulty if identification of anatomical structures with absolute certainty or unusual duress associated with attempts at dissection, then conversion is a feasible option. Studies investigating laparoscopic-to-open cholecystectomies also cite male gender, number of co-morbidities, age and surgeon experience as potential risk factors [54, 55, 56, 57].

Operative Technique

The right subcostal incision (Kocher's incision) is preferred by most surgeon's as it provides excellent exposure and access to the gallbladder [58]. Alternatively, an upper abdominal midline incision can be utilized. The length of the incision is dictated by the comfort level of the surgeon in most cases. The "Mini-lap cholecystectomy" is a modification of the Kocher's incision; it utilizes an (approximately) 4 cm incision which is typically one third to one half the length of a traditional Kocher's incision. The advantages derived include less scarring and post-operative pain; the challenges associated with performing the procedure from a smaller incision are considerable however. The "Mini-lap" technique is generally preferred by more experienced surgeons for these reasons.

The abdomen is opened in layers with electrocautery. Special attention to hemostasis should be applied when dissecting through the muscle layers. Once the peritoneum is incised and the abdominal cavity entered the liver and gallbladder are inspected carefully. Self-retaining retractors are useful in allowing the hands of the surgeons to be free, but care must be taken to ensure that the retractor blades do not cause damage to the liver or bowel; laparotomy tapes folded into pads work nicely in this respect. The right lobe of the liver overlying the gallbladder fossa (along Cantlie's line) should be gently retracted cranially to expose the gallbladder. Judicious placement of oro- or naso-gastric tubes will decompress the stomach and assist in its retraction. Laparotomy tapes can be used for packing to keep small bowel, hepatic flexure of the colon, stomach and omentum outside of the immediate operating field. As with any procedure, adequate exposure is a key to success.

The gallbladder may require decompression to allow for easier manipulation and prevention of accidental bile spillage. This can be easily performed by insertion of the decompressing needle into the body of the organ. Moist packs should be placed around the gallbladder to catch any potential bile spillage. Following decompression, a clamp or stitch is placed on the artificial orifice created to limit further seepage.

There are two approaches to removing the gallbladder – the "Dome-down" technique and the "Critical View" technique. The latter adheres to the same principles as in laparoscopic cholecystectomy and is considered advantageous for the reasons that it adds familiarity to the procedure for the surgeon who may otherwise be accustomed to the minimally-invasive approach, and it allows for identification of anatomical structures prior to dissection. However, scarred gallbladders that are adherent to surrounding structures may make this approach just as difficult via an open incision as they would have done via laparoscopy. In these circumstances, the "Dome-down" technique is prudent. The performance of the "Critical view" technique follows the same sequence as previously described with the exception that a retrieval bag is not necessary.

The "Dome-down" technique entails dissecting the gallbladder off of its bed before identifying and addressing the vessels and cystic duct. It is a technique that can also be applied laparoscopically. The fundus of the gallbladder is grasped with a Kelly clamp and a plane of dissection is started between the gallbladder and the underlying gallbladder fossa of the liver. The length of the mesenteric attachment of the gallbladder dictates the ease of this dissection as well as the presence or absence of chronic inflammation and scar tissue. Electrocautery is appropriate for the dissection to minimize bleeding. With continuous gentle traction on the gallbladder, the plane of dissection is carried toward the neck of the organ with care taken during this approach to identify the vital structures of the cystic artery and cystic duct. A right-angled forceps is an invaluable tool during dissection as it allows for blunt dissection of the tissue before cauterization; this reduces the risk of inadvertent injury to ductal or vascular tissue. The cystic artery, once encountered, is ligated and transected. Hemostatic clips or 2/0 Vicryl suture are both appropriate. Special consideration should be afforded to the vessel prior to ligation to ensure that it is indeed the cystic vessel and not an aberrant hepatic vessel. Following transection of the cystic artery, the cystic duct is identified using blunt dissection and isolated from its surrounding tissue. Meticulous attention is applied to ensure the duct is not mis-identified to prevent inadvertent injury to the hepatic ducts or

CBD. The cystic duct should be ligated with hemoclips or sutures similar to the cystic artery, however it should be double-ligated on the proximal end to cater for possible slippage and to prevent egress of gallstones into the CBD. The duct is divided sharply following ligation and any additional attachments on the gallbladder are removed so that the organ can be extracted.

Occasionally, the gallbladder is extremely scarred and adherent to its fossa. In such instances, dissection of the required plane can become extremely difficult. A sub-total cholecystectomy can be performed in these circumstances, leaving a small portion of the gallbladder wall that is adherent to the liver parenchyma. This reduces the risk of damage to the hepatic tissue and subsequent bleeding while maintaining the integrity of the procedure [59, 60]. Apart from avoiding dissection of the gallbladder tissue adherent to its fossa, the cystic duct may be difficult to isolate and separate. The orifice of the duct should identified from an intra-luminal approach and then ligated with a 3/0 absorbable suture. No further attempts should be made to dissect the duct as this may lend itself to iatrogenic injuries to adjacent structures. The mucosa of all gallbladder tissue being left in-situ should be ablated with the electrocautery to reduce the likelihood of post-operative biloma. Many surgeons would advocate oversewing of residual tissue as well to minimize this complication. Additionally, post-operative drainage is appropriate in such circumstances.

Following removal of the gallbladder, a final inspection of the operative field is performed to ensure hemostasis. If bile spillage occurred, or if gangrenous tissue was present, copious irrigation is performed prior to beginning closure. In such cases, consideration may be given to drain placement. There has been much discussion regarding the placement of drains, with the general consensus being that they are not routinely required. In circumstances where drainage is desired, closed-suction drains are preferred and the goal is early removal post-operatively to limit drain-associated morbidity [61, 62].

Troublesome bleeding from hepatic parenchyma may be addressed by topical coagulants, packing or laser coagulation when the electrocautery device is inadequate. Severe or persistent bleeding should be controlled prior to closure. Intra-operative cholangiography can be performed via the stump of the cystic duct following removal of the gallbladder. A full discussion on the details of this procedure is outside the scope of this chapter.

Closure of the abdominal wall should be performed in layers. Failure to perform adequate closure will predispose the patient to incisional hernia. The peritoneum, Scarpa's fascia, muscle layers and skin should be approximated and closed adequately to prevent this complication.

In cases of gangrene or severe spillages, a case can be made for non-closure or partial closure of the skin in anticipation of post-operative wound infection. In cases of non-infected bile spillage, this precaution is seldom necessary. Injection of local anesthetic during wound closure improves pain control post-operatively. We routinely admit these patients for overnight observation and pain control.

Complications

The myriad of potential complications following open cholecystectomy mirrors those encountered during laparoscopy. Injury to the bile ducts, bleeding and retained stones are all managed similarly. Unique to the open approach is a higher incidence of incisional hernias

[63]. This may lend itself to long-term morbidity associated with the procedure. Meticulous technique during closure reduces the likelihood of this complication. Open procedures are associated with higher incidences of post-operative pain and delayed return to normal function [64, 65].

This can be overcome with appropriate adjustment to analgesia regimens as well as aggressive ambulation and rehabilitation. The potential sequelae of delayed ambulation include the feared outcomes of venous thrombo-embolism. Patients should be stratified according to their risk status and managed accordingly with either mechanical or chemical thrombo-prophylaxis or combinations thereof.

Minilaparotomy Cholecystectomy (MLC)

Although the advantages of laparoscopic cholecystectomy (LC) over open cholecystectomy (OC) are well established, MLC offers many of the same benefits as LC [66, 67]. In fact, MLC reduced postoperative pain, hospital stay, resulted in quicker recovery and provided better patient satisfaction when compared to OC[68]. Pre-operative evaluation is the same as for LC and OC.

Operative Technique

The procedure is performed under General Anesthesia, through a transverse 3-6 cm right subcostal incision placed over the lateral half of the rectus abdominis and extending into the external oblique. All layers, anterior rectus sheath, lateral half of rectus abdominis, posterior rectus sheath and the adjacent external, internal obliques and transversus abdominis, are incised down to the peritoneum using diathermy. It is also possible to do a rectus sparing exposure where, when the anterior rectus is incised, the muscle is mobilised and drawn medially in order to expose and incise the posterior rectus sheath. When the peritoneum is opened, a laparotomy pack is completely inserted into the abdomen, between the liver cephalad and the gut caudally, using the left index finger as a guide. If there is an acute aortic inflammatory mass, the index finger is used to peel the omentum off the tense gall bladder before inserting the pack. A narrow deep retractor is placed cephalad and caudad exposing the area between the duodenum and liver (Figure 5).

A long curved artery forceps is used to grasp and pull Hartmann's pouch upward and laterally. Dissection of the cystic duct and cystic artery are done as for an OC; clips are used to secure these before dividing them. The gall bladder is then dissected off the liver using diathermy although some surgeons have suggested that it can be safely peeled off with a finger [69].

Thus, dissection is done as for OC but through a much smaller incision (Figure 6), using narrow retractors, long instruments aided by a fibreoptic headlight and 3.5 x loupe magnification. No drains or nasogastric tubes are used. The incision is closed in layers along with infiltration of 20 ml of .25% bupivacaine into the sheath and muscle under vision. Opiods such as morphine or NSAIDS are used for postoperative analgesia as needed. Oral fluids are introduced as soon as the patient is fully awake since intravenous fluids are not routinely used. Usually patients are discharged with 24 hours.

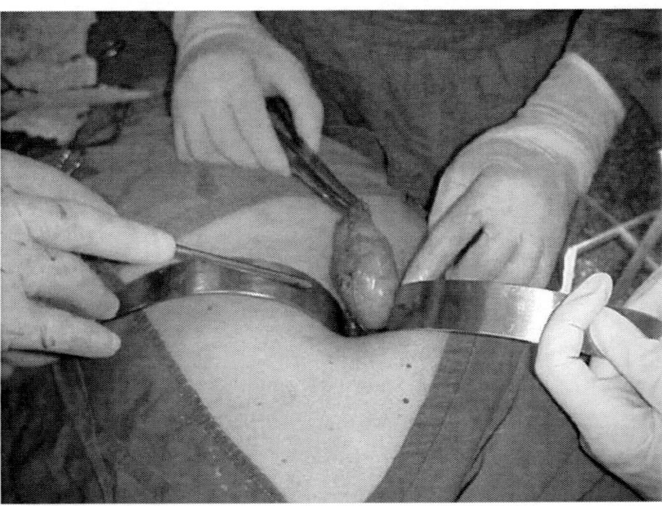

Figure 5. Extraction of gallbladder from the minilaparotomy incision.

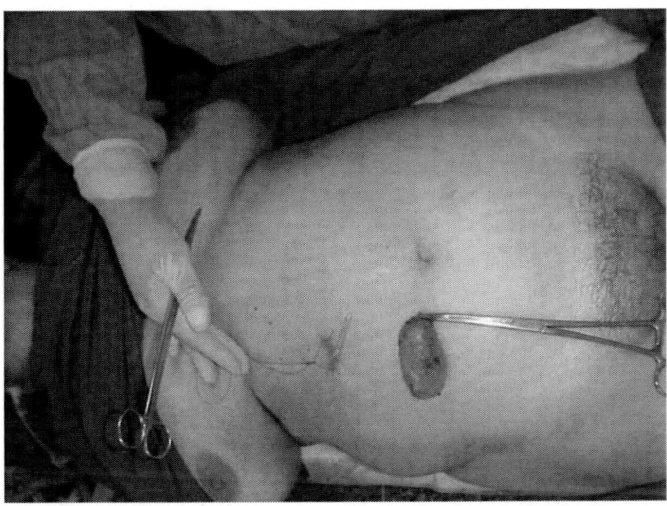

Figure 6. Comparison of the gallbladder (specimen) to the surgical incision for minilaparotomy cholecystectomy.

Discussion

MLC can be performed with the same instruments and using essentially the same technique as OC. It is therefore does not require additional equipment, specialized training and certification for its performance. In addition, it can be safely performed for acute cholecystitis, empyema, gall bladder masses or mucocele in shorter time than LC [70]. Thus, while the superiority of LC over OC is well established, evidence for its advantages over MLC has been poor and the result of randomized controlled trials conflicting [66-67, 71-73]. In certain circumstances where populations are small, the number of cases limited, the cost of instrumentation prohibitive, expertise in equipment servicing is lacking and operating room time is restricted, MLC may be advantageous over LC [70, 74]. Mastery of MLC may also have the benefit that when conversion is needed during LC, one can proceed with MLC and still provide similar benefits of LC to the patient.

Conclusion

Gallbladder disease has posed challenges to surgeons for centuries, and especially with the obesity pandemic, gives little promise of relenting. Possessing anatomy that has been extensively studied and described, and being introduced to the young surgeon at the burgeoning stages of training, it can be underestimated in its capacity for surgical complications. The techniques described in this chapter do not begin exhaust the repertoire of skills utilized for extrication of this organ, however they do provide a solid base from which an enterprising and diligent surgeon can build. Ultimately, adherence to sound surgical technique and principles will be the most invaluable tools in any surgeon`s armamentarium.

Acknowledgments

Photos courtesy of Dr Etwar McBean, Providence Hospital, Washington, DC and Professor Vijay Naraynsingh, University of the West Indies, St Augustine, Trinidad.

References

[1]   Traverso LW. Carl Langenbuch and the first cholecystectomy. *Am. J. Surg.* 1976 Jul; 132 (1):81-2.

[2]   van Gulik, TM.Neth. Langenbuch's cholecystectomy, once a remarkably controversial operation. *J. Surg.* 1986 Oct; 38(5):138-41.

[3]   Soper NJ. Cholecystectomy: from Langenbuch to natural orifice transluminal endoscopic surgery. *World J. Surg.* 2011 Jul; 35(7):1422-7.

[4]   Jani K, Rajan PS, Sendhilkumar K, Palanivelu C.J. Twenty years after Erich Muhe: Persisting controversies with the gold standard of laparoscopic cholecystectomy. *Minim. Access Surg.* 2006 Jun;2(2):49-58.

[5]   Hussain A. Difficult Laparoscopic Cholecystectomy: *Current Evidence and Strategies of Management.Surg Laparosc Endosc. Percutan. Tech.* 2011 Aug; 21(4):211-7.

[6]   Schirmer BD, Winters KL, Edlich RF. Cholelithiasis and cholecystitis. *J. Long Term Eff. Med. Implants.* 2005;15(3):329-38.

[7]   Benarroch-Gampel J, Boyd CA, Sheffield KM, Townsend CM Jr, Riall TS. Overuse of CT in patients with complicated gallstone disease. *J. Am. Coll Surg.* 2011 Oct; 213(4):524-30.

[8]   Kohut M, Nowakowska-Duława E, Marek T, Kaczor R, Nowak A. Accuracy of linear endoscopic ultrasonography in the evaluation of patients with suspected common bile duct stones. *Endoscopy.* 2002 Apr; 34(4):299-303.

[9]   Bortoff GA, Chen MY, Ott DJ, Wolfman NT, Routh WD. Gallbladder stones: imaging and intervention..*Radiographics.* 2000 May-Jun; 20(3):751-66.

[10] Lu J, Guo CY, Xu XF, Wang XP, Wan R. Efficacy of intraductal ultrasonography in the diagnosis of non-opaque choledocholith. *World J. Gastroenterol.* 2012 Jan 21; 18(3):275-8.

[11] Linghu EQ, Cheng LF, Wang XD, Wang ZQ, Yang YS, Li W, Cai FC, Wang HZ, Du H, Meng JY. Intraductal ultrasonography and endoscopic retrograde cholangiography in diagnosis of extrahepatic bile duct stones: a comparative study. *Hepatobiliary Pancreat. Dis. Int.* 2004 Feb; 3(1):129-32.

[12] Steinert R, Nestler G, Sagynaliev E, Müller J, Lippert H, Reymond MA. Laparoscopic cholecystectomy and gallbladder cancer. *J. Surg. Oncol.* 2006 Jun 15; 93(8):682-9.

[13] Laurence JM, Tran PD, Richardson AJ, Pleass HC, Lam VW. Laparoscopic or open cholecystectomy in cirrhosis: a systematic review of outcomes and meta-analysis of randomized trials. *HPB* (Oxford). 2012 Mar; 14(3):153-61.

[14] Urban L, Eason GA, ReMine S, Bogard B, Magisano J, Raj P, Pratt D, Brown T. Laparoscopic cholecystectomy in patients with early cirrhosis. *Curr. Surg.* 2001 May; 58(3):312-315.

[15] Ikard RW. Combining laparoscopic cholecystectomy and (peri) umbilical herniorrhaphy. *Am. Surg.* 1995 Apr; 61(4):304-5.

[16] Ergul Z, Ersoy E, Kulacoglu H, Olcucuoglu E, Devay AO, Gundogdu H. A simple modified technique for repair of umbilical hernia in patients undergo laparoscopic cholecystectomy. Report of 10 cases. *G Chir.* 2009 Oct; 30(10):437-9.

[17] de Bakker JK, Dijksman LM, Donkervoort SC. Safety and outcome of general surgical open and laparoscopic procedures during pregnancy. *Surg. Endosc.* 2011 May; 25(5):1574-8.

[18] Dan D, Seetahal S, Harnanan D, Singh Y, Hariharan S, Naraynsingh V. Laparoscopic cholecystectomy in sickle cell disease patients: does operating time matter? *Int. J. Surg.* 2009 Feb; 7(1):70-3.

[19] Garg PK, Teckchandani N, Hadke NS, Chander J, Nigam S, Puri SK. Alteration in coagulation profile and incidence of DVT in laparoscopic cholecystectomy. *Int. J. Surg.* 2009 Apr;7(2):130-5.

[20] Ahmad G, O'Flynn H, Duffy JM, Phillips K, Watson A. Laparoscopic entry techniques. *Cochrane Database Syst. Rev.* 2012 Feb 15;2:CD006583.

[21] Minervini A, Davenport K, Pefanis G, Keeley FX Jr, Timoney AG. Prospective study comparing the bladeless optical access trocar versus Hasson open trocar for the establishment of pneumoperitoneum in laparoscopic renal procedures. *Arch. Ital. Urol. Androl.* 2008 Sep; 80(3):95-8.

[22] Vettoretto N, Saronni C, Harbi A, Balestra L, Taglietti L, Giovanetti M. Critical view of safety during laparoscopic cholecystectomy. *JSLS.* 2011 Jul-Sep; 15(3):322-5.

[23] Bessa SS, Al-Fayoumi TA, Katri KM, Awad AT. Clipless laparoscopic cholecystectomy by ultrasonic dissection. *J. Laparoendosc. Adv. Surg. Tech A.* 2008 Aug; 18(4):593-8.

[24] Imrie CW. An inexpensive laparoscopic gallbladder retrieval bag. *Surg. Endosc.* 1999 Mar; 13(3):313.

[25] Rolton DJ, Lovegrove RE, Dehn T. Use of a sterile glove as a retrieval bag in laparoscopic surgery. *Ann. R. Coll. Surg. Engl.* 2009 Jul;91(5):440.

[26] Weber A, Vázquez JA, Valencia S, Cueto J. Retrieval of specimens in laparoscopy using reclosable zipper-type plastic bags: a simple, cheap, and useful method. *Surg. Laparosc. Endosc.* 1998 Dec; 8(6):457-9.

[27] Bunting DM. Port-site hernia following laparoscopic cholecystectomy. *JSLS.* 2010 Oct-Dec; 14(4):490-7.

[28] Barry M, Winter DC. Laparoscopic port site hernias: any port in a storm or a storm in any port? *Ann. Surg.* 2008 Oct;248(4):687-9.

[29] Mohandas S, John AK. Role of intra operative cholangiogram in current day practice. *Int. J. Surg.* 2010;8(8):602-5.

[30] Livraghi L, Berselli M, Bianchi V, Latham L, Farassino L, Cocozza E. Glove technique in single-port access laparoscopic surgery: results of an initial experience. *Minim. Invasive Surg.* 2012; 2012:415430.

[31] Han HJ, Choi SB, Kim WB, Lee JS, Boo YJ, Song TJ, Suh SO, Choi SY. Surgical stress response and clinical outcomes of single port laparoscopic cholecystectomy: prospective nonrandomized study. *Am. Surg.* 2012 Apr; 78(4):485-91.

[32] Koo EJ, Youn SH, Baek YH, Roh YH, Choi HJ, Kim YH, Jung GJ. Review of 100 cases of single port laparoscopic cholecystectomy. *J. Korean Surg. Soc.* 2012 Mar; 82(3):179-84.

[33] Nicholson T, Travis S, Ettles D, Dyet J, Sedman P, Wedgewood K, Royston C. Hepatic artery angiography and embolization for hemobilia following laparoscopic cholecystectomy. *Cardiovasc. Intervent. Radiol.* 1999 Jan; 22(1):20-4.

[34] Azurin DJ, Go LS, Maslack M, Kirkland ML. Bile leak following laparoscopic cholecystectomy. *J. Laparoendosc. Surg.* 1995 Aug;5(4):233-6.

[35] Barkun AN, Rezieg M, Mehta SN, Pavone E, Landry S, Barkun JS, Fried GM, Bret P, Cohen A. Postcholecystectomy biliary leaks in the laparoscopic era: risk factors, presentation, and management. McGill Gallstone Treatment Group. *Gastrointest Endosc.* 1997 Mar; 45(3):277-82.

[36] Mac Fayden BV, Vecchio R, Ricardo A. Bile duct injuries after Laparoscopic cholecystectomy. The United States experience. *Surg. Endosc.* 1998;12: 315-321.

[37] Flum D, Dellinger E, Chaedle A et al. Intra-operative Cholangiography and the Risk of Common Bile Duct Injury during laparoscopic cholecystectomy. *J. Am. Med. Assoc.* 2003; 289:1639-1644.

[38] Archer SB, Brown DW, Smith CD, Branum GD, Hunter JG. Bile duct injury during laparoscopic cholecystectomy: results of a national survey. *Ann. Surg.* 2001 Oct;234(4):549-59.

[39] Honda G, Iwanaga T, Kurata M, Watanabe F, Satoh H, Iwasaki K. The critical view of safety in laparoscopic cholecystectomy is optimized by exposing the inner layer of the subserosal layer. *J. Hepatobiliary Pancreat. Surg.* 2009; 16(4):445-9.

[40] Ausania F, Holmes LR, Ausania F, Iype S, Ricci P, White SA. Intraoperative cholangiography in the laparoscopic cholecystectomy era: why are we still debating? *Surg. Endosc.* 2012 May; 26(5):1193-200.

[41] Dageforde LA, Landman MP, Feurer ID, Poulose B, Pinson CW, Moore DE. A Cost-Effectiveness Analysis of Early vs Late Reconstruction of Iatrogenic Bile Duct Injuries. *J. Am. Coll Surg.* 2012 Apr 9.

[42] Stewart L, Way LW. Laparoscopic bile duct injuries: timing of surgical repair does not influence success rate. A multivariate analysis of factors influencing surgical outcomes. *HPB* (Oxford). 2009 Sep; 11(6):516-22.

[43] Tabone LE, Sarker S, Fisichella PM, Conlon M, Fernando E, Yi S, Luchette FA. To 'gram or not'? Indications for intraoperative cholangiogram. *Surgery.* 2011 Oct; 150(4):810-9.

[44] Zhang WJ, Xu GF, Wu GZ, Li JM, Dong ZT, Mo XD. Laparoscopic exploration of common bile duct with primary closure versus T-tube drainage: a randomized clinical trial. *J. Surg. Res.* 2009 Nov;157(1):e1-5.

[45] Laursen HB, Kannerup AS, Oxlund H, Yasuda Y, Funch-Jensen P, Rokkjaer M, Mortensen FV. T-tube drainage stimulates the healing of choledocho-choledochostomies. An experimental study in pigs. *J. Hepatobiliary Pancreat. Surg.* 2008;15(6):622-6.

[46] Navez B, Ungureanu F, Michiels M, Claeys D, Muysoms F, Hubert C, Vanderveken M, Detry O, Detroz B, Closset J, Devos B, Kint M, Navez J, Zech F, Gigot JF; The Belgian Group for Endoscopic Surgery (BGES) and the Hepatobiliary and Pancreatic Section (HBPS) of the Royal Belgian Society of Surgery. Surgical management of acute cholecystitis: results of a 2-year prospective multicenter survey in Belgium. *Surg. Endosc.* 2012 Mar 10.

[47] Kim RS, Itriago FP, Rosser Jr JC, Redan JA. Don't Fear Adhesions: Safe Approaches for Reoperative Minimally Invasive Surgery. *Surg. Technol. Int.* 2012 Dec 1;XXI: 147-155.

[48] Eldar S, Sabo E, Nash E, Abrahamson J, Matter I. Laparoscopic cholecystectomy for the various types of gallbladder inflammation: a prospective trial. *Surg. Laparosc. Endosc.* 1998 Jun; 8(3):200-7.

[49] Stefanidis D, Bingener J, Richards M, Schwesinger W, Dorman J, Sirinek K. Gangrenous cholecystitis in the decade before and after the introduction of laparoscopic cholecystectomy. *JSLS.* 2005 Apr-Jun; 9(2):169-73.

[50] Mazer LM, Losada HF, Chaudhry RM, Velazquez-Ramirez GA, Donohue JH, Kooby DA, Nagorney DM, Adsay NV, Sarmiento JM. Tumor Characteristics and Survival Analysis of Incidental Versus Suspected Gallbladder Carcinoma. *J. Gastrointest. Surg.* 2012 May 9.

[51] Foster JM, Hoshi H, Gibbs JF, Iyer R, Javle M, Chu Q, Kuvshinoff B. Gallbladder cancer: Defining the indications for primary radical resection and radical re-resection. *Ann. Surg. Oncol.* 2007 Feb; 14(2):833-40.

[52] Coburn NG, Cleary SP, Tan JC, Law CH. Surgery for gallbladder cancer: a population-based analysis. *J. Am. Coll Surg.* 2008 Sep; 207(3):371-82.

[53] Kano N, Takeshi A, Kusanagi H, Watarai Y, Mike M, Yamada S, Mishima O, Uwafuji S, Kitagawa M, Watanabe H, Kitahama S, Matsuda S, Endo S, Gremillion D. Current surgical training: simultaneous training in open and laparoscopic surgery. *Surg. Endosc.* 2010 Dec; 24(12):2927-9.

[54] Kaafarani HM, Smith TS, Neumayer L, Berger DH, Depalma RG, Itani KM. Trends, outcomes, and predictors of open and conversion to open cholecystectomy in Veterans Health Administration hospitals. *Am. J. Surg.* 2010 Jul;200(1):32-40.

[55] Zehetner J, Leidl S, Wuttke ME, Wayand W, Shamiyeh A. Conversion in laparoscopic cholecystectomy in low versus high-volume hospitals: is there a difference? *Surg. Laparosc. Endosc. Percutan. Tech.* 2010 Jun;20(3):173-6.

[56] Shamiyeh A, Danis J, Wayand W, Zehetner J. A 14-year analysis of laparoscopic cholecystectomy: conversion--when and why? *Surg. Laparosc. Endosc. Percutan. Tech.* 2007 Aug; 17(4):271-6.

[57] Genc V, Sulaimanov M, Cipe G, Basceken SI, Erverdi N, Gurel M, Aras N, Hazinedaroglu SM. What necessitates the conversion to open cholecystectomy? A retrospective analysis of 5164 consecutive laparoscopic operations. *Clinics* (Sao Paulo). 2011; 66(3):417-20.

[58] Dorfman S, Rincón A, Shortt H. Cholecystectomy via Kocher incision without peritoneal closure. *Invest. Clin.* 1997 Mar; 38(1):3-7.

[59] Nakajima J, Sasaki A, Obuchi T, Baba S, Nitta H, Wakabayashi G. Laparoscopic subtotal cholecystectomy for severe cholecystitis. *Surg. Today.* 2009; 39(10):870-5.

[60] Di Carlo I, Pulvirenti E, Toro A, Corsale G. Modified subtotal cholecystectomy: results of a laparotomy procedure during the laparoscopic era. *World J. Surg.* 2009 Mar; 33(3):520-5.

[61] Thrumurthy SG, Shetty VD, Ward JB, Pursnani KG, Mughal MM. Peritonitis from an abdominal wall biloma: a unique reason to avoid prophylactic surgical drainage. *Ann. R. Coll. Surg. Engl.* 2011 Oct;93(7):e144-6.

[62] Gurusamy KS, Samraj K. Routine abdominal drainage for uncomplicated open cholecystectomy. *Cochrane Database Syst. Rev.* 2007 Apr 18;(2):CD006003.

[63] Sanz-López R, Martínez-Ramos C, Núñez-Peña JR, Ruiz de Gopegui M, Pastor-Sirera L, Tamames-Escobar S. Incisional hernias after laparoscopic vs open cholecystectomy. *Surg. Endosc.* 1999 Sep;13(9):922-4.

[64] Lengyel BI, Panizales MT, Steinberg J, Ashley SW, Tavakkoli A. Laparoscopic cholecystectomy: What is the price of conversion? *Surgery.* 2012 Apr 11.

[65] Cagir B, Rangraj M, Maffuci L, Ostrander LE, Herz BL. A retrospective analysis of laparoscopic and open cholecystectomies. *J. Laparoendosc. Surg.* 1994 Apr;4(2): 89-100.

[66] Keus F, de Jong, J Goszen HG, Larrhoven CJHM. Laparoscopic versus open cholecystectomy for patients with symptomatic cholecystolithiasis. Cochrane Database Syst Rev. 2006, Issue 4. Art. No: CD 006231. *DOI* 10.1002/14651858. CD006231.

[67] Keus F, de Jong, J Goszen HG, Larrhoven CJHM. Systematic review: open, small-incision or laparoscopic cholecystectomy for symptomatic cholecystolithiasis. *Aliment. Pharmacol. Ther.* 2009; 29, 359 -78.

[68] Ledet WP. Ambulatory cholecystectomy without disability. *Arch. Surg.* 1990; 125: 1434-5.

[69] Chalkoo M, Ahangar S, Durrani A.M. , Chalkoo S, Shah M. J., Bashir M I.Mini-lapcholecystectomy: Modifications and innovations in technique. International Journal of Surgery 2010; 8 (2): 112- 117.

[70] Naraynsingh V, Singh Y, Remy T, Hariharan S, Dan D. Minilaparotomy cholecystectomy – An appropriate alternative to laparoscopic cholecystectomy in developing nations. *Tropical Gastroenterology* 2010; 31 (4): 312 – 316.

[71] McGinn FP, Miles AJG, Uglow M, Ozmen M, Terzi C, Humby M. Randomized trial of laparoscopic cholecystectomy and mini cholecystectomy. *Br. J. Surg* 1995; 82: 1374 -7.

[72] Ros A, Gustafsson L, Drook H, Nordgren CE, Thorell A, Wallin G, et al. Laparoscopic cholecystectomy versus mini-laparotomy cholecystectomy. A prospective randomized single-blind study. *Ann. Surg.* 2001; 234: 741-9.

[73] Keus F, Werner JEM, Gooszen HG, Oostvogel HJM, van Larrhoven CJ. Randomized clinical trial of small-incision and laparoscopic cholecystectomy in patients with symptomatic cholecystolithiasis. *Arch. Surg.* 2008; 143 : 371 – 7.

[74] Sharma AK, Rangan HK, Choubey RP. Mini-lap cholecystectomy: a viable alternative ot laparoscopic cholecystectomy for the third world. *Aust. NZ J. Surg.* 1998; 68: 774-7.

In: Cholecystectomies
Editors: Miyu Akiyama and Satomi Kunomasu

ISBN: 978-1-62257-890-0
© 2013 Nova Science Publishers, Inc.

Chapter III

Iatrogenic Bile Duct Injuries After Cholecystectomy

F. Ruiz-Gómez[1], J. M. Ramia[2,], J. E. Quiñones-Sampedro[2], J. C. Palomo-Sánchez[1] and J. García-Parreño[2]*

[1]Department of Surgery, Hospital Virgen de la Luz,
Cuenca, Spain
[2]Hepato-Pancreato-Biliary Surgical Unit, Department of Surgery,
Hospital Universitario de Guadalajara,
Guadalajara, Spain

Iatrogenic Bile duct injuries (IBDI) are complex clinical situations usually caused by surgeons in healthy patients, and are associated with significant morbidity and low, but no negligible, mortality [1]. IBDI can result from surgery (cholecystectomy, liver transplants and other procedures) or non-surgical procedures (tumour ablative therapies [RF], liver biopsies, TIPS or external radiation therapy) [2].

Most of IBDI occurs performing a cholecystectomy. Since Carl Langebuch performed the first open cholecystectomy in 1882 until now [3, 4], IBDI has been an inherent complication of this surgery due to the surgeon's perceptive error. Laparoscopic cholecystectomy (LC) has led to a decrease in postoperative pain and hospital stay, but unfortunately has increased some complications such as IBDI [5]. In a meta-analysis of more than 78 747 LCs, the IBDI incidence ranged from 0.36%-0.47% [6].

For treating IBDI correctly, high level of scrutiny in the intraoperative and immediate postoperative phases is required [7], and also a multidisciplinary approach between surgeons, radiologists and gastroenterologists to offer the patient the best initial diagnosis, the best treatment options and better management of complications and follow-up is needed [8, 9].

This chapter is intended to describe the current status of the literature on this type of injury and its therapeutic management.

---

[*] Correspondence: J. M. Ramia, Chief of HPB Surgical Unit. Department of Surgery. Personal address: General Moscardo 26, 5-1, Madrid 28020. Spain. Phone: 0034616292056. E-mail: jose_ramia@hotmail.com.

A. Classifications

Different classifications of IBDI have been proposed, based on the anatomical level of the injury or the procedures need to be taken, but remarkably none have assessed factors such as sepsis, the patient's haemodynamic status or comorbidities. The presence of associated vascular lesions, that occur generally in IBDI which are more proximal to the liver hilum and its clinical impact is only considered in the classifications of Hannover [10-11] Lau, [12] Kapoor [13] and Stewart-Way [14] but not in those of Strasberg [15], Bismuth [16], Neuhaus [17], Csendes [18], McMahon [19], Siewert [20], Frattaroli [21], Amsterdam [22] or Cannon [23]. None of these classifications is accepted as a universal standard that reduces its clinical usefullness. The most commonly used are those of Strasberg (Figure 1 and 2) and Bismuth.

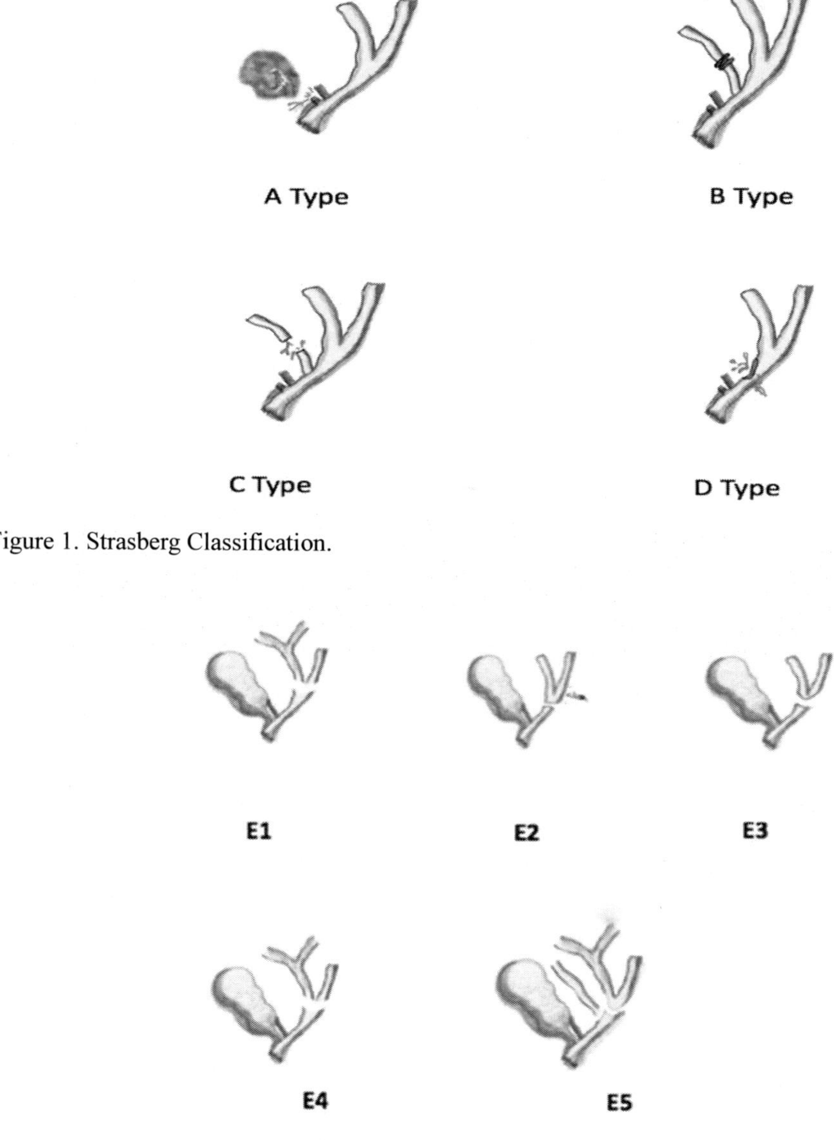

Figure 1. Strasberg Classification.

Figure 2. Strasberg Classification.

B. Risk Factors

1. *Age/sex:* male and elderly patients have an increased risk of IBDI [24].
2. *Congenital malformations:* partial liver agenesis [25], and liver Segment IV Hypoplasia [26] has been described as a risk factor.
3. *Acute cholecystitis:* IBDI is 3 times more frequent in LC due to acute cholecystitis with an incidence between 0.77%-5.0%, and is the most important predisposing factor for IBDI [27-32].
4. *Hidden cystic duct syndrome*: When the infundibulum is dissected to identify the cystic duct in the infundibular technique, the hepatocholedochus may be confused with a falsely identified cystic duct and sectioned. This is more likely in the presence of acute or chronic inflammation, large stones impacted in the infundibulum, adhesions between the gallbladder and choledochus [33-36].
5. *Anatomical anomalies of the biliary tract (BT):* Anomalously, the cystic duct can bind to the bile duct (BD) very near to the location of the segmental sectoral ducts. It may drain into a sectoral duct, as well as in the convergence of anterior and posterior sectoral ducts [37]. The confluence between the cystic duct and the main BD may be angular (75%), parallel (20%) or spiral (5%). With a parallel implementation, it is possible to thermally damage the exterior of the BD when dissecting due to its proximity [38].
6. *LC perceptive error and conversion to open surgery:* Although the infundibulum technique is a good option for open surgery, when a cholecysto- choledochal fistula is suspected, this technique may lead to injuring the bile duct in laparoscopic surgery [38]. An emphasis on appropriate conversions to open cholecystectomy may help reduce the risk of IBDI [39].
7. *Type of approach*: IBDI due to LC is more serious and complex due to its more proximal location, its frequent association with vascular injury and the associated thermal mechanism [40-42]. In Single Incision Laparoscopic Cholechystectomy, the complication rate may be as high as 16.6 %.No learning curves are established for these scarless techniques [43-45].
8. *Experience of the surgeon*: although experience is essential to prevent high morbidity with any surgery, in LC the learning curve does not seem to be the most important factor for diminishing IBDI rate [46-48], but growing experience of the multidisciplinary team, improve long term results of bile duct injury repair [49]. Surgical residency Program did not affect the rate of IBDI but increases the rate of conversion [50].

C. Preventive Measures

There are many techniques for preventing IBDI: use of a 30° degree camera, avoiding using thermocoagulation near the main BD, meticulous dissection and conversion to open surgery when the anatomy is uncertain [51, 52].

Navigation principles have been copied to reduce IBDI. For open cholecystectomy, there is the fundus first technique. In LC, the reference point is the Groove of Rouviere [53].

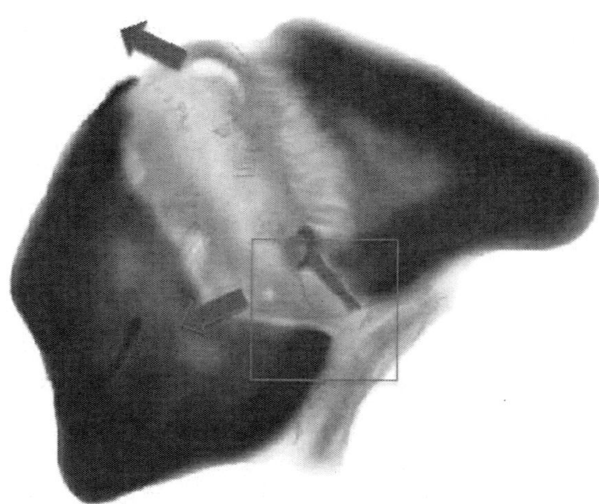

Figure 3. Critical view.

Since the main cause of IBDI is misidentification of the main BD, or an aberrant duct like the cystic duct, the surgeon must have a way to identify the artery and cystic duct [54].

The following are among the methods used:

1. *Tri-structure method:* During LC, the CD, common hepatic duct and common bile duct must be identified [55].
2. *Fischer method:* Consists of completely separating the gallbladder from the gallbladder bed from the bottom towards the infundibulum, as in open surgery, until it hangs from the artery and the cystic duct. This is especially difficult in intrahepatic or very swollen vesicles [56]. Separating the gallbladder from the liver bed also tends to bleed more, due to it not having been previously linked to the cystic artery.
3. *Infundibular technique:* Consists of identifying the cystic duct where it joins the infundibulum of gallbladder. It is currently the most widely used technique in most centres. It has the drawback of not preventing IBDI in patients with hidden cystic duct syndrome. Thus, different groups consistently recommend the use of intraoperative cholangiography (IOC) with this type of technique [38].
4. *Strasberg Critical View Technique:* Consists of the dissection and removal of Calot's triangle to expose the artery and cystic duct, thereby exposing the base of the liver. Once this view has been achieved, theses structures can only correspond to the duct and cystic artery (Figure 3) [30]. For aberrant ducts or cases of very swollen vesicles, it is suggested that the inner layer of the subserosa be exposed, which optimises the critical view [57].
5. *Cholangiography:* Since the Argentinian, Pablo Mirizzi, introduced the first intraoperative cholangiography (IOC) to the present day, its benefit for preventing IBDI has been debated [58]. IOC can help prevent IBDI in at least 3 ways [59]:
    1. It shows the diversity of the biliary tree and its abnormalities.
    2. It helps the surgeon to identify patients at risk of IBDI due to abnormal anatomy.
    3. It allows IBDI to be identified and repaired, if it has occurred.
    IOC has proven to be cost-effective, especially if used by less experienced surgeons or if there are risk factors [60]. Other studies do not accept that IOC prevents the

incidence of IBDI and highlight the increase in total surgery time [61, 62]. Currently, there are no randomised trials supporting the use of IOC [63]. Although protective effects of IOC against IBDI continue to be controversial [64-66], the undeniable fact that IOC does reduce the cost of litigation will likely get more routine IOC by economic reasons [67].

6. *Intraoperative laparoscopic ultrasound:* its advantages in preventing IBDI were highlighted in a recent multi-centre study. However, it is another method which is very expensive and often not available in hospitals. It does not completely replace IOC but has a promising future [68, 69]

D. Diagnosis

A high level of suspect must be maintained to diagnose IBDI [70]. There are three possible scenarios [71]:

1. Intraoperative diagnosis (<50%).
2. Immediate post-operative diagnosis: patients who are not clinically well during the first 48hrs after surgery, or with bile in the abdominal drainage. It may be accompanied by cholestasis [72, 73].
3. Patients diagnosed late with symptoms of cholangitis or obstructive jaundice.

Ultrasound can show fluid collections and dilation of the bile duct, but it does not reveal the full path of the BD or other related injuries. Computed tomography (CT) with contrast is therefore recommended as an initial diagnostic study. Taken with the information from ultrasound, it can assess the level of injury, associated vascular damage or liver atrophy-hypertrophy [74]. Scanning with iminodiacetic acid (HIDA scan) helps to diagnose bile leaks, but does not mark the limits of the injury and the biliary anatomy [75], MR cholangiography identifies any need for ERCP due to leakage of small biliary radicals or cystic duct stump leak, and gives information on the presence or absence of choledocholithiasis [76, 77]. MR cholangiography with manganese is a non-invasive method which is efficient in the diagnosis of IBDI, but requires larger series to evaluate it [78]. The level of IBDI in the biliary tree can be seen by cholangiography using percutaneous colangiography (PTCA) or ERCP. In cases of lesions proximal to the hilum, with transaction or presence of an aberrant duct, ERCP cannot draw the biliary tree correctly, requiring anterograde cholangiography by PTCA [79].

Perhaps in the next years, Hyperespectral Cholangiography and near-infrared fluorescente cholangiography, may help in the intraoperative assesment of biliary anatomy [80-83].

E. Therapeutic Approach

Treatment of IBDI is complex and multidisciplinary. The following factors need to be known: the type of injury, the patient's clinical condition, associated vascular damage, local hospital factors, etc. Some general comments on non-surgical and surgical treatment are briefly described below, especially regarding hepatojejunostomy (HJ). Subsequently, treatment according to the Strasberg types is defined. Endoscopic treatment for Strasberg type A injuries is also expanded upon.

1. Non-surgical Treatment (Endoscopic and Interventional Radiology)

The multimodal treatment of IBDI includes endoscopic treatment and interventional radiology. Percutaneous interventional radiology techniques require bilioenteric continuity. They are less invasive and may be more appropriate in patients who are not candidates for surgery, or in those whose anatomy makes it technically very difficult to use endoscopic instrumentation [84]. The development of covered self-expanding stents, specifically designed to be removed later, may soon change the management of benign strictures [85].

2. Surgical Treatment

There are 3 independent prognostic parameters for surgical treatment of IBDI which involve poor postoperative outcome and a higher rate of complications [86]:

1. Proximal IBDI: technically much more complex to repair and usually associated with vascular injury [87].
2. Repair in the acute phase: For acute IBDI, immediate repair is the best option if the patient's haemodynamic status and septic conditions allow it [88] There is no evidence to support early or deferred repair when IBDI is identified days after the injury [89]. Although there is great difference in cost and quality of live in early repair by a hepatobiliary surgeon [90].
3. Late referral to a tertiary centre: biliary reconstruction in a reference centre by an experienced surgeon in IBDI has a better success rate as well as shorter hospital stay, morbidity and mortality. The moment of referral to a tertiary centre may affect biliary reconstruction surgery when this is performed [86, 91], but timing of repair , it Is not a key factor in outcome success in comparison with erradication of intraabdominal infection, use of correct technique, performed by anexperienced hepatobiliary surgeon [92].

Surgical Technique

The bilioenteric anastomosis which offers the best results is Roux-en-Y HJ. The defunctionalised loop guarantees the absence of intestinal reflux into the BD, and prevents ascending cholangitis. The hepatoduodenal anastomosis has an increased anastomotic tension, a macroscopic reflux of food at the biliary tree level and the possibility of developing a high debit biliary fistula [93]. The most common errors related to repair failures and bilioenteric anastomosis are the lack of complete mucosal apposition between the BD and the intestine and the use of poorly absorbable suture material [94]. The use of a transanastomotic stent is not universal. Placing it proximally so as not go through the repair has been suggested [95,

96]. Using a redundant proximal loop attached to the wall to make it easier to perform percutaneous radiological monitoring has also been suggested [97-100].

There are experimental animal studies for IBDI using ringed Gore-Tex vascular prostheses [100], magnetic stents [101], fibrin glue products [102], vesicular flaps [103], expended polytetrafluorothylene patch [104], tissue-engineered bioabsorbable polymer patch [105] and isolated gastric tube flap [106] as a substitute for bile duct.

There are two complications that require liver transplantation (LT): IBDI associated with repeat episodes of cholangitis and chronic cholestasis with secondary biliary cirrhosis and IBDI associated with lesions of the hepatic hilar vessels (severe vascular injury) [107-108], especially the hepatic artery, which could lead to a fulminant hepatic failure [109]. There are few articles on LT secondary to IBDI [108-115]. A liver transplantation in these patients is technically more complex for the following reasons: intra-abdominal adhesions, sclerosis of the hepatic pedicle, severe portal hypertension and associated coagulopathy [116]. The higher incidence of IBDI due to LC suggests that the indication of LT will increase in the future [117].

Techniques According to the Strasberg IBDI Classification

Type A: Endoscopic treatment (papillotomy+prosthesis) for cystic duct (CD) bile leakage is very efficient [118] However, if the leakage is more proximal, the percentage of clinical resolution is lower [119]. The differences in the basal pressure or intraductal pressure , the cystic duct length and BD diameter may explain the differences in outcomes [120] There are no comparative data to define the optimal number of stents, their size, configuration (straight or pigtail), length and withdrawal time [121]. There is no difference between the use of stents passing through the leak (leak bridging) or reductions that only decompress and reduce the transpapillary pressure gradient [122]. Although in some centres these lesions are addressed in the immediate postoperative period through exploratory laparoscopy and repositioning of clips or Luschka duct suturing, there is currently no comparative study to compare the endoscopic and laparoscopic approaches in this scenario. Japanese authors had use endoscopic Nasobiliary Drainage as inicial treatment, before any use of endoscopic stent treatment to manage cystic duct leaks [123].

Type B: Treatment as A type. We have to suspect Sectorial Duct IBDI in patients with bile leak when ERCP is interpreted as normal or when bile leak persists after Endoscopic stent placed for a theoretical Strasberg A lesion [124].

Type C: there is no continuity with the main BD so the use of a prosthesis would not be effective. If the duct is small, it can be linked, developing into atrophy or leading to cholangitis episodes [125]. If there is a duct of greater calibre (2 or more segments), it should be reconstructed by HJ. Biliary reconstruction in an aberrant right sectorial with respect to the main BD has greater occurrences of stenosis and long-term colangitis [126]. Liver resection should be reserved for the failure of a previous HJ or if symptoms are persistent [127].

Type D: Can be addressed as follows:

- *Primary closure with absorbable suture and a subhepatic drain.* The placement of a T tube has been associated with an increased amount of late stenosis in transplanted patients [128]. It therefore seems prudent to avoid placing a foreign body in a non-dilated BT [63].

- *End-end anastomosis*: This depends on a number of factors, such as the presence of intact proximal and distal ends, similarity in diameter between the ends, lesions less than 1 cm. in length and no excessive tension or signs of infection or inflammation. The advantages are its simplicity and the preservation of the length of the BD, but approximately 50% is stenotic during follow-up. A reinforcement has been described using a patch from the umbilical vein and round ligament adipose tissue [129-131].
- *Hepatojejunostomy*: this is the most used and safest method.

Bilioenteric anastomosis with side-to-side anastomosis is better as it preserves the blood supply better and minimises the dissection behind the ducts [132]. It is recommended to perform HJ on the extrahepatic portion of the left hepatic duct (LHD) at the base of segment IV, with side-to-side anastomosis between the LHD and Roux-en-Y jejunum. This technique was described by Hepp and is called the Hepp-Coinaud technique in reference to the extrahepatic anatomical description of the LHD described by Coinaud [133].

Type E: the HJ described for type D lesions is the ideal technique for injuries E1, E2 and E3. Those lesions located above the bifurcation (E4) or that may affect the sectoral branches of the right side (E5) cannot be repaired with this technique, as only the left hepatic duct system can drain.

- *E1 and E2*: Another technique applied for these patients was described 23 years ago and renamed as the bile duct growing factor by Mercado et al., in honour of the term coined by Starzl in vascular anastomosis [134, 135, 136]. It consists of the anastomosis of the anterior face of the common and left hepatic duct into a jejunal loop. It is an alternative technique for the reconstruction of a thin CHD, less than 4 mm, provided that the hepatic confluence is preserved.
- *E4 and E5*: in these cases, the anastomosis is technically more demanding, especially if there is a wide break between the BD and left duct and the stenosis extends longitudinally to a sectorial duct. It is generally associated with vascular damage, liver atrophy, cholangitis and previous attempts at repair. In this context, hepatectomy is recommended before a liver transplantation [137]. Hepatectomy is much more likely after an injury to the right Hepatic Artery associated with a high rather than a low biliary injury [138]. Two subgroups of patients can be distinguished: those with injury-induced liver necrosis and those with liver atrophy following long term cholangitis [139-140].

Strasberg et al. described the extra-Glissonian approach for these lesions, based on intrahepatic dissection of the right and left pedicle confluence; the descent of so-called the "hilar plate" [141]. The surgeon has to puncture both pedicles with a fine needle until finding the BD, make an opening as wide as possible and perform side-to-side anastomosis. Exposure of an adequate length of the posterior sectoral duct may be limited by the position of the right anterior sectorial portal vein. It is also important not to devascularise the anterior right hepatic artery [137, 142]. Partial resection of segments IV and V has also been described to allow a better anastomosis [143], although other groups believe that the mobilisation of the hilar plate is enough to repair it [136, 144].

F. Late IBDI Complications

1. Biliary Strictures

Early strictures are usually related to aspects of the surgical procedure. Late strictures are related to inflammatory phenomena and fibrosis due to biliary leaks or secondary to ischaemia due to associated vascular injury. Vascular injury is associated with 61% of primary biliary-enteric repair failures. Stenosis after HJ anastomosis is between 9%-25% [146, 147].

Treatment of these strictures usually begins by PTCA and transhepatic drainage to resolve cholangitis. The "rendez-vous" technique can facilitate therapeutic management for these patients [149-151]. If radiologic dilation fails, performing a new HJ is the solution. Interventional radiology treatment has similar results to surgery, but with less morbidity and mortality [148].

2. Portal Hypertension

The incidence of biliary stricture and portal hypertension in patients with IBDI is between 15%-20%. [152, 153]. The surgical mortality rate in these cases reaches 23%-46% [154]. Portal hypertension in IBDI may be due to: prolonged biliary obstruction, portal injury during cholecystectomy, inflammatory portal vein thrombosis or coexistence with previous liver disease (cirrhosis) [155]. The most accepted treatment is balloon dilatation, and use of a stent [37]. If this fails, a venovenous bypass and a new HJ could be performed [156]. LT is the best option in patients with cirrhosis.

3. Secondary Biliary Cirrhosis (SBC)

The incidence of portal hypertension and SBC in IBDI is approximately 8% [157]. The presence of cirrhosis during repair leads to increased morbidity and mortality [158]. SBC needs 7.1 years to develop with a benign stenosis, 4.6 years with choledocholithiasis and 0.8 years in malignant stenosis [159].

4. Vasculobiliary Injury (VBI)

VBI is a combined injury to bile duct and any liver vessel (hepatic artery and /or portal vein). [38, 160]. Right Hepatic artery is the vessel most usually injured [35]. Portal vein or common or proper hepatic artery are less common lesions but have very serious effects even with liver infarction [161]. Univariate and multivariate analyses have shown that associated vascular injury is a risk factor for the development of postoperative biliary complications [162-165].

The extrahepatic BD and the main intrahepatic BD have arterial blood flow only. There are 3 levels of irrigation: the supplying arteries, the marginal arteries and the epicholedochal plexus. The part of the plexus around the confluence of the right and left hepatic ducts is termed the hilar plexus [160, 166, 167]. In type E injuries, there is a deprivation of blood flow from the gastroduodenal and pancreatodudoenal artery, with the flow depending on the hepatic artery only [168].

If the diagnosis is intraoperative, vascular reconstruction can be performed with an end-to-end anastomosis [42]. Postoperatively, the portal flow and retrograde flow to the lesion should be studied by angiography. Special caution for avoiding vascular insjury has to be taken, when fundus-down cholecystectomy is performed in the presence of severe inflammation [169]

G. Quality of Life

To date there have been only 4 studies in the literature on the quality of life after IBDI with varying results [170-173]. The most recent papers claims that quality of life is not affected in patients who survive IBDI [174].

H. Legal Responsibility

In the context of IBDI, the cornerstone of medical negligence rests on whether the standards of care have been met. A surgeon who does not use or misuses the accepted identification methods within this context will be legally less protected [54].

National Surgical Societies should hold consensus conferences to define LC standards. In November 2006, the Dutch Laparoscopic Society prepared and implemented a protocol recommending the analogue or digital recording of the critical safety view before the transection of the duct and cystic artery. These images are of great interest in the postoperative period and for the treatment of possible complications [175]. Remember that no surgeon is immune from the risk for IBDI, IBDI ranks among the leading sources of medical malpractise claims against surgeons worldwide [176].

References

[1]   Mercado MA, Chan C, Orozco H, Tielve M, Hinojosa CA. Acute bile duct injury. The need for a high repair. *Surg. Endosc.* 2003; 17:1351-5.

[2]   Shah JN. Bile duct injuries. The clinician's guide to pancreatobiliary disorder. Thorafore, NJ: SLACK Incorporated; 2006:69-90.

[3]   Traverso LW. Carl Langenbuch and the first cholecystectomy. *Am. J. Surg.* 1976; 132:81-2.

[4] Mühe E. Laparoscopic cholecystectomy − late results. *Langenbecks Arch. Chir. Suppl. Kongressbd.* 1991; 416-23.

[5] Sicklick JK, Camp MS, Lillemoe KD, Melton GB, Yeo CJ, Campbell KA, et al. Surgical management of bile duct injuries sustained during laparoscopic cholecystectomy: perioperative results in 200 patients. *Ann. Surg.* 2005; 241:786-92.

[6] Shea JA, Healey MJ, Berlin JA, Clarke JR, Malet PF, Staroscik RN et al. Mortality and complications associated with laparoscopic cholecystectomy. A meta-analysis. *Ann. Surg.* 1996; 224:609-20.

[7] Lillemoe KD. Evaluation of suspected bile duct injuries. *Surg. Endosc.* 2006; 20: 1638-43.

[8] Nuzzo G, Giuliante F, Giovannini I, Murazio M, D'Acapito F, Ardito F, et al. Advantages of multidisciplinary management of bile duct injuries occurring during cholecystectomy. *Am. J. Surg.* 2008;195:763-9.

[9] Lau WY, Lai EC, Lau SH Management of bile duct injury after laparoscopic cholecystectomy: a review. *ANZ J. Surg.* 2010; 80:75-81.

[10] Bektas H, Schrem H, Winny M, Klempnauer J. Surgical treatment and outcome of iatrogenic bile duct lesions after cholecystectomy and the impact of different clinical classification systems. *Br. J. Surg.* 2007; 94: 1119-27.

[11] Bektas H, Kleine M, Tamac A, Klempnauer J, Schrem H. Clinical application of the Hannover classification for iatrogenic bile duct lesions. *HPB Surg.* 2011; 2011: 612384.

[12] Lau WY, Lai EC. Classification of iatrogenic bile duct injury. *Hepatobiliary Pancreat. Dis. Int.* 2007; 6:459-63.

[13] Kapoor VK. New classification of acute bile duct injuries. *Hepatobiliary Pancreat. Dis. Int.* 2008; 7:555-6.

[14] Stewart L, Robinson TN, Lee CM, Liu K, Whang K, Way W. Right hepatic artery injury associated with laparoscopic bile duct injury: incidence, mechanism, and consequences. *J. Gastrointest. Surg.* 2004;8:523-30.

[15] Strasberg SM, Hertl M, Soper NJ. An analysis of the problem of biliary injury during laparoscopic cholecystectomy. *J. Am. Coll. Surg.* 1995;180:101-25.

[16] Bismuth H. Postoperative strictures of the bile ducts. In: Blumgart LH, editor. The Biliary Tract V. New York, NY: Churchill-Livingstone; 1982. p. 209-8.

[17] Neuhaus P, Schmidt SC, Hintze RE, Adler A, Veltzke W, Raakow R, et al. Classification and treatment of bile duct injuries after laparoscopic cholecystectomy. *Chirurg.* 2000;71:166-73.

[18] Csendes A, Navarrete C, Burdiles P, Yarmuch J. Treatment of common bile duct injuries during laparoscopic cholecystectomy: endoscopic and surgical management. *World J. Surg.* 2001;25:134651.

[19] McMahon AJ, Fullarton G, Baxter JN, O'Dwyer PJ. Bile duct injury and bile leakage in laparoscopic cholecystectomy. *Br. J. Surg.* 1995;82:307-13.

[20] Siewert JR, Ungeheuer A, Feussner H. Bile duct lesions in laparoscopic cholecystectomy. *Chirurg.* 1994;65:748-57.

[21] Frattaroli FM, Reggio D, Guadalaxara A, Illomei G, Pappalardo G. Benign biliary strictures: a review of 21 years of experience. *J. Am. Coll. Surg.* 1996;183:506-13.

[22] Bergman JJ, Van den Brink GR, Rauws EA, De Wit L, Obertop H, Huibregtse K, et al. Treatment of bile duct lesions after laparoscopic cholecystectomy. *Gut.* 1996;38:141-7.

[23] A novel classification system to address financial impact and referral decisions for bile duct injury in laparoscopic cholecystectomy.Cannon RM, Brock G, Buell JF. *HPB Surg.* 2011;2011:371245.

[24] Waage A, Nilsson M. Iatrogenic bile duct injury: a population- based study of 152 776 cholecystectomies in the Swedish Inpatient Registry. *Arch. Surg.* 2006;141:1207-13.

[25] Fields RC, Heiken JP, Strasberg SM. Biliary injury after laparoscopic cholecystectomy in a patient with right liver agenesis: case report and review of the literature. *J. Gastrointest. Surg.* 2008;12:1577-81.

[26] Liver segment IV hypoplasia as a risk factor for bile duct injury.Mercado MA, Franssen B, Arriola JC, Garcia-Badiola A, Arámburo R, Elnecavé A, Cortés-González R. *J. Gastrointest. Surg.* 2011 Sep;15(9):1589-93.

[27] Kerin MJ, Gorey TF. Biliary injuries in the laparoscopic era. *Eur. J. Surg.* 1994;160: 195-201.

[28] Ooi LL, Goh YC, Chew SP, Tay KH, Foo E, Low CH, et al. Bile duct injuries during laparoscopic cholecystectomy: a collective experience of four teaching hospitals and results of repair. *Aust. N. Z. J. Surg.* 1999;69:844-6.

[29] Adamsen S, Hansen OH, Funch-Jensen P, Schulze S, Stage JG, Wara P. Bile duct injury during laparoscopic cholecystectomy: a prospective nationwide series. *J. Am. Coll. Surg.* 1997;184:571-8.

[30] Strasberg SM. Avoidance of biliary injury during laparoscopic cholecystectomy. *J. Hepatobiliary Pancreat. Surg.* 2002;9:543-7.

[31] Russell JC, Walsh SJ, Mattie AS, Lynch JT. Bile duct injuries, 1989-1993. A statewide experience. Connecticut Laparoscopic Cholecystectomy Registry. *Arch. Surg.* 1996; 131:382-8.

[32] Kitano S, Matsumoto T, Aramaki M, Kawano K. Laparoscopic cholecystectomy for acute cholecystitis. *J. Hepatobiliary Pancreat. Surg.* 2002;9:534-7.

[33] Strasberg SM, Eagon CJ, Drebin JA. The "hidden cystic duct" syndrome and the infundibular technique of laparoscopic cholecystectomy−the danger of the false infundibulum. *J. Am. Coll. Surg.* 2000;191:661-7.

[34] Chapman WC, Abecassis M, Jarnagin W, Mulvihill S, Strasberg SM. Bile duct injuries 12 years after the introduction of laparoscopic cholecystectomy. *J. Gastrointest. Surg.* 2003;7:412-6.

[35] Davidoff AM, Pappas TN, Murray EA, Hilleren DJ, Johnson RD, Baker ME, et al. Mechanisms of major biliary injury during laparoscopic cholecystectomy. *Ann. Surg.* 1992; 215:196-202.

[36] Martin RF, Rossi RL. Bile duct injuries. Spectrum, mechanisms of injury, and their prevention. *Surg. Clin. North Am.* 1994;74:781-803.

[37] Colovic RB. Isolated segmental, sectoral and right hepatic bile duct injuries. *World J. Gastroenterol.* 2009;15:1415-9.

[38] Strasberg SM. Error traps and vasculo-biliary injury in laparoscopic and open cholecystectomy. *J. Hepatobiliary Pancreat. Surg.* 2008;15:284-92.

[39] Does increased experience with laparoscopic cholecystectomy yield more complex bile duct injuries? Chuang KI, Corley D, Postlethwaite DA, Merchant M, Harris HW. *Am. J. Surg.* 2012 Apr;203(4):480-7.

[40] Fletcher DR, Hobbs MS, Tan P, Valinsky LJ, Hockey RL, Pikora TJ, et al. Complications of cholecystectomy: risks of the laparoscopic approach and protective

effects of operative cholangiography: a population-based study. *Ann. Surg.* 1999;229: 449-57.

[41] Targarona EM, Marco C, Balagué C, Rodriguez J, Cugat E, Hoyuela C, et al. How, when, and why bile duct injury occurs. A comparison between open and laparoscopic cholecystectomy. *Surg. Endosc.* 1998;12:322-6.

[42] De Santibáñes E, Ardiles V, Pekolj J. Complex bile duct injuries: management. HPB (Oxford). 2008;10:4-12.

[43] Tacchino R, Greco F, Matera D.Single-incision laparoscopic cholecystectomy: surgery without a visible scar. *Surg. Endosc.* 2009 Apr;23(4):896-9.

[44] Lau KN, Sindram D, Agee N, Martinie JB, Iannitti DA Bile duct injury after single incision laparoscopic cholecystectomy.. *JSLS.* 2010 Oct-Dec;14(4):587-91.

[45] Iatrogenic combined bile duct and right hepatic artery injury during single incision laparoscopic cholecystectomy.Chiruvella A, Sarmiento JM, Sweeney JF, Lin E, Davis SS Jr. *JSLS.* 2010 Apr-Jun;14(2):268-71.

[46] Woods MS, Traverso LW, Kozarek RA, Tsao J, Rossi RL, Gough D, et al. Characteristics of biliary tract complications during laparoscopic cholecystectomy: a multi-institutional study. *Am. J. Surg.* 1994;167:27-33.

[47] Calvete J, Sabater L, Camps B, Verdú A, Gomez-Portilla A, Martín J, et al. Bile duct injury during laparoscopic cholecystectomy: myth or reality of the learning curve? *Surg. Endosc.* 2000;14:608-11.

[48] Archer SB, Brown DW, Smith CD, Branum GD, Hunter JG. Bile duct injury during laparoscopic cholecystectomy: results of a national survey. *Ann. Surg.* 2001;234: 549-58.

[49] Mercado MÁ, Franssen B, Dominguez I, Arriola-Cabrera JC, Ramírez-Del Val F, Elnecavé-Olaiz A, Arámburo-García R, García A. Transition from a low: to a high-volume centre for bile duct repair: changes in technique and improved outcome HPB (Oxford). 2011 Nov;13(11):767-73.

[50] Harrison VL, Dolan JP, Pham TH, Diggs BS, Greenstein AJ, Sheppard BC, Hunter JG. Bile duct injury after laparoscopic cholecystectomy in hospitals with and without surgical residency programs: is there a difference? *Surg. Endosc.* 2011 Jun;25(6): 1969-74.

[51] Hunter JG. Laser or electrocautery for laparoscopic cholecystectomy? *Am. J. Surg.* 1991;161:345-9.

[52] Troidl H. Disasters of endoscopic surgery and how to avoid them: error analysis. *World J. Surg.* 1999;23:846-55.

[53] Hugh TB. New strategies to prevent laparoscopic bile duct injury—surgeons can learn from pilots. *Surgery.* 2002;132:826-35.

[54] Strasberg SM. Biliary injury in laparoscopic surgery: part 1. Processes used in determination of standard of care in misidentification injuries. *J. Am. Coll. Surg.* 2005;201:598-603.

[55] Wang DC, Dong YH, Chen Z, Wu SS, Bi XG, DI WD, et al. Value of identification of cystic duct, common bile duct, and common hepatic duct in prevention of bile duct injury during laparoscopic cholecystectomy. Zhonghua Yi Xue Za Zhi. 2009;89:406-8.

[56] Fischer JE. Is damage to the common bile duct during laparoscopic cholecystectomy an inherent risk of the operation? *Am. J. Surg.* 2009;197:829-32.

[57] Honda G, Iwanaga T, Kurata M, Watanabe F, Satoh H, Iwasaki K. The critical view of safety in laparoscopic cholecystectomy is optimized by exposing the inner layer of the subserosal layer. *J. Hepatobiliary Pancreat. Surg.* 2009;16:445-9.

[58] Mirrizzi PL. La cholangiografía durante las operaciones de las vías biliares. *Bol. Soc. Cir. Buenos Aires.* 1932;16:1133.

[59] Traverso LW. Intraoperative cholangiography lowers the risk of bile duct injury during cholecystectomy. *Surg. Endosc.* 2006;20:1659-61.

[60] Flum DR, Flowers C, Veenstra DL. A cost-effectiveness analysis of intraoperative cholangiography in the prevention of bile duct injury during laparoscopic cholecystectomy. *J. Am. Coll. Surg.* 2003;196:385-93.

[61] Hugh TB. New strategies to prevent laparoscopic bile duct injury—surgeons can learn from pilots. *Surgery.* 2002;132: 826-35.

[62] Wright KD, Wellwood JM. Bile duct injury during laparoscopic cholecystectomy without operative cholangiography. *Br. J. Surg.* 1998;85:191-4.

[63] Connor S, Garden OJ. Bile duct injury in the era of laparoscopic cholecystectomy. *Br. J. Surg.* 2006;93:158-68.

[64] Hamad MA, Nada AA, Abdel-Atty MY, Kawashti AS Major biliary complications in 2, 714 cases of laparoscopic cholecystectomy without intraoperative cholangiography: a multicenter retrospective study. *Surg. Endosc.* 2011 Dec;25(12):3747-51.

[65] Ammori MB, Al-Dabbagh AK Laparoscopic cholecystectomy without intraoperative cholangiography.. *J. Laparoendosc. Adv. Surg. Tech. A.* 2012 Mar;22(2):146-51.

[66] Ford JA, Soop M, Du J, Loveday BP, Rodgers M. Systematic review of intraoperative cholangiography in cholecystectomy. *Br. J. Surg.* 2012 Feb;99(2):160-7.

[67] Ausania F, Holmes LR, Ausania F, Iype S, Ricci P, White SA Intraoperative cholangiography in the laparoscopic cholecystectomy era: why are we still debating?. *Surg. Endosc.* 2012 May;26(5):1193-200.

[68] Machi J, Johnson JO, Deziel DJ, Soper NJ, Berber E, Siperstein A, et al. The routine use of laparoscopic ultrasound decreases bile duct injury: a multicenter study. *Surg. Endosc.* 2009;23:384-8.

[69] Hashimoto M, Matsuda M, Watanabe G Intraoperative ultrasonography for reducing bile duct injury during laparoscopic cholecystectomy.. *Hepatogastroenterology.* 2010 Jul-Aug;57(101):706-9.

[70] De Wit LT, Rauws EA, Gouma DJ. Surgical management of iatrogenic bile duct injury. *Scand. J. Gastroenterol. Suppl.* 1999;230:89-94.

[71] Mercado MA, Chan C, Orozco H, Tielve M, Hinojosa CA. Acute bile duct injury. The need for a high repair. *Surg. Endosc.*2003;17:1351-5.

[72] Lillemoe KD. Evaluation of suspected bile duct injuries. *Surg. Endosc.* 2006;20: 1638-43.

[73] Andrei VE, Schein M, Margolis M, Rucinski JC, Wise L. Liver enzymes are commonly elevated following laparoscopic cholecystectomy: is elevated intra-abdominal pressure the cause? *Dig. Surg.* 1998;15:256-9.

[74] Blumgart LH. Hilar and intrahepatic biliary enteric anastomosis. *Surg. Clin. North Am.* 1994;74:845-63.

[75] McPartland KJ, Pomposelli JJ. Iatrogenic biliary injuries: classification, identification, and management. *Surg. Clin. North Am.* 2008;88:1329-43.

[76] Khalid TR, Casillas VJ, Montalvo BM, Centeno R, Levi JU. Using MR cholangiopancreatography to evaluate iatrogenic bile duct injury. *AJR Am. J. Roentgenol.* 2001;177:1347-52.

[77] Yeh TS, Jan YY, Tseng JH, Hwang TL, Jeng LB, Chen MF. Value of magnetic resonance cholangiopancreatography in demonstrating major bile duct injuries following laparoscopic cholecystectomy. *Br. J. Surg.* 1999;86:181-4.

[78] Hirano Y, Tatsuzawa Y, Shimizu J, Kinoshita S, Kawaura Y, Takahashi S. Efficacy of multi-slice computed tomography cholangiography before laparoscopic cholecystectomy. *ANZ J. Surg.* 2006;76:693-5.

[79] Pawa S, Al-Kawas FH. ERCP in the management of biliary complications after cholecystectomy. *Curr. Gastroenterol. Rep.* 2009;11:160-6.

[80] Nieuwenhuijs VB, van Buuren L, Hulscher JB, de Jong JS, van Dam GM Intraoperative assessment of biliary anatomy for prevention of bile duct injury: a review of current and future patient safety interventions.Buddingh KT, *Surg. Endosc.* 2011 Aug;25(8): 2449-61.

[81] Figueiredo JL, Siegel C, Nahrendorf M, Weissleder R. Intraoperative near-infrared fluorescent cholangiography (NIRFC) in mouse models of bile duct injury.. *World J. Surg.* 2010 Feb;34(2):336-43.

[82] Ishizawa T, Bandai Y, Ijichi M, Kaneko J, Hasegawa K, Kokudo N Fluorescent cholangiography illuminating the biliary tree during laparoscopic cholecystectomy.. *Br. J. Surg.* 2010 Sep;97(9):1369-77.

[83] Matsui A, Tanaka E, Choi HS, Winer JH, Kianzad V, Gioux S, Laurence RG, Frangioni JV. Real-time intra-operative near-infrared fluorescence identification of the extrahepatic bile ducts using clinically available contrast agents. *Surgery.* 2010 Jul;148(1):87-95.

[84] Misra S, Melton GB, Geschwind JF, Venbrux AC, Cameron JL, Lillemoe KD. Percutaneous management of bile duct strictures and injuries associated with laparoscopic cholecystectomy: a decade of experience. *J. Am. Coll. Surg.* 2004;198: 218-26.

[85] Ramos-De la Medina A, Misra S, Leroy AJ, Sarr MG.Management of benign biliary strictures by percutaneous interventional radiologic techniques (PIRT). *HPB* (Oxford). 2008;10:428-32.

[86] De Reuver PR, Grossmann I, Busch OR, Obertop H, Van Gulik TM, Gouma DJ. Referral pattern and timing of repair are risk factors for complications after reconstructive surgery for bile duct injury. *Ann. Surg.* 2007;245:763-70.

[87] Bilge O, Bozkiran S, Ozden I, Tekant Y, Acarli K, Alper A, et al. The effect of concomitant vascular disruption in patients with iatrogenic biliary injuries. *Langenbecks Arch. Surg.* 2003;388:265-9.

[88] Mercado MA, Chan C, Orozco H, Tielve M, Hinojosa CA. Acute bile duct injury. The need for a high repair. *Surg. Endosc.* 2003;17:1351-5.

[89] Mercado MA. Early versus late repair of bile duct injuries. *Surg. Endosc.* 2006; 20: 1644-7.

[90] Dageforde LA, Landman MP, Feurer ID, Poulose B, Pinson CW, Moore DE A Cost-Effectiveness Analysis of Early vs Late Reconstruction of Iatrogenic Bile Duct Injuries.. *J. Am. Coll. Surg.* 2012 Jun;214(6):919-27.

[91] Barros F, Fernandes RA, de Oliveira ME, Pacheco LF, Martinho JM. The influence of time referral in the treatment of iatrogenic lesions of biliary tract. *Rev. Col. Bras. Cir.* 2010 Dec;37(6):407-12.

[92] Stewart L, Way LW. Laparoscopic bile duct injuries: timing of surgical repair does not influence success rate. A multivariate analysis of factors influencing surgical outcomes. *HPB* (Oxford). 2009 Sep;11(6):516-22.

[93] Mercado MA, Chan C, Salgado-Nesme N, López-Rosales F. Intrahepatic repair of bile duct injuries. A comparative study. *J. Gastrointest. Surg.* 2008;12:364-8.

[94] Frilling A, Li J, Weber F, Frühauf NR, Engel J, Beckebaum S, et al. Major bile duct injuries after laparoscopic cholecystectomy: a tertiary center experience. *J. Gastrointest. Surg.* 2004;8: 679-85.

[95] Sutherland F, Launois B, Stanescu M, Campion JP, Spiliopoulos Y, Stasik C. A refined approach to the repair of postcholecystectomy bile duct strictures. *Arch. Surg.* 1999; 134:299-302.

[96] Mercado MA, Chan C, Orozco H, Cano-Gutiérrez G, Chaparro JM, Galindo E, et al. To stent or not to stent bilioenteric anastomosis after iatrogenic injury: a dilemma not answered? *Arch. Surg.* 2002;137:60-3.

[97] Al-Ghnaniem R, Benjamin IS. Long-term outcome of hepaticojejunostomy with routine access loop formation following iatrogenic bile duct injury. *Br. J. Surg.* 2002;89: 1118-24.

[98] Gibson RN, Collier NA, Speer TG, Sherson ND. Percutaneous transjejunal biliary intervention: 10-year experience with access via Roux-en-Y loops. *Radiology.* 1998; 206:883-4.

[99] Barrow PJ, Siriwardena AK. Outcome of hepaticojejunostomy without access loop for repair of iatrogenic bile duct injury at laparoscopic cholecystectomy. *J. Hepatobiliary Pancreat. Surg.* 2007;14:374-6.

[100] Gómez NA, Alvarez LR, Mite A, Andrade JP, Alvarez JR, Vargas PE, et al. Repair of bile duct injuries with Gore-Tex vascular grafts: experimental study in dogs. *J. Gastrointest. Surg.* 2002;6:116-20.

[101] Li J, Lü Y, Qu B, Zhang Z, Liu C, Shi Y, et al. Application of a new type of sutureless magnetic biliary-enteric anastomosis stent for one-stage reconstruction of the biliary-enteric continuity after acute bile duct injury: an experimental study. *J. Surg. Res.* 2008; 148:136-42.

[102] Kram HB, Garces MA, Klein SR, Shoemaker WC. Common bile duct anastomosis using fibrin glue. *Arch. Surg.* 1985;120:1250-6.

[103] Mortensen FV, Ishibashi T, Hojo N, Yasuda Y. A gallbladder flap for reconstruction of the common bile duct. An experimental study on pigs. *J. Hepatobiliary Pancreat. Surg.* 2004;11:112-5.

[104] Schanaider A, Pannain VL, Müller LC, Maya MC Expanded polytetrafluoroethylene in canine bile duct injury: a critical analysis.. *Acta Cir. Bras.* 2011 Aug;26(4):247-52.

[105] Aikawa M, Miyazawa M, Okamoto K, Toshimitsu Y, Torii T, Okada K, Akimoto N, Ohtani Y, Koyama I, Yoshito I A novel treatment for bile duct injury with a tissue-engineered bioabsorbable polymer patch.. *Surgery.* 2010 Apr;147(4):575-80.

[106] Helmy AA, Hamad MA, Aly AM, Sherif T, Hashem M, El-Sers DA, Semieka M Novel technique for biliary reconstruction using an isolated gastric tube with a vascularized

pedicle: a live animal experimental study and the first clinical case.. *Ann. Surg. Innov. Res.* 2011 Oct 10;5:8.

[107] Schmidt SC, Langrehr JM, Hintze RE, Neuhaus P. Long-term results and risk factors influencing outcome of major bile duct injuries following cholecystectomy. *Br. J. Surg.* 2005;92:76-82.

[108] Nordin A, Mäkisalo H, Isoniemi H, Halme L, Lindgren L, Höckerstedt K. Iatrogenic lesion at cholecystectomy resulting in liver transplantation. *Transplant. Proc.* 2001;33: 2499-500.

[109] Fernández JA, Robles R, Marín C, Sánchez-Bueno F, Ramírez P, Parrilla P. Laparoscopic iatrogeny of the hepatic hilum as an indication for liver transplantation. *Liver Transpl.* 2004;10:147-52.

[110] Loinaz C, González EM, Jiménez C, García I, Gómez R, González-Pinto I, et al. Long-term biliary complications after liver surgery leading to liver transplantation. *World J. Surg.* 2001;25:1260-3.

[111] Oncel D, Ozden I, Bilge O, Tekant Y, Acarli K, Alper A, et al. Bile duct injury during cholecystectomy requiring delayed liver transplantation: a case report and literature review. *Tohoku J. Exp. Med.* 2006;209:355-9.

[112] Robertson AJ, Rela M, Karani J, Steger AC, Benjamin IS, Heaton ND. Laparoscopic cholecystectomy injury: an unusual indication for liver transplantation. *Transpl. Int.* 1998;11:449-51.

[113] De Santibañes E, Ardiles V, Gadano A, Palavecino M, Pekolj J, Ciardullo M. Liver transplantation: the last measure in the treatment of bile duct injuries. *World J. Surg.* 2008;32:1714-21.

[114] Ardiles V, McCormack L, Quiñonez E, Goldaracena N, Mattera J, Pekolj J, Ciardullo M, de Santibañes Experience using liver transplantation for the treatment of severe bile duct injuries over 20 years in Argentina: results from a National Survey. E. *HPB (Oxford).* 2011 Aug;13(8):544-50.

[115] Yan JQ, Peng CH, Shen BY, Zhou GW, Yang WP, Chen YJ, Li HW. Liver transplantation as a treatment for complicated bile duct injury.. *Hepatogastroenterology.* 2011 Jan-Feb;58(105):8-13.

[116] De Santibañes E, Pekolj J, McCormack L, Nefa J, Mattera J, Sivori J et al. Liver transplantation for the sequelae of intra- operative bile duct injury. *HPB* 2002;4:111-5.

[117] De Santibañes E, Sívori J, Pekolj J, Ciardullo M, Sendin R, Beveraggi E. Lesiones de vía biliar, secundarias a colecistectomía laparoscópica. *Rev. Arg. Cir.* 1996;70:208-18.

[118] Fatima J, Barton JG, Grotz TE, Geng Z, Harmsen WS, Huebner M, Baron TH, Kendrick ML, Donohue JH, Que FG, Nagorney DM, Farnell MB Is there a role for endoscopic therapy as a definitive treatment for post-laparoscopic bile duct injuries?. *J. Am. Coll. Surg.* 2010 Oct;211(4):495-502.

[119] Weber A, Feussner H, Winkelmann F, Siewert JR, Schmid RM, Prinz C. Long-term outcome of endoscopic therapy in patients with bile duct injury after cholecystectomy. *J. Gastroenterol. Hepatol.* 2009;24:762-9.

[120] Marks JM, Ponsky JL, Shillingstad RB, Singh J. Biliary stenting is more effective than sphincterotomy in the resolution of biliary leaks. *Surg. Endosc.* 1998;12:327-30.

[121] Rauws EA, Gouma DJ. Endoscopic and surgical management of bile duct injury after laparoscopic cholecystectomy. *Best Pract. Res. Clin. Gastroenterol.* 2004;18:829-46.

[122] Bjorkman DJ, Carr-Locke DL, Lichtenstein DR, Ferrari AP, Slivka A, Van Dam J, et al. Postsurgical bile leaks: endoscopic obliteration of the transpapillary pressure gradient is enough. *Am. J. Gastroenterol.* 1995;90:2128-33.

[123] Ichiya T, Maguchi H, Takahashi K, Katanuma A, Osanai M, Kin T Endoscopic management of laparoscopic cholecystectomy-associated bile duct injuries.. *J. Hepatobiliary Pancreat. Sci.* 2011 Jan;18(1):81-6.

[124] Li J, Frilling A, Nadalin S, Radunz S, Treckmann J, Lang H, Malago M, Broelsch CE Surgical management of segmental and sectoral bile duct injury after laparoscopic cholecystectomy: a challenging situation.. *J. Gastrointest. Surg.* 2010 Feb;14(2): 344-51.

[125] Pottakkat B, Vijayahari R, Prasad KV, Sikora SS, Behari A, Singh RK, et al. Surgical management of patients with post- cholecystectomy benign biliary stricture complicated by atrophy-hypertrophy complex of the liver. *HPB* (Oxford). 2009;11:125-9.

[126] Chapman WC, Halevy A, Blumgart LH, Benjamin IS. Postcholecystectomy bile duct strictures. Management and outcome in 130 patients. *Arch. Surg.* 1995;130:597-602.

[127] Nishio H, Kamiya J, Nagino M, Uesaka K, Kanai M, Sano T, et al. Right hepatic lobectomy for bile duct injury associated with major vascular occlusion after laparoscopic cholecystectomy. *J. Hepatobiliary Pancreat. Surg.* 1999;6:427-30.

[128] Thethy S, Thomson BNJ, Pleass H, Wigmore SJ, Madhavan K, Akyol M, et al. Management of biliary tract complications after orthotopic liver transplantation. *Clin. Transplant.* 2004;18:647-53.

[129] Watanabe M, Yamazaki K, Tsuchiya M. i wsp: Use of an opened umbilical vein patch for the reconstruction of the injured biliary tract. *J. Hepatobiliay Pancreat. Surg.* 2007; 14:270-5.

[130] Cai JX, Liu FX, Ying DJ. Pedicle umbilical vein flap for repairing the bile duct (in Chinese). *J. Pract. Surg.* 1990; 10:663-4.

[131] Ying D.J., Ho G.T., Cai J.X. Anatomic bases of the vascularized hepatic teres ligament flap. *Surg. Radiol. Anat.* 1997;19:293-4.

[132] Winslow ER, Fialkowski EA, Linehan DC, Hawkins WG, Picus DD, Strasberg SM. "Sideways": results of repair of biliary injuries using a policy of side-to-side hepatico-jejunostomy. *Ann. Surg.* 2009;249:426-34.

[133] Hepp J. Hepaticojejunostomy using the left biliary trunk for iatrogenic biliary lesions: the French connection. *World J. Surg.* 1985;9:507-11.

[134] Machado MC, Da Cunha JE, Bacchella T. A modified technique for surgical repair of cicatricial stenosis of the bile duct. *Surg. Gynecol. Obstet.* 1986;162:282-4.

[135] Mercado MA, Orozco H, Chan C, Quezada C, Barajas-Olivas A, Borja-Cacho D, et al. Bile duct growing factor: an alternate technique for reconstruction of thin bile ducts after iatrogenic injury. *J. Gastrointest. Surg.* 2006;10:1164-9.

[136] Starzl TC, Iwatsuki S, Shaw BW. A growth factor in fine vascular anastomoses. *Surg. Gynecol. Obstet.* 1984;159:164-5.

[137] Laurent A, Sauvanet A, Farges O, Watrin T, Rivkine E, Belghiti J. Major hepatectomy for the treatment of complex bile duct injury. *Ann. Surg.* 2008;248:77-83.

[138] Truant S, Boleslawski E, Lebuffe G, Sergent G, Pruvot FR Hepatic resection for post-cholecystectomy bile duct injuries: a literature review.. *HPB* (Oxford). 2010 Jun;12(5): 334-41.

[139] Li J, Frilling A, Nadalin S, Broelsch CE, Malago M Timing and risk factors of hepatectomy in the management of complications following laparoscopic cholecystectomy.. *J. Gastrointest. Surg.* 2012 Apr;16(4):815-20.

[140] Mercado M, Sánchez N, Ramírez-Del Val F, Cerón R, Urencio J, Domínguez I. [Indications of hepatectomy for iatrogenic biliary injury.].. *Rev. Gastroenterol. Mex.* 2010 Jan-Mar;75(1):22-9.

[141] Strasberg SM, Picus DD, Drebin JA. Results of a new strategy for reconstruction of biliary injuries having an isolated right- sided component. *J. Gastrointest. Surg.* 2001;5: 266-74.

[142] Mercado MA, Chan C, Salgado-Nesme N, López-Rosales F. Intrahepatic repair of bile duct injuries. A comparative study. *J. Gastrointest. Surg.* 2008;12:364-8.

[143] Mercado MA, Chan C, Orozco H, Villalta JM, Barajas-Olivas A, Eraña J, et al. Long-term evaluation of biliary reconstruction after partial resection of segments IV and V in iatrogenic injuries. *J. Gastrointest. Surg.* 2006;10:77-82.

[144] Thomson BN, Parks RW, Madhavan KK, Garden OJ. Liver resection and transplantation in the management of iatrogenic biliary injury. *World J. Surg.* 2007; 31:2363-9.

[145] Koffron A, Ferrario M, Parsons W, Nemcek A, Saker M, Abecassis M. Failed primary management of iatrogenic biliary injury: incidence and significance of concomitant hepatic arterial disruption. *Surgery.* 2001;130:722-8.

[146] Lillemoe KD, Melton GB, Cameron JL, Pitt HA, Campbell KA, Talamini MA, et al. Postoperative bile duct strictures: management and outcome in the 1990s. *Ann. Surg.* 2000; 232:430-41.

[147] Costamagna G, Pandolfi M, Mutignani M, Spada C, Perri V. Long-term results of endoscopic management of postoperative bile duct strictures with increasing numbers of stents. *Gastrointest. Endosc.* 2001;54:162-8.

[148] Vitale GC, Tran TC, Davis BR, Vitale M, Vitale D, Larson G. Endoscopic management of postcholecystectomy bile duct strictures. *J. Am. Coll. Surg.* 2008;206:918-23.

[149] Grönroos JM. Unsuccessful endoscopic stenting in iatrogenic bile duct injury: remember rendezvous procedure. *Surg. Laparosc. Endosc. Percutan. Tech.* 2007;17: 186-9.

[150] Shlansky-Goldberg RD, Ginsberg GG, Cope C. Percutaneous puncture of the common bile duct as a rendezvous procedure to cross a difficult biliary obstruction. *J. Vasc. Interv. Radiol.* 1995;6:943-6.

[151] Calvo MM, Bujanda L, Heras I, Cabriada JL, Bernal A, Orive V, et al. The rendezvous technique for the treatment of choledocholithiasis. *Gastrointest. Endosc.* 2001;54: 511-3.

[152] Blumgart LH, Kelley CJ, Benjamin IS. Benign bile duct stricture following cholecystectomy: critical factors in management. *Br. J. Surg.* 1984;71:836-43.

[153] Chapman WC, Halevy A, Blumgart LH, Benjamin IS. Postcholecystectomy bile duct strictures: Management and outcome in 130 patients. *Arch. Surg.* 1995;130:597-604.

[154] Kelley CJ, Benjamin IS, Blumgart LH. Portal hypertension and post-cholecystectomy biliary strictures. *Dig. Surg.* 1986;3:292-6.

[155] Agarwal AK, Gupta V, Singh S, Agarwal S, Sakhuja P. Management of patients of postcholecystectomy benign biliary stricture complicated by portal hypertension. *Am. J. Surg.* 2008;195:421-6.

[156] Chaudhary A, Dhar P, Sarin SK, Sachdev A, Agarwal AK, Vij JC, et al. Bile duct obstruction due to portal biliopathy in extrahepatic portal hypertension: surgical management. *Br. J. Surg.* 1998;85:326-9.

[157] Braasch JW, Bolton JS, Rossi RL. A technique of biliary tract reconstruction with complete follow-up in 44 consecutive cases. *Ann. Surg.* 1981;194:635-8.

[158] Röthlin MA, Löpfe M, Schlumpf R, Largiadèr F. Long-term results of hepaticojejunostomy for benign lesions of the bile ducts. *Am. J. Surg.* 1998;175:22-6.

[159] Scobie BA, Summerskill WH. Hepatic cirrhosis secondary to obstruction of the biliary system. *Am. J. Dig. Dis.* 1965;10:135-46.

[160] Strasberg SM, Helton WS An analytical review of vasculobiliary injury in laparoscopic and open cholecystectomy.. *HPB* (Oxford). 2011 Jan;13(1):1-14.

[161] Pulitanò C, Parks RW, Ireland H, Wigmore SJ, Garden OJ Impact of concomitant arterial injury on the outcome of laparoscopic bile duct injury.. *Am. J. Surg.* 2011 Feb;201(2):238-44.

[162] Gupta N, Solomon H, Fairchild R, Kaminski DL. Management and outcome of patients with combined bile duct and hepatic artery injuries. *Arch. Surg.* 1998;13.

[163] Bachellier P, Nakano H, Weber JC, Lemarque P, Oussoultzoglou E, Candau C, et al. Surgical repair after bile duct and vascular injuries during laparoscopic cholecystectomy: when and how? *World J. Surg.* 2001;25:1335-45.

[164] Majno PE, Prêtre R, Mentha G, Morel P. Operative injury to the hepatic artery. Consequences of a biliary-enteric anastomosis and principles for rational management. *Arch. Surg.* 1996;131:211-5.

[165] Buell JF, Cronin DC, Funaki B, Koffron A, Yoshida A, Lo A, et al. Devastating and fatal complications associated with combined vascular and bile duct injuries during cholecystectomy. *Arch. Surg.* 2002;137:703-8.

[166] Stapleton GN, Hickman R, Terblanche J. Blood supply of the right and left hepatic ducts. *Br. J. Surg.* 1998;85:202-7.

[167] Vellar ID. The blood supply of the biliary ductal system and its relevance to vasculobiliary injuries following cholecystectomy. *Aust. N. Z. J. Surg.* 1999;69:816-20.

[168] Testa G, Malagò M, Broelseh CE. Complications of biliary tract in liver transplantation. *World J. Surg.* 2001;25:1296-9.

[169] Strasberg SM, Gouma DJ. 'Extreme' vasculobiliary injuries: association with fundus-down cholecystectomy in severely inflamed gallbladders. *HPB* (Oxford). 2012 Jan; 14(1):1-8.

[170] Boerma D, Rauws EA, Keulemans YC, Bergman JJ, Obertop H, Huibregtse K, et al. Impaired quality of life 5 years after bile duct injury during laparoscopic cholecystectomy: a prospective analysis. *Ann. Surg.* 2001;234:750-7.

[171] Moore DE, Feurer ID, Holzman MD, Wudel LJ, Strickland C, Gorden DL, et al. Long-term detrimental effect of bile duct injury on health-related quality of life. *Arch. Surg.* 2004;139:476-81.

[172] Sarmiento JM, Farnell MB, Nagorney DM, Hodge DO, Harrington JR. Quality-of-life assessment of surgical reconstruction after laparoscopic cholecystectomy-induced bile duct injuries: what happens at 5 years and beyond? *Arch. Surg.* 2004;139:483-8.

[173] Melton GB, Lillemoe KD, Cameron JL, Sauter PA, Coleman J, Yeo CJ. Major bile duct injuries associated with laparoscopic cholecystectomy: effect of surgical repair on quality of life. *Ann. Surg.* 2002;235:888-95.

[174] Hogan AM, Hoti E, Winter DC, Ridgway PF, Maguire D, Geoghegan JG, et al. Quality of life after iatrogenic bile duct injury: a case control study. *Ann. Surg.* 2009;249:292-5.

[175] Wauben LS, Goossens RH, Van Eijk DJ, Lange JF. Evaluation of protocol uniformity concerning laparoscopic cholecystectomy in the Netherlands. *World J. Surg.* 2008; 32:613-20.

[176] Berney CR. Major common bile duct injury and risk of litigation: a surgeon's perspective. *Am. J. Surg.* 2011.

Chapter IV

Bile Duct Injury Following Cholecystectomy: Prevention, Management, and Outcome

Takahisa Fujikawa[*] *Hisatsugu Maekawa*
and Akira Tanaka
Department of Surgery, Kokura Memorial Hospital,
Kitakyushu, Fukuoka, Japan

Abstract

Background: Bile duct injury (BDI) following cholecystectomy is a severe and potentially life-threatening complication associated with significant morbidity and mortality and high rates of medical malpractice litigation. With the small number of patients having BDI recognized in each center, a prospective comparative study is difficult to perform.

Methods: A review of the English language literature listed on Medline database, concerning BDI following cholecystectomy, was performed.

Results: Although a rate of BDI following cholecystectomy is recently stabilized at 0.1-0.7% in the literature, higher incidence of BDI is reported to be occurred in the setting of laparoscopic approach. In addition, BDI following laparoscopic cholecystectomy often involves complete disruption and excision of bile ducts, and may be associated with hepatic artery injuries. Factors which have been associated with BDI include surgeon experience, patient age, male sex, and acute cholecystitis. The safety of cholecystectomy requires careful dissection and correct identification of the relevant anatomy to ensure the "critical view of safety" prior to dividing any structures. Increasing evidence suggests that prompt recognition and diagnosis of BDI directly affect outcome, and that it should be managed by an experienced hepatobiliary surgeon. Since patients

[*] Corresponding author: Takahisa Fujikawa, MD, PhD, FACS, Department of Surgery, 3-2-1 Asano, Kokurakita-ku, Kitakyushu, Fukuoka 802-8555, Japan. Tel.: 81-93-511-2000, Fax: 81-93-511-3240; E-mail: fujikawa-t@kokurakinen.or.jp.

with BDI may require long-term follow-up due to possible delayed biliary stricture, the outcome and quality of life after BDI remains poor.

Conclusion: Although it can and should be regarded as preventable, bile duct injury following cholecystectomy is still one of the most severe and complicated events especially in the era of laparoscopic cholecystectomy. A great effort must continue to be taken to highlight seriousness of this catastrophic complication and to reduce its incidence.

Keywords: Laparoscopic cholecystectomy, bile duct injury, prevention, outcome, management

Introduction

Bile duct injury (BDI) following cholecystectomy is a severe and potentially life-threatening complication. Before laparoscopic cholecystectomy (LC) was introduced, the incidence of BDIs reduced and stabilized at approximately 0.1-0.3% [1, 2]. LC has currently replaced open surgery and became the new gold standard in the treatment of symptomatic cholecystolithiasis [3-9]. During the surgical learning curve for this new technique, there was an initial rise in the reports of BDIs [10], and numerous reports have demonstrated that the incidence of BDIs has now stabilized but they still occurred more frequently during LC at the rate of 0.3-0.7% [11-17] (Table 1). BDI following cholecystectomy is an iatrogenic catastrophe which is associated with significant perioperative morbidity and mortality [18, 19], reduced long-term survival [14] and quality of life [20, 21]. There is a significant increase in healthcare expenses associated with the complication, and this is a common reason for medical malpractice litigation [4, 22]. The optimal management depends on the timing of recognition of injury, the extent of BDI, the patient's condition, and the availability of experienced hepatobiliary surgeons. Patients who suffered from BDI following cholecystectomy have impaired quality of life and continue to have a higher risk of dying as compared with those who have an uncomplicated surgery [4, 22]. With the small number of patients and the difference of presentation in BDIs in each center, a prospective study is difficult to proceed for the prevention or management of BDIs. Thus, only case series and experiences were published in the medical literature. The aim of this paper is to discuss BDI after cholecystectomy, with reference to its prevention, management and outcome.

Prevention

BDI should be regarded as preventable, but from the fact that one-third of BDI happen after the surgeon has performed more than 200 [23], most surgeons think that it is regarded unavoidable [24]. It has been suggested that the main cause of BDI is misidentification of biliary anatomy, as well as inexperience for cholecystectomy [2, 25]. Several local risk factors that predispose to BDI have been reported including acute cholecystitis, Mirizzi's syndrome, bleeding in Calot's triangle, severely scarred or shrunken gall bladder, and abnormal biliary anatomy [3-9]. However, we should understand that more than half of BDIs occurred during the "easy" LC performed by an inexperienced surgeon [3].

Table 1. Reported data concerning rate of bile duct injuries and subsequent mortality

Reports	Year	Rate of BDIs in LC (rate in OC)	Mortality after LC (mortality after OC)	Mortality after repair of BDI
Cohen [12]	1996	0.9% (0.3%)	0.3% (0.2%)	-
Russell [17]	1996	0.11% (0.06%)	-	-
Richardson [16]	1996	0.4% (-)	-	-
Adamsen [11]	1997	0.7% (-)	0.0001% (-)	-
Flecher [13]	1999	0.29% (0.15%)	-	-
Flum [15]	2003	0.5% (-)	0% (-)	-
Mirza [90]	1997	-	-	3.7%
Lillemoe [88]	2000	-	-	0%
Reuver [61]	2007	-	-	0.2%
Mercado [89]	2008	-	-	0.6%

*Abbreviations: BDI; bile duct injury, LC; laparoscopic cholecystectomy, OC; open cholecystectomy.

Table 2. Recommended basic assessment and techniques to avoid major bile duct injuries during laparoscopic cholecystectomy

Preoperative assessment:
■ Recognition of biliary anomary or variation
■ Recognition of degree of acute/chronic inflammation (cf. acute cholecystitis, Mirizzi's syndrome, or shrunken gallbladder)
■ Recognition of impaired medical condition (cf. liver cirrhosis, use of antithrombotics)
Intraoperative techniques:
- sufficient exposure of Calot's triangle (gaining "critical view of safety")
- dissection close to the gallbladder-cystic duct junction
- avoidance of unnecessary dissection close to the common hepatic duct
- avoidance of electrocautery close to the common hepatic duct
- avoidance of blind application of clips
- delineation of biliary anatomy by intraopeative cholangiography if needed
− - conversion to an open approach when encountered uncertain anatomy

Table 2 shows recommended basic assessment and techniques to avoid BDIs during LC. In addition to appropriate preoperative assessment of biliary anatomy and patients' medical condition, it is generally accepted that some basic and important techniques are needed to avoid BDIs during LC including sufficient exposure of Calot's triangle (gaining the "critical view of safety"), avoidance of diathermy close to the hepatic duct, and conversion to an open surgery when uncertain anatomy was recognized [26-29]. Three quarters of BDIs are not recognized at the time of injury [2, 25].

Therefore, correct interpretation of the anatomy is of paramount importance, and wrong or incomplete dissection of Calot's triangle may result in misidentification of the cystic duct, which causes major BDIs [26, 29, 30]. The "critical view of safety" has been accepted as the most important concept to gain a sufficient view of Calot's triangle before transecting the cystic duct [27]. However, in cases of highly inflamed gallbladders, it is often hard to achieve a critical view of safety, because Calot's triangle is likely to be solid and cannot be expanded.

Some landmarks including cystic lymph node, gall bladder neck, Hartman's pouch, and Rouviere's sulcus have been advocated for identifying the cystic duct and safe dissection [31]. Although it may be distorted and is carefully identified in patients with atrophic cholecystitis or adhesions around cystic duct, Hartman's pouch is often used as a landmark as it is easily visualized and connects gallbladder to cystic duct [32].

Hugh et al. recommends identifying Rouviere's sulcus as a fixed extra-biliary point ventral to the right portal pedicle, and dissection ventral to this sulcus and extending this dissection as far as possible up the gallbladder fossa both posteriorly and anteriorly allows the hepatobiliary triangle to open out [25].

Strasberg et al. suggested that misidentification of the common bile duct (CBD) as cystic duct can be attributed to the direction of traction on the gallbladder in superior direction rather than laterally bringing the cystic duct and CBD into alignment, thus it is essential to retract the gallbladder in lateral direction when clipping or dividing the cystic duct [28]. Honda et al. recommended exposing the inner layer of the subserosal layer (ss-i) to achieve the "critical view of safety" in case of severe acute cholecystitis [30].

In case of difficult cholecystectomy resulting from severe cholecystitis, extensive adhesions, and fibrosed and obliterated Calot's triangle, early conversion from LC to open surgery is strongly advised [28]. The conversion rates during LC vary from 3.6 to 13.9% [3, 9, 33]. The common indication for conversion includes technical difficulties, uncontrolled bleeding, difficulty in dissecting the Calot's triangle, CBD stones, and bile duct injuries [9, 28, 33]. It is again highly recommended not to hesitate to convert to open surgery in the event of uncertainty of anatomical landmarks and failure to progress after a reasonable period of dissection.

Misuse of cautery in dissecting the Calot's triangle may cause serious BDI with loss of ductal tissue due to thermal necrosis [28]. Once the serosa of the gall bladder is opened, blunt dissection by forceps may be performed instead of cautery in Calot's triangle [9]. It is very important not to use cautery to cut the cystic duct particularly when titanium clips are placed on the cystic duct as titanium clips conduct electric current well and may lead to thermal necrosis of the cystic duct stump or adjacent bile duct.

It is appropriate that short bursts of minimal amount of energy to dissect or secure hemostasis are always applied [9, 28]. Dissection in the presence of acute inflammation and scarred tissue may result in significant bleeding which masks the visualization of the biliary anatomy [9, 28]. Bleeding in such situation is adequately managed by maintaining a calm composure in addition to compressing the bleeding point and adjoining tissue with atraumatic forceps for several minutes, thus the hemorrhage is usually controlled and then clips can be placed accurately once good exposure is obtained [9, 28].

The role of routine intraoperative cholangiography (IOC) to avoid BDI remains controversial [3, 23, 34]. There is no randomized controlled trial to determine the effect of IOC on the occurrence of BDI. Some reports demonstrated good results for LC without routine IOC performance, though others report its use to decrease the incidence of BDI or its early intraoperative detection [3, 9, 13, 15, 23, 25, 34-36]. Although all are subject to bias, three population-based studies have shown a reduction in risk of BDI if surgeons perform routine IOC [13, 15, 35]. Flum et al. examined the outcome in more than 1.5 million LC and demonstrated that failure to perform an IOC increased the risk of BDI by 1.5-7 times, which remained even when adjusted for surgeon and patient factors [15]. Routine use of IOC is also reported to be cost-effective, with maximum efficiency achieved when used by inexperienced surgeons or when complex disease is encountered [37].

On the other hand, the disadvantage of IOC includes the need for surgical experience, the prolongation of the operative time and the need for interpretation by an experienced radiologist [9]. It is also argued that BDI is not prevented by IOC, and that only meticulous dissection and correct interpretation of anatomy will avoid this complication [25, 36].

Despite this controversy, there is reasonable evidence to show that IOC can identify BDI at the time of surgery. Archer et al. demonstrated that 81% of BDI were detected at the time of initial injury when IOC was carried out compared with only 45% when it was not performed [23]. This includes a significant suggestion for the patient given the improved outcome by performing early appropriate repair [19].

Last but not least, it is also important to analyze the effect of surgeons characteristics on risk of BDI. Inadvertent injuries of bile duct are reported to occur due to casual approach, overconfidence, and ignorance of difficult situations [9, 38, 39].

Massarweh et al. suggested that the surgical community is working to create a safety culture by better training and standard use of safety measures when even a rare event such as BDI are encountered [38]. The proper methods include incorporating modules that simulate potential intraoperative errors in judgment and stress safe decision making and emphasize use of proved safety measures that are likely to be helpful.

Diagnosis

Delay in diagnosis is associated with an increase in serious complications and an adverse outcome [40]. Therefore, recognition of BDI at the time of cholecystectomy is of outmost importance, and it allows an opportunity for the hepatobiliary surgeon to assess its severity and to manage properly. However, given that most injuries are not recognized during the initial operation, a high index of suspicion is required in patients who become unwell in the early postoperative period [41, 42]. Although early classical symptoms of BDI include jaundice, biloma, bile peritonitis, sepsis, multiple organ failure, external biliary fistula, cholangitis, and liver abscess [5, 6, 8, 9, 41, 43], initial symptoms may be nonspecific [40, 44]. After discharge, patients frequently reappear only a few days later with classical symptoms and signs. The median delay in diagnosis is 1–2 weeks, but it may be months or years for delayed symptoms of recurrent cholangitis resulting from biliary stricture [43, 44]. If the biliary stricture is not appropriately managed, intrahepatic lithiasis, secondary biliary cirrhosis, portal hypertension, and finally catastrophic end stage liver disease are likely to occur [6, 7]. These complications may be associated with mortality rate of almost 5% if it is not properly managed [45]. LC is also associated with a higher risk of vascular injury to the hepatic artery and portal vein which further increases the mortality [46].

BDI may present in the same way as less serious complications of cholecystectomy, thus initial management must be dictated by the clinical presentation. Abnormal liver function test showing cholestasis to suggest BDI should be investigate further. However, these tests may be normal or mildly elevated in such cases like bile leakage. Abdominal ultrasonography and computed tomography (CT) is the initial investigation of choice and they may show fluid collection within the right subhepatic space as well as a proximal dilated biliary structure in patients with complete division of CBD [47]. Consequently, further investigation is warranted in the evaluation of the cause of this collection or suspected obstruction. Magnetic resonance cholangiography (MRC) provides a noninvasive diagnostic investigation that gives sufficient delineation of the biliary anatomy, but it can miss minor bile leakage.

Endoscopic retrograde cholangiography (ERC) and percutaneous transhepatic cholangiography (PTC) are likely to demonstrate the presence of bile leak and often provide the level of duct laceration or transaction [47-49]. Additionally, ERC and PTC provide a therapeutic option in the setting of BDI and sphincterotomy, biliary drainage and/or endobiliary stenting may be considered [48-50].

Once referred to hepatobiliary specialist for management, an assessment of vascular anatomy is mandatory as vascular injury is presented in 26-32% of BDI patients [51-53]. The less invasive CT angiography or magnetic resonance angiography is preferable to invasive angiography and should exclude injury to both the arterial and portal venous systems and the presence of pseudoaneurysms that may follow sepsis or intraabdominal bleeding. Vascular assessment is specifically important if surgeons attempted to repair BDI during cholecystectomy or if the level of BDI is more proximal, because these cases may be associated with damage to the right hepatic artery [52, 53]. In cases of delayed biliary stricture, it is requisite to assess the quality of the obstructed liver. Hepatocellular atrophy may develop in the presence of long-term obstruction of the biliary system and be associated with the development of liver fibrosis or cirrhosis [54].

The difficulty in management and outcome of BDI vary case by case and are highly dependent on the type of injury and its location. Consequently, a classification involving therapeutic and prognostic implications is requisite [55]. Several classifications of BDI have been proposed, but none is accepted as a universal standard [28, 43, 56, 57]. Table 3 demonstrates summary of proposed classifications of BDI by Bismuth, Strasberg, and Lau [28, 55, 56]. Strictures involving the CBD or common hepatic duct (CHD) may be less technically difficult to repair and may recur less frequently than those involving more proximal biliary system.

Table 3. Proposed classifications of bile duct injuries

Classification (year)	Bismuth [56] (1982)	Strasberg [28] (1995)	Lau [55] (2007)
Bile leak from cystic duct or terminal small ducts	-	Type A	Type 1
Bile leak from CBD/CHD	-	Type D	Type 2[#]
Transection of CBD/CHD	-	-	Type 3[#]
Transection of RHD/PHD	-	Type C	Type 4[#]
Low CHD stricture (CHD stump >2cm)	Type I	Type E1	-
Low CHD stricture (CHD stump<2cm)	Type II	Type E2	-
Hilar stricture but confluence intact	Type III	Type E3	-
Hilar stricture with disruption of confluence	Type IV	Type E4	-
Involvement of PHD (with or without CBD/CHD stricture)	Type V	Type E5/B	-
BDI associated with vascular injuries	-	-	Type 5

[#]Each type was subdivided into injuries without tissue loss (A) and with tissue loss (B).

[*]Abbreviations: CBD; common bile duct, CHD; common hepatic duct, RHD; right hepatic duct, PHD; right posterior hepatic duct, BDI; bile duct injury.

The Bismuth classification, which is one of the most classical classification system of BDI and originated from the era of open cholecystectomy, is based on the most distal level at which healthy biliary mucosa at the proximal site of the injury is available for anastomosis [56] (Table 3). This classification is intended to choose the most appropriate technique for repair and has a good correlation with the final outcome after repair [56, 58]. McMahon et al. suggested that BDIs can be divided into laceration, transection or excision, and stricture, and the level of stricture can further be graded according to the Bismuth classification [59]. They also proposed a subdivision into major and minor BDI since minor injury can be managed by simple suture repair with/without insertion of a T-tube, and major BDI usually requires hepaticojejunostomy [59]. However, the Bismuth and the McMahon classifications cannot include the whole spectrum of possible BDIs. BDIs following LC tend to be more severe than in open surgery.

Strasberg et al. made Bismuth classification much more comprehensive by including various types of laparoscopic extrahepatic BDIs [28]. Strasberg classification of laparoscopic BDIs is stratified from type A to type E, and type E are further subdivided into E1 to E5 according to the Bismuth classification (Table 3). The outcome of patients with major BDIs combined with arterial disruptions was suggested to be worse than in those with an intact vascular system [53, 60]. None of the early proposed classifications allow for the documentation of an associated vascular injury. Lau et al. proposed another classification to overcome the problems associated with several previous classifications mentioned above, which include BDIs associated with vascular injury [48, 55] (Table 3). This classification may have some advantages including both preventive measures and management being instituted for each type. Thus, several classifications of BDI have been proposed so far, but none is accepted as a universal standard due to its own limitation.

Management

Management depends on the timing of recognition of injury and the type, extent and level of the injury. It may be considered as intraoperative, early and delayed. Table 4 demonstrates summary of recommended management in each stage of BDI according to its type and severity.

There are increasing reports supporting the importance of early referral to a tertiary care hospital which can provide a multidisciplinary approach to treat BDI [61, 62]. Biliary anatomy should be sufficiently investigated before any attempt at surgical repair [63]. It is also indicated that biliary reconstruction is best performed by a hepatobiliary specialist surgeon [14, 63].

Stewart et al. reported in a review of 88 patients with BDI after LC that only 17% of BDI repairs were successful in those performed by a primary surgeon compared with 94% of those performed by a biliary specialist surgeon, and the hospital stay was three times longer [63]. The morbidity and mortality of those treated by a primary and by a biliary surgeon were 58% and 1.6% versus 4% and 0%, respectively.

Flum et al. also showed the adjusted hazard of death during follow-up was 11% greater if BDI repair was done by a primary surgeon [15]. Heise et al. identified that the number of attempted repairs before referral was a significant prognostic factor of poor outcome [64].

Table 4. Recommended management in each type of bile duct injury

Type of injury	Early management	Delayed management
Minor duct injury	# Conversion to laparotomy # Control with suturing # Drain subhepatic space	# Drain intraabdominal collection # Control sepsis # Biliary drainage
Partial injury of CBD/CHD	# Conversion to laparotomy # Repair small laceration # Drain subhepatic space	# Same as minor duct injury # Laparotomy, repair and drainage
Transection of CBD/CHD	# Conversion to laparotomy # HJ # Drain subhepatic space	# Same as minor duct injury # HJ when sepsis controlled
Transection of RHD/PHD	# Conversion to laparotomy # RHJ or PHJ # Drain subhepatic space	# Same as minor duct injury # RHJ/PHJ when sepsis controlled # liver resection if HJ impossible
BDI associated with vascular injuries	# Conversion to laparotomy # Reconstruction of vessels # Reconstruction of bile ducts # ligate duct and vessels and wait for delayed treatment if reconstruction impossible	# Same as minor duct injury # Follow up if asymptomatic # HJ, liver resection, or liver transplant if symptomatic

*Abbreviations: CBD; common bile duct, CHD; common hepatic duct, RHD; right hepatic duct, PHD; right posterior hepatic duct, BDI; bile duct injury, HJ; hepaticojejunostomy, RHJ; anastomosis of right hepatic duct to jejunum, PHJ; anastomosis of right posterior hepatic duct to jejunum.

Intraoperative Management

If a bile leak from a bile duct is identified especially within the proximal gallbladder fossa or hilum, a major injury should be suspected. In such situations during laparoscopic approach, prompt conversion to open laparotomy with cholangiography should be performed to determine if an injury is present and to define the nature of the injury.

Also, one should first call for help and consult an experienced hepatobiliary surgeon, since it is reported that outcome is improved when an experienced hepatobiliary surgeon managed BDIs [14, 63]. If such assistance is unavailable, transfer of the patient should be considered after adequate drainage is achieved. Injudicious attempts at exploration of the bile leak by laparoscopic means or at open operation should be avoided as further extension of BDI into the intrahepatic ducts or subsequent damage to the arterial supply can occur. Interpretation of IOR is particularly important and failure to identify the right posterior hepatic duct (PHD) should warn the surgeon to the possibility of a concomitant segmental injury.

Ligation of a significant isolated segmental branch may result in obstructive cholangitis in the sacrificed branch, hepatic abscess and prolonged biliary fistula. If IOR demonstrates a presence of major BDI, biliary reconstruction, mostly hepaticojejunostomy, is required. A choledocho- or hepaticoduodenostomy should be avoided since revision is often necessary because of recurrent cholangitis [65].

Early Postoperative Management

Primary repair of a major duct injury may be successfully performed if done within the first few days. The surgeon should identify the entire biliary tree before repair and assess any associated vascular injury, particularly in the presence of a proximal injury [52]. Bilioenteric anastomosis (mostly hepaticojejunostomy) with healthy mature tissue has been advocated in a non-infected environment [66].

Despite increasing evidence that early repair is associated with a shorter duration of treatment and subsequent improved quality of life [20, 63], the timing of intervention remains controversial [67, 68]. Chaudhary et al. demonstrated that repair within the first 3 weeks is associated with an increased risk of failure, although they did not mention how many repairs were performed by an experienced surgeon [69]. In contrast, Thomson et al. have recently reported that among 64 patients who had not undergone prior repair, 22 underwent repair within the first 2 weeks of injury and only one required further surgical intervention [70]. On the other hand, 74% of 50 patients undergoing repair by the primary surgeon required further surgery subsequently. If the criteria for a successful anastomosis cannot be met, as in the event of disruption of the confluence with an associated vascular injury, or significant diathermy injury, or surrounding sepsis, it may be wise to delay repair and establish a controlled fistula.

Delayed Postoperative Management

Initial management of patients with delayed diagnosis of BDI is directed at controlling sepsis, drainage of bilomas or abscesses, establishing biliary drainage and obtaining the correct diagnosis, type and extent of BDI. Broad-spectrum parenteral antibiotics covering the common biliary pathogens should be started. Intra-abdominal collection or abscess should be percutaneously drained. Endoscopic or percutaneous biliary drainage should be established. Nutritional support should be maintained during subsequent anatomical delineation and definitive repair [71, 72]. Biliary reconstruction in the presence of peritonitis may lead to a worse outcome in BDI patients [73]. Once sepsis is controlled, there is no rush to proceed with surgical intervention for BDI. The inflammation, scar formation and development of fibrosis take several weeks to cool down. Reconstruction of the biliary system is preferably performed electively after an interval of at least 6-8 weeks.

Minor Duct Injury

A bile leak has been reported more commonly after LC than open cholecystectomy and usually occurs due to an injury of a minor duct. The cystic duct stump and small peripheral right hepatic ducts (RHDs) within the liver bed account for most injuries of this type. Cystic stump leaks can occur by failure of clip application, slipping of the clips, necrosis of the cystic duct stump due to cautery injury or cystic stump blow-out due to an obstructing CBD stone. Endoscopic management by sphincterotomy and drainage by insertion of a nasobiliary drain or internal biliary stent decreases the intraductal pressure, and diverts the bile flow away from the site of bile leak [50, 74-77]. Most reports recommended biliary stent insertion rather than sphincterotomy, because biliary stent covers the leakage point, as well as reduces the intraductal pressure, and supports BDI patients to heal early. Although this endoscopic management is effective in patients suffering from bile leak, there is no comprehensive data to indicate the most effective therapy. In patients with intraabdominal fluid collections, percutaneous drainage of these collections should be performed to avoid abdominal abscess formation.

Partial Injury of CBD/CHD

For a bile leak from partial injuries of CBD/CHD, the most preferable option of treatment is primary closure with fine absorbable sutures and subhepatic drainage after conversion to laparotomy. T-tube placement in this situation is still controversial. Experience in liver transplantation has shown that a T-tube placed within a choledocho-choledochostomy is associated with a significantly higher stricture rate than with repair without a T-tube (25% versus 11%) [78]. It may be preferable to avoid a foreign body in a non-dilated damaged duct. Biliary drainage by endoscopic stenting or sphincterotomy can be performed in case of postoperative bile leak and have a 57–70% chance of successful management [43, 63, 79]. If the defect from injury is large, the defect should be treated in the same fashion as in complete ductal transection.

Complete Transection of CBD/CHD

End-to-end anastomosis of the transected duct is rarely achievable without tension, even with additional mobilization of the duodenum. Stewart et al. reported that a rate of recurrent stricture after end-to-end repair of BDI during LC was 100% [63]. A Roux-en-Y hepaticojejunostomy is the best procedure for the majority of major BDIs. For cautery injury to the bile duct, the anastomosis should be made more proximally close to the confluence of the bile ducts to avoid delayed stricture as a consequence to coagulation injury to the collateral network of blood vessels supplying the CBD/CHD [48, 49].

Injury of RHD/LHD/PHD

If cholangiography demonstrates a major RHD or LHD injury, in which a correct diagnosis is usually achieved easily, reconstruction in the form of a hepaticojejunostomy is mandatory. Liver resection should be reserved in case of failed management of surgical duct reconstruction [48, 49]. On the other hand, PHD injury represents not only a diagnostic but also a therapeutic dilemma. Because of the small size of the injured ducts, the diagnosis of PHD injury is difficult in most cases. The main clue to manage an isolated PHD injury is recognition. Cholangiogram may not detect any bile leak and show 'normal' biliary structures. Recognition of absence in part of the RHD tree is the key to diagnosis. Based on the cholangiogram, the involved duct was accessed by either endoscopic or percutaneous approach. External or internal drainage allows prompt control of biliary leakage, eliminates sepsis and allows optimal timing of elective biliary reconstruction [48]. Surgical reconstruction is performed to the isolated PHD as a Roux-en-Y hepaticojejunostomy.

BDI Associated with Vascular Injuries

The rate of vascular injuries in patients with BDIs during cholecystectomy is 16.7-47%, and the transection of the right hepatic artery is the most frequent type since the right hepatic artery is close to the CHD [51, 57, 80-83]. The right hepatic artery usually traverses posteriorly (80% to 90%) to the duct. Unlike biliary injury, the right hepatic artery injury is often failed to diagnose because it is rare to develop early severe complications, and therefore remains unnoticed in most patients. Hepatic artery ligation is usually tolerated without any sequelae thanks to the portal flow and the supply of other collateral arteries. With regard to the impact of concomitant vascular injury to the hepatic duct, it has been reported that the presence of vascular injury is associated with increased intraoperative bleeding during repair, more difficult reconstruction and higher incidence of anastomotic stricture due to duct ischemia [84-86]. Secondary biliary cirrhosis resulting from persisting biliary stricture, as well as liver atrophy or necrosis due to hepatic ischemia, may need to be managed by liver resection or even liver transplantation. In the setting when this situation happens during cholecystectomy and becomes promptly recognized, some authors suggested to try to repair the vascular injury if possible [81, 82]. However, other authors suggested not to attempt to reconstruct the injured right hepatic artery and just to ignore it regardless of the timing of recognition or repair, since the complications following artery ligation in a normal liver have been usually unremarkable [48, 60].

Outcome

The goal of surgical repair of BDI is the restoration of a functional bile duct and the prevention of short- and long-term complications including biliary stricture with recurrent cholangitis and secondary biliary cirrhosis [5, 7, 45]. Long-term follow-up is required in case of BDI, as delayed and recurrent complications are not uncommon. Bottger et al. reported that about a third of recurrent strictures occurred within the first 3 years, and at least 10 years of follow-up is recommended [65]. More recent study reported by Al-Ghnaniem et al. demonstrated that 60% of patients with BDI had no further problems during 6-year follow-up period after hepaticojejunostomy, but the rest having further episodes of recurrent cholangitis requiring intervention [87]. The probability of developing ongoing symptoms was directly related to the level of injury, and those with more severe injuries presented earlier with recurrent problems, usually within the first 2 years. The overall long-term success rate when performed in specialized center is more than 90% and the mortality rate was 0-3.7% [53, 61, 88-90] (Table 4). It is reported that the factor that influence the long-term outcome after hepaticojejunostomy include the presence of active peritonitis at the time of repair, the combination of bile duct and vascular injury, the level of injury above the biliary bifurcation, and the number of previous operations [7, 46, 61, 88, 90].

Despite the excellent functional and anatomical results that can be achieved by early referral and appropriate primary repair, the effect of BDI on patient's quality of life remains worrisome. Boerma et al. assessed the outcome in 89 patients who had undergone BDI repair mostly by endoscopic approach, and demonstrated that a type of minor duct injury was paradoxically associated with a poorer quality of life [20]. Melton et al. have also shown that BDI patients who are involved in litigation have a poorer quality of life, and the patients in this study were often treated by endoscopic or percutaneous stenting [91]. In a more recent series in which surgical reconstruction was predominantly used, the quality of life of BDI patients was equivalent to that of the general population [92]. Thus, we should take into account the quality of life as well as the long-term outcome when patients suffering from BDI are managed.

Conclusion

Laparoscopic cholecystectomy has become the treatment of choice for symptomatic gallstone diseases, and it is associated with an increase in incidence of bile duct injury. Although it can and should be regarded as preventable, bile duct injury following cholecystectomy is still one of the most severe and complicated events especially in the era of laparoscopic cholecystectomy. After an appropriate diagnosis and assessment, the patient with bile duct injury should be immediately referred to an experienced hepatobiliary surgeon for the management. A proximal hepaticojejunostomy is the preferred treatment of choice for most patients, and long-term follow-up is requisite. A great effort must continue to be taken to highlight seriousness of this catastrophic complication and to reduce its incidence.

References

[1] Gharaibeh, K. I., Ammari, F., Al-Heiss, H., Al-Jaberi, T. M., Qasaimeh, G. R., Bani-Hani, K., et al. Laparoscopic cholecystectomy for gallstones: a comparison of outcome between acute and chronic cholecystitis. *Ann. Saudi Med.* 2001;21(5-6):312-316.

[2] Olsen, D. O. Bile duct injuries during laparoscopic cholecystectomy: a decade of experience. *J. Hepatobiliary Pancreat. Surg.* 2000;7(1):35-39.

[3] Giger, U., Ouaissi, M., Schmitz, S. F., Krahenbuhl, S., Krahenbuhl, L. Bile duct injury and use of cholangiography during laparoscopic cholecystectomy. *Br. J. Surg.* 2011;98(3):391-396.

[4] Gossage, J. A., Forshaw, M. J. Prevalence and outcome of litigation claims in England after laparoscopic cholecystectomy. *Int. J. Clin. Pract.* 2010;64(13):1832-1835.

[5] Kapoor, V. K. Management of bile duct injuries: a practical approach. *Am. Surg.* 2009;75(12):1157-1160.

[6] Nuzzo, G., Giuliante, F., Giovannini, I., Ardito, F., D'Acapito, F., Vellone, M., et al. Bile duct injury during laparoscopic cholecystectomy: results of an Italian national survey on 56 591 cholecystectomies. *Arch. Surg.* 2005;140(10):986-992.

[7] Schmidt, S. C., Langrehr, J. M., Hintze, R. E., Neuhaus, P. Long-term results and risk factors influencing outcome of major bile duct injuries following cholecystectomy. *Br. J. Surg.* 2005;92(1):76-82.

[8] Shamiyeh, A., Wayand, W. Laparoscopic cholecystectomy: early and late complications and their treatment. *Langenbecks Arch. Surg.* 2004;389(3):164-171.

[9] Zha, Y., Chen, X. R., Luo, D., Jin, Y. The prevention of major bile duct injures in laparoscopic cholecystectomy: the experience with 13,000 patients in a single center. *Surg. Laparosc. Endosc. Percutan. Tech.* 2010;20(6):378-383.

[10] Huang, Z. Q., Huang, X. Q. Changing patterns of traumatic bile duct injuries: a review of forty years experience. *World J. Gastroenterol.* 2002;8(1):5-12.

[11] Adamsen, S., Hansen, O. H., Funch-Jensen, P., Schulze, S., Stage, J. G., Wara, P. Bile duct injury during laparoscopic cholecystectomy: a prospective nationwide series. *J. Am. Coll. Surg.* 1997;184(6):571-578.

[12] Cohen, M. M., Young, W., Theriault, M. E., Hernandez, R. Has laparoscopic cholecystectomy changed patterns of practice and patient outcome in Ontario? *CMAJ.* 1996;154(4):491-500.

[13] Fletcher, D. R., Hobbs, M. S., Tan, P., Valinsky, L. J., Hockey, R. L., Pikora, T. J., et al. Complications of cholecystectomy: risks of the laparoscopic approach and protective effects of operative cholangiography: a population-based study. *Ann. Surg.* 1999;229(4):449-457.

[14] Flum, D. R., Cheadle, A., Prela, C., Dellinger, E. P., Chan, L. Bile duct injury during cholecystectomy and survival in medicare beneficiaries. *JAMA.* 2003;290(16):2168-2173.

[15] Flum, D. R., Dellinger, E. P., Cheadle, A., Chan, L., Koepsell, T. Intraoperative cholangiography and risk of common bile duct injury during cholecystectomy. *JAMA.* 2003;289(13):1639-1644.

[16] Richardson, M. C., Bell, G., Fullarton, G. M. Incidence and nature of bile duct injuries following laparoscopic cholecystectomy: an audit of 5913 cases. West of Scotland Laparoscopic Cholecystectomy Audit Group. *Br. J. Surg.* 1996;83(10):1356-1360.

[17] Russell, J. C., Walsh, S. J., Mattie, A. S., Lynch, J. T. Bile duct injuries, 1989-1993. A statewide experience. Connecticut Laparoscopic Cholecystectomy Registry. *Arch. Surg.* 1996;131(4):382-388.

[18] Moossa, A. R., Mayer, A. D., Stabile, B. Iatrogenic injury to the bile duct. Who, how, where? *Arch. Surg.* 1990;125(8):1028-1030; discussion 1030-1021.

[19] Savader, S. J., Lillemoe, K. D., Prescott, C. A., Winick, A. B., Venbrux, A. C., Lund, G. B., et al. Laparoscopic cholecystectomy-related bile duct injuries: a health and financial disaster. *Ann. Surg.* 1997;225(3):268-273.

[20] Boerma, D., Rauws, E. A., Keulemans, Y. C., Bergman, J. J., Obertop, H., Huibregtse, K., et al. Impaired quality of life 5 years after bile duct injury during laparoscopic cholecystectomy: a prospective analysis. *Ann. Surg.* 2001;234(6):750-757.

[21] Moore, D. E., Feurer, I. D., Holzman, M. D., Wudel, L. J., Strickland, C., Gorden, D. L., et al. Long-term detrimental effect of bile duct injury on health-related quality of life. *Arch. Surg.* 2004;139(5):476-481; discussion 481-472.

[22] Kern, K. A. Malpractice litigation involving laparoscopic cholecystectomy. Cost, cause, and consequences. *Arch. Surg.* 1997;132(4):392-397; discussion 397-398.

[23] Archer, S. B., Brown, D. W., Smith, C. D., Branum, G. D., Hunter, J. G. Bile duct injury during laparoscopic cholecystectomy: results of a national survey. *Ann. Surg.* 2001;234(4):549-558; discussion 558-549.

[24] Francoeur, J. R., Wiseman, K., Buczkowski, A. K., Chung, S. W., Scudamore, C. H. Surgeons' anonymous response after bile duct injury during cholecystectomy. *Am. J. Surg.* 2003;185(5):468-475.

[25] Hugh, T. B. New strategies to prevent laparoscopic bile duct injury--surgeons can learn from pilots. *Surgery.* 2002;132(5):826-835.

[26] Hunter, J. G. Avoidance of bile duct injury during laparoscopic cholecystectomy. *Am. J. Surg.* 1991;162(1):71-76.

[27] Strasberg, S. M. Avoidance of biliary injury during laparoscopic cholecystectomy. *J. Hepatobiliary Pancreat. Surg.* 2002;9(5):543-547.

[28] Strasberg, S. M., Hertl, M., Soper, N. J. An analysis of the problem of biliary injury during laparoscopic cholecystectomy. *J. Am. Coll. Surg.* 1995;180(1):101-125.

[29] Troidl, H. Disasters of endoscopic surgery and how to avoid them: error analysis. *World J. Surg.* 1999;23(8):846-855.

[30] Honda, G., Iwanaga, T., Kurata, M., Watanabe, F., Satoh, H., Iwasaki, K. The critical view of safety in laparoscopic cholecystectomy is optimized by exposing the inner layer of the subserosal layer. *J. Hepatobiliary Pancreat. Surg.* 2009;16(4):445-449.

[31] Singh, K., Ohri, A. Anatomic landmarks: their usefulness in safe laparoscopic cholecystectomy. *Surg. Endosc.* 2006;20(11):1754-1758.

[32] Van Eijck, F. C., van Veen, R. N., Kleinrensink, G. J., Lange, J. F. Hartmann's gallbladder pouch revisited 60 years later. *Surg. Endosc.* 2007;21(7):1122-1125.

[33] Machi, J. Laparoscopic ultrasonography: an additional method for potentially preventing biliary tract injury. *Surg. Endosc.* 2008;22(3):802-803.

[34] Lo, C. M., Fan, S. T., Liu, C. L., Lai, E. C., Wong, J. Early decision for conversion of laparoscopic to open cholecystectomy for treatment of acute cholecystitis. *Am. J. Surg.* 1997;173(6):513-517.

[35] Flum, D. R., Koepsell, T., Heagerty, P., Sinanan, M., Dellinger, E. P. Common bile duct injury during laparoscopic cholecystectomy and the use of intraoperative cholangiography: adverse outcome or preventable error? *Arch. Surg.* 2001;136(11):1287-1292.

[36] Wright, K. D., Wellwood, J. M. Bile duct injury during laparoscopic cholecystectomy without operative cholangiography. *Br. J. Surg.* 1998;85(2):191-194.

[37] Flum, D. R., Flowers, C., Veenstra, D. L. A cost-effectiveness analysis of intraoperative cholangiography in the prevention of bile duct injury during laparoscopic cholecystectomy. *J. Am. Coll. Surg.* 2003;196(3):385-393.

[38] Massarweh, N. N., Devlin, A., Symons, R. G., Broeckel Elrod, J. A., Flum, D. R. Risk tolerance and bile duct injury: surgeon characteristics, risk-taking preference, and common bile duct injuries. *J. Am. Coll. Surg.* 2009;209(1):17-24.

[39] Way, L. W., Stewart, L., Gantert, W., Liu, K., Lee, C. M., Whang, K., et al. Causes and prevention of laparoscopic bile duct injuries: analysis of 252 cases from a human factors and cognitive psychology perspective. *Ann. Surg.* 2003;237(4):460-469.

[40] Lee, C. M., Stewart, L., Way, L. W. Postcholecystectomy abdominal bile collections. *Arch. Surg.* 2000;135(5):538-542; discussion 542-534.

[41] Abdel Wahab, M., El-Ebiedy, G., Sultan, A., El-Ghawalby, N., Fathy, O., Gad El-Hak, N., et al. Postcholecystectomy bile duct injuries: experience with 49 cases managed by different therapeutic modalities. *Hepatogastroenterology*. 1996;43(11):1141-1147.

[42] De Wit, L. T., Rauws, E. A., Gouma, D. J. Surgical management of iatrogenic bile duct injury. *Scand. J. Gastroenterol. Suppl.* 1999;230(89-94.

[43] Keulemans, Y. C., Bergman, J. J., de Wit, L. T., Rauws, E. A., Huibregtse, K., Tytgat, G. N., et al. Improvement in the management of bile duct injuries? *J. Am. Coll. Surg.* 1998;187(3):246-254.

[44] Carroll, B. J., Birth, M., Phillips, E. H. Common bile duct injuries during laparoscopic cholecystectomy that result in litigation. *Surg. Endosc.* 1998;12(4):310-313; discussion 314.

[45] Diamantis, T., Tsigris, C., Kiriakopoulos, A., Papalambros, E., Bramis, J., Michail, P., et al. Bile duct injuries associated with laparoscopic and open cholecystectomy: an 11-year experience in one institute. *Surg. Today*. 2005;35(10):841-845.

[46] Strasberg, S. M., Helton, W. S. An analytical review of vasculobiliary injury in laparoscopic and open cholecystectomy. *HPB* (Oxford). 2010;13(1):1-14.

[47] Lohan, D., Walsh, S., McLoughlin, R., Murphy, J. Imaging of the complications of laparoscopic cholecystectomy. *Eur. Radiol.* 2005;15(5):904-912.

[48] Lau, W. Y., Lai, E. C., Lau, S. H. Management of bile duct injury after laparoscopic cholecystectomy: a review. *ANZ J. Surg.* 2010;80(1):75-81.

[49] Machado, N. O. Biliary complications postlaparoscopic cholecystectomy: mechanism, preventive measures, and approach to management: a review. *Diagn. Ther. Endosc.* 2011;2011(ID967017):1-9.

[50] Sandha, G. S., Bourke, M. J., Haber, G. B., Kortan, P. P. Endoscopic therapy for bile leak based on a new classification: results in 207 patients. *Gastrointest. Endosc.* 2004;60(4):567-574.

[51] Buell, J. F., Cronin, D. C., Funaki, B., Koffron, A., Yoshida, A., Lo, A., et al. Devastating and fatal complications associated with combined vascular and bile duct injuries during cholecystectomy. *Arch. Surg.* 2002;137(6):703-708; discussion 708-710.

[52] Koffron, A., Ferrario, M., Parsons, W., Nemcek, A., Saker, M., Abecassis, M. Failed primary management of iatrogenic biliary injury: incidence and significance of concomitant hepatic arterial disruption. *Surgery*. 2001;130(4):722-728; discussion 728-731.

[53] Stewart, L., Robinson, T. N., Lee, C. M., Liu, K., Whang, K., Way, L. W. Right hepatic artery injury associated with laparoscopic bile duct injury: incidence, mechanism, and consequences. *J. Gastrointest. Surg.* 2004;8(5):523-530; discussion 530-521.

[54] Johnson, S. R., Koehler, A., Pennington, L. K., Hanto, D. W. Long-term results of surgical repair of bile duct injuries following laparoscopic cholecystectomy. *Surgery*. 2000;128(4):668-677.

[55] Lau, W. Y., Lai, E. C. Classification of iatrogenic bile duct injury. Hepatobiliary *Pancreat. Dis. Int.* 2007;6(5):459-463.

[56] Bismuth, H. Postoperative strictures of the bile ducts. In: Blumgart, L. H. (ed.). *The Biliary Tract* V. New York, NY: Churchill-Livingstone, 1982; 209-18.

[57] Schmidt, S. C., Settmacher, U., Langrehr, J. M., Neuhaus, P. Management and outcome of patients with combined bile duct and hepatic arterial injuries after laparoscopic cholecystectomy. *Surgery*. 2004;135(6):613-618.

[58] Bismuth, H., Majno, P. E. Biliary strictures: classification based on the principles of surgical treatment. *World J. Surg.* 2001;25(10):1241-1244.

[59] McMahon, A. J., Fullarton, G., Baxter, J. N., O'Dwyer, P. J. Bile duct injury and bile leakage in laparoscopic cholecystectomy. *Br. J. Surg.* 1995;82(3):307-313.

[60] Tzovaras, G., Dervenis, C. Vascular injuries in laparoscopic cholecystectomy: an underestimated problem. *Dig. Surg.* 2006;23(5-6):370-374.

[61] De Reuver, P. R., Rauws, E. A., Bruno, M. J., Lameris, J. S., Busch, O. R., van Gulik, T. M., et al. Survival in bile duct injury patients after laparoscopic cholecystectomy: a multidisciplinary approach of gastroenterologists, radiologists, and surgeons. *Surgery.* 2007;142(1):1-9.

[62] Sicklick, J. K., Camp, M. S., Lillemoe, K. D., Melton, G. B., Yeo, C. J., Campbell, K. A., et al. Surgical management of bile duct injuries sustained during laparoscopic cholecystectomy: perioperative results in 200 patients. *Ann. Surg.* 2005;241(5):786-792; discussion 793-785.

[63] Stewart, L., Way, L. W. Bile duct injuries during laparoscopic cholecystectomy. Factors that influence the results of treatment. *Arch. Surg.* 1995;130(10):1123-1128; discussion 1129.

[64] Heise, M., Schmidt, S. C., Adler, A., Hintze, R. E., Langrehr, J. M., Neuhaus, P. [Management of bile duct injuries following laparoscopic cholecystectomy]. *Zentralbl. Chir.* 2003;128(11):944-951.

[65] Bottger, T., Junginger, T. Long-term results after surgical treatment of iatrogenic injury of the bile ducts. *Eur. J. Surg.* 1991;157(8):477-480.

[66] Schol, F. P., Go, P. M., Gouma, D. J. Outcome of 49 repairs of bile duct injuries after laparoscopic cholecystectomy. *World J. Surg.* 1995;19(5):753-756; discussion 756-757.

[67] Gazzaniga, G. M., Filauro, M., Mori, L. Surgical treatment of iatrogenic lesions of the proximal common bile duct. *World J. Surg.* 2001;25(10):1254-1259.

[68] Gouma, D. J., Obertop, H. Management of bile duct injuries: treatment and long-term results. *Dig. Surg.* 2002;19(2):117-122.

[69] Chaudhary, A., Chandra, A., Negi, S. S., Sachdev, A. Reoperative surgery for postcholecystectomy bile duct injuries. *Dig. Surg.* 2002;19(1):22-27.

[70] Thomson, B. N., Parks, R. W., Madhavan, K. K., Wigmore, S. J., Garden, O. J. Early specialist repair of biliary injury. *Br. J. Surg.* 2006;93(2):216-220.

[71] Connor, S., Garden, O. J. Bile duct injury in the era of laparoscopic cholecystectomy. *Br. J. Surg.* 2006;93(2):158-168.

[72] Kamiya, S., Nagino, M., Kanazawa, H., Komatsu, S., Mayumi, T., Takagi, K., et al. The value of bile replacement during external biliary drainage: an analysis of intestinal permeability, integrity, and microflora. *Ann. Surg.* 2004;239(4):510-517.

[73] Goykhman, Y., Kory, I., Small, R., Kessler, A., Klausner, J. M., Nakache, R., et al. Long-term outcome and risk factors of failure after bile duct injury repair. *J. Gastrointest. Surg.* 2008;12(8):1412-1417.

[74] Eisenstein, S., Greenstein, A. J., Kim, U., Divino, C. M. Cystic duct stump leaks: after the learning curve. *Arch. Surg.* 2008;143(12):1178-1183.

[75] Pinkas, H., Brady, P. G. Biliary leaks after laparoscopic cholecystectomy: time to stent or time to drain. Hepatobiliary Pancreat *Dis. Int.* 2008;7(6):628-632.

[76] Ryan, M. E., Geenen, J. E., Lehman, G. A., Aliperti, G., Freeman, M. L., Silverman, W. B., et al. Endoscopic intervention for biliary leaks after laparoscopic cholecystectomy: a multicenter review. *Gastrointest. Endosc.* 1998;47(3):261-266.

[77] Tzovaras, G., Peyser, P., Kow, L., Wilson, T., Padbury, R., Toouli, J. Minimally invasive management of bile leak after laparoscopic cholecystectomy. *HPB* (Oxford). 2001;3(2):165-168.

[78] Thethy, S., Thomson, B., Pleass, H., Wigmore, S. J., Madhavan, K., Akyol, M., et al. Management of biliary tract complications after orthotopic liver transplantation. *Clin. Transplant.* 2004;18(6):647-653.

[79] Llach, J., Bordas, J. M., Elizalde, J. I., Enrico, C., Gines, A., Pellise, M., et al. Sphincterotomy in the treatment of biliary leakage. *Hepatogastroenterology.* 2002;49(48):1496-1498.

[80] Alves, A., Farges, O., Nicolet, J., Watrin, T., Sauvanet, A., Belghiti, J. Incidence and consequence of an hepatic artery injury in patients with postcholecystectomy bile duct strictures. *Ann. Surg.* 2003;238(1):93-96.

[81] Bachellier, P., Nakano, H., Weber, J. C., Lemarque, P., Oussoultzoglou, E., Candau, C., et al. Surgical repair after bile duct and vascular injuries during laparoscopic cholecystectomy: when and how? *World J. Surg.* 2001;25(10):1335-1345.

[82] Gupta, N., Solomon, H., Fairchild, R., Kaminski, D. L. Management and outcome of patients with combined bile duct and hepatic artery injuries. *Arch. Surg.* 1998;133(2):176-181.

[83] Jamil, L. H., Krause, K. R., Chengelis, D. L., Jury, R. P., Jackson, C. M., Cannon, M. E., et al. Endoscopic management of early upper gastrointestinal hemorrhage following laparoscopic Roux-en-Y gastric bypass. *Am. J. Gastroenterol.* 2008;103(1):86-91.

[84] De Santibanes, E., Ardiles, V., Gadano, A., Palavecino, M., Pekolj, J., Ciardullo, M. Liver transplantation: the last measure in the treatment of bile duct injuries. *World J. Surg.* 2008;32(8):1714-1721.

[85] Laurent, A., Sauvanet, A., Farges, O., Watrin, T., Rivkine, E., Belghiti, J. Major hepatectomy for the treatment of complex bile duct injury. *Ann. Surg.* 2008;248(1): 77-83.

[86] Thomson, B. N., Parks, R. W., Madhavan, K. K., Garden, O. J. Liver resection and transplantation in the management of iatrogenic biliary injury. *World J. Surg.* 2007;31(12):2363-2369.

[87] Al-Ghnaniem, R., Benjamin, I. S. Long-term outcome of hepaticojejunostomy with routine access loop formation following iatrogenic bile duct injury. *Br. J. Surg.* 2002;89(9):1118-1124.

[88] Lillemoe, K. D., Melton, G. B., Cameron, J. L., Pitt, H. A., Campbell, K. A., Talamini, M. A., et al. Postoperative bile duct strictures: management and outcome in the 1990s. *Ann. Surg.* 2000;232(3):430-441.

[89] Mercado, M. A., Chan, C., Salgado-Nesme, N., Lopez-Rosales, F. Intrahepatic repair of bile duct injuries. A comparative study. *J. Gastrointest. Surg.* 2008;12(2):364-368.

[90] Mirza, D. F., Narsimhan, K. L., Ferraz Neto, B. H, Mayer, A. D., McMaster, P., Buckels, J. A. Bile duct injury following laparoscopic cholecystectomy: referral pattern and management. *Br. J. Surg.* 1997;84(6):786-790.

[91] Melton, G. B., Lillemoe, K. D., Cameron, J. L., Sauter, P. A., Coleman, J., Yeo, C. J. Major bile duct injuries associated with laparoscopic cholecystectomy: effect of surgical repair on quality of life. *Ann. Surg.* 2002;235(6):888-895.

[92] Sarmiento, J. M., Farnell, M. B., Nagorney, D. M., Hodge, D. O., Harrington, J. R. Quality-of-life assessment of surgical reconstruction after laparoscopic cholecystectomy-induced bile duct injuries: what happens at 5 years and beyond? *Arch. Surg.* 2004;139(5):483-488; discussion 488-489.

ISBN: 978-1-62257-890-0
© 2013 Nova Science Publishers, Inc.

Chapter V

Cholecystectomy in Patients with Suspected Choledocholithiasis: Endoscopic-Laparoscopic Management

Luis R. Rábago, Ana Olivares, Inmaculada Chico and Alejandro Ortega
Gastroenterology Department, Hospital Severo Ochoa,
Leganés, Madrid, Spain

Abstract

In the treatment of patients with symptomatic cholelithiasis and possible choledocholithiasis (CBDS) there is not an algorithm that is fully accepted. Therefore the management of these patients depends upon the availability, capability and skill of the surgical and endoscopic teams involved in the process. There is consensus to perform preoperative ERCP if the patient can be classified as a high risk for CBDS following the ASGE guideline 2010. There is also complete agreement to not perform any other diagnostic or therapeutic radiologic or endoscopic studies if the patient has a low risk of CBDS. However when the patient has an intermediate risk of CBDS, and in order to avoid risky and unnecessary procedures (such as preoperative ERCP) there are a range of therapeutic options available to use (Intraoperative ERCP, Postoperative ERCP, Laparoscopic management of CBDS) whenever an intraoperative cholangiography (IOC) shows the CBDS. Magnetic resonance cholangiopancreatography (MRC) for imaging the biliary tract and endoscopic ultrasound (EUS) are very helpful to diagnose CBDS in this setting. However not every hospital in the world has these facilities available and nor have they easy or timely access to them. It is important to know that in spite of the fact of their availability there are patients with contradictory radiological and clinical results (normal MRCP with persistently pathologic liver tests not justifiable by other reasons). In these cases we can use IOC during Laparoscopic Cholecistectomy as a definitive radiological test to determine whether or not it will be necessary to use Intraoperative or postoperative ERCP or laparoscopic management of CBDS. Postoperative ECP is a good choice with some drawbacks such as it is a two-stage treatment that in case of failure can be followed by another surgical operation. The laparoscopic management of CBDS is a single–stage treatment which needs a very good and experienced surgical team, and in order to reach this skill it requires a long learning curve. Intraoperative ERCP has the advantage of being a single-stage treatment that can be used all over the world, that has a significant success rate, an easy learning curve, low morbidity involving a shorter hospital stay and lower costs than the two-stage treatments (postoperative and preoperative ERCP). Intraoperative ERCP is also a good salvage treatment when preoperative ERCP fails or when total laparoscopic management is not successful thereby avoiding open cholecystectomies. It also has some drawbacks such as the need for good coordination between surgical and endoscopic teams and that cholecistectomy must be practically completed before the ERCP is performed.

Introduction

Biliary lithiasis is a frequent entity with a high rate of occurrence in our society of 10% - 15%, although it depends on various factors such as age [1-2], gender (more frequent in women), diet, obesity and certain illnesses. Up to 80% of cases will remain asymptomatic. However, in symptomatic patients, the estimated probability of clinical recurrence within the following two years is approximately 65%, and the annual complication rate is 1%-2% (pancreatitis, cholecystitis and obstruction of the bile duct).

Asymptomatic patients are usually diagnosed by chance during the performance of an abdominal x-ray, generally an abdominal ultrasound (US).

Abdominal pain (biliary colic) is the most frequent symptom of cholelithiasis. It is caused by the temporary obstruction of the cystic duct or the sphincter of Oddi by a calculus migrating from the gallbladder. The abdominal pain is located in the epigastrium or in the right hypochondrium, occasionally spreading to the scapular region or right shoulder. The pain usually starts suddenly and does not fluctuate. Abdominal ultrasound (US) is a fundamental diagnostic technique during acute episodes, since it enables biliary lithiasis to be detected with a sensitivity and specificity of over 95% [3]. When biliary colic is strongly suspected and the ultrasound yields negative results, other diagnostic techniques may be used such as abdominal CT scan, magnetic resonance cholangiography (MRC) or endoscopic ultrasound (EUS), which has shown sensitivity of 96% and specificity of 86% in diagnosing microlithiasis [4].

When symptomatic biliary lithiasis is diagnosed, the study must be completed to rule out the association of symptomatic choledocholithiasis (CBDS). Between 7% and 20% of cholecystectomies resulting from symptomatic biliary lithiasis present calculi in the main bile duct [5], and 2%-4% of patients on whom cholecystectomies have been performed present CBDS following the intervention [5].

Preoperative Diagnosis of CBDS

Endoscopic Retrograde Cholangiopancreatography (ERCP) was traditionally considered the benchmark diagnostic/therapeutic method in diagnosing CBDS, but its invasive nature and significant morbidity have questioned its role in diagnosing the pancreatobiliary disease, and, therefore, it has been gradually substituted by other non-invasive diagnostic techniques.

Abdominal ultrasound (US) presents low sensitivity in the diagnosis of CBDS (13%-55%) [6], but its universal availability, safety and low cost make it the number one diagnostic technique of choice. Other alternative radiological techniques show better diagnostic performance, such as helical computed tomography (CT) with a sensitivity of 80%, and magnetic resonance cholangiography (MRC) in particular, which are diagnostic alternatives with better diagnostic performance, although they are more expensive.

MRC has facilitated the non-invasive study of the bile duct with a sensitivity of 85%-92% and a specificity of 93%-97% for diagnosing CBDS [7]. Its sensitivity decreases when the calculi measure less than 6 mm and during episodes of acute pancreatitis.

Endoscopic Ultrasound (EUS) is also a very accurate diagnostic technique in the diagnosis of CBDS (sensitivity of 91%-97% and specificity of 100%) [8-9], although its minimally-invasive nature, the fact that it is operator-dependent and its variable availability continue to curtail its use, [10] although it has greater sensitivity than MRC in the detection of microlithiasis [9].

In recent decades, numerous indices have been developed to quantify the risk of presentation of CBDS in a particular patient, thereby enabling those who require a more extensive additional radiological assessment using EUS, MRC, or a therapeutic diagnostic technique such as ERCP prior to the performance of laparoscopic cholecystectomy, to be more appropriately selected. Clinical criteria (jaundice, recent history of pancreatitis, cholecystitis), analytical criteria (elevation of total bilirubin, elevation of cytolytic and cholestatic enzymes)and ultrasonographic criteria (dilated bile duct or visualisation of repletion defects in the bile duct) have been used and combined as preoperative screening methods for CBDS. In spite of the multitude of scores published attempting to assess the risk of CBDS, none have been implemented in a general manner. In fact, only 27%-54% of patients selected with suspected CBDS ultimately have calculi. [11-12].

In 2001, and more recently in 2010, the American Society for Gastrointestinal Endoscopy (ASGE) published a review of the pros and cons of each preoperative screening method used to detect CBDS [13]. It proposed a scoring system to categorise CBDS risk into high, intermediate and low and also devised a diagnostic and therapeutic algorithm for its management.

The high risk group would include patients with symptomatic cholelithiasis, total bilirubin > 4 mg/dL, ascending cholangitis, the presence of intracholedochal calculi, or those with a dilated bile duct and total bilirubin of more than 1.8 mg/dL. For patients > 55 years, alterations in liver biochemistry other than bilirubin or with a recent history of biliary pancreatitis would have intermediate risk. If they do not present with any of these criteria, the patients have low CBDS risk.

The diagnostic and therapeutic algorithm of the high-risk group will require preoperative ERCP followed by cholecystectomy (LC) due to the high prevalence of CBDS in this group, whereas the low risk group will only require laparoscopic cholecystectomy without any subsequent preoperative diagnostic tests.

The intermediate risk group will benefit from the use of MRC or EUS in order to confirm or rule out the existence of CBDS, and, therefore, allow the patient to be reclassified into the high- or low-risk group and proceed accordingly. However, despite the use of various scores to assess the risk of CBDS and of different sophisticated radiological techniques such as MRC or EUS, there is a small number of patients with important clinical/radiological discordance (e.g. persistence of abnormal liver function test with increased levels of GGT and/or GPT] and abnormal US findings [such as a dilated bile duct], with normal MRC or EUS findings. In these cases and in order to prevent preoperative ERCP from being performed, Intraoperative Cholangiography (IOC) could be of great clinical use.

For this specific group of intermediate risk patients, various therapeutic/endoscopic/surgical options are available: a) single-stage treatment (LC with laparoscopic bile duct clearance, exclusive surgical treatment, or LC with IOC and intraoperative ERCP), or b) a two-stage endoscopic/surgical treatment (preoperative ERCP followed by LC or LC with IOC and postoperative ERCP). At present, there is no unanimous consensus regarding the most appropriate therapeutic management in these cases and the decision depends mainly on each group's level of experience in the various options [14], and their degree of commitment in order to prevent preoperative ERCP from being performed when there are not enough indications to do so.

Endoscopic/Surgical Management of CBDS

For many decades, open cholecystectomy was the gold standard for the treatment of patients with CBDS and today, it is still used as the salvage treatment for a small number of patients that present complications during LC, or in others where endoscopic/surgical treatment fails to resolve CBDS.

Choledochotomy with or without transduodenal sphincteroplasty and exploration of the common bile duct, or choledochoduodenostomy have been the most widely surgical techniques used in this respect. However, their systematic use has become obsolete over the past ten years in relation to the development of LC and mainly endoscopic, but also laparoscopic treatment of the common bile duct pathology. Open cholecystectomy (OC) does not only condition aesthetic changes in relation to the presence and length of the abdominal scar and its long-term consequences, it also has significant postoperative morbidity that increases considerably when surgical techniques are added such as choledochotomy, transduodenal sphincteroplasty, exploration of the common bile duct or choledochoduodenostomy [15].

Other therapeutic strategies are currently available using endoscopic treatment: two-stage management (preoperative ERCP followed by LC), a widely used option that is not exempt from complications, including post-ERCP pancreatitis, the possibility of performing explorations unnecessarily without ultimately detecting CBDS and the possibility of cannulation failure. Alternatively, intraoperative ERCP during LC (rendez-vous) is an attractive option, which in theory lowers the risk of morbidity associated with ERCP, in particular the post-ERCP pancreatitis, and shorter hospital stay, and provides comparable success rate of bile duct clearance [16].

Preoperative ERCP Followed by LC Two-Stage Treatment

At present, preoperative ERCP followed by LC is the option that is universally accepted for patients with symptomatic cholelithiasis and CBDS evidenced by any of the aforementioned radiological techniques, or for patients that can be classified as at high risk for CBDS [13]. The exception would be patients with significant surgical risk, either due to their age or the co-existence of serious systemic diseases, which might only be treated through endoscopic bile duct clearance.

In the case of failed preoperative ERCP, other endoscopic/surgical or surgical therapeutic alternatives could be attempted (consulting more widely-experienced centres of reference, intraoperative ERCP vs laparoscopic management of CBDS, with open cholecystectomy as the ultimate salvage option).

ERCP was introduced in the 1970s as a treatment for residual or recurrent CBDS, with a success rate of over 85%-90%, immediate severe morbidity of 2.5%-11%, and mortality of 0.5%-3.7%. [17]

The biliary cannulation rate is over 95%, due to improvements in endoscopic techniques (duodenoscopes, accessories, hydrophilic guidewires and the use of precut techniques), and these are being carried out by endoscopists who have become increasingly experienced in performing a growing number of endoscopic procedures (more than 50-100 procedures each year). After selective biliary cannulation and endoscopic sphincterotomy (ES), the bile duct is cleared with the help of various basic cleaning accessories (Fogarty balloons and/or dormia baskets). The gallstones are removed in 80% of cases. Transpapillary mechanical lithotripsy and papillary or bile duct dilation using biliary dilators of various calibres (CRE by Boston Scientific) are second line resources which increase the success rates to over 90%. Lastly, electrohydraulic or laser lithotripsy with the help of choledochoscopes fragment large stones, which can then be removed endoscopically in almost every case [18].

In order to reduce ERCP morbidity, to begin with, it should not be performed if indications are doubtful (low probability of CBDS). It is therefore essential to obtain an accurate diagnosis of CBDS either preoperatively or intraoperatively, aided by IOC.

The second strategy which has shown to be effective is the temporary placement of plastic prophylactic pancreatic stents in patients at high risk for post-ERCP pancreatitis (sphincter of Oddi dysfunction, history of previous post-ERCP pancreatitis, difficult bile duct cannulation with multiple pancreatic duct injections) [19].

When CBDS of the bile duct cannot be eliminated completely, plastic biliary stents are also used to reduce the risk of post-ERCP cholangitis [20], and, accordingly, the need for urgent decompression using percutaneous approaches or surgery. The biliary stents also allow the CBDS to be finally extracted, followed by a second attempt of ERCP 8-12 weeks later due to shrinkage of the stones [20].

Under exceptional circumstances, in patients with a very high surgical risk, a limited life expectancy and complex calculi, the stents may be left in definitively for palliative reasons, although they entail an annual cholangitis risk of 10%.[21]

LC in this group of patients should be performed as early as possible, once the ES has been performed and the bile duct cleared, thereby preventing the onset of post-ERCP acute cholecystitis [22], which has reached a rate of 4-8.6% in some reports [22-23].

One disadvantage described in performing preoperative sphincterotomy followed by LC is that it has shown a greater reconversion rate to OC (open cholecystectomy) compared to LC that did not require a sphincterotomy to be performed previously [24-27]. The reasons have not been clarified. The area surrounding the gallbladder and hepatoduodenal ligament appears to become inflamed, which would hamper the performance of LC.

Laparoscopic Management of CBDS (Single-Stage Treatment)

Laparoscopic surgery of CBDS was introduced over 15 years ago [28]and various surgical groups have shown that it has a high success rate,[2, 29-33] and is just as efficient and safe as pre- or postoperative ERCP associated with LC[33] , thereby avoiding the need to perform additional procedures,. Nevertheless, its technical difficulties, its long and difficult learning curve and the need for the allocation of technical resources (high-quality fluoroscopy and choledochoscopes), which are not available at many operating theatres, has curtailed its expansion [34].

During the laparoscopic treatment of CBDS, the first surgical step involves the transcystic exploration and extraction of the common bile duct stones [35-38]. Most of the stones (66%-93%) are eliminated in this manner using wash-outs, balloons or Dormia baskets in order to extract the small stones through the cystic duct or the papilla. All of these manoeuvres have difficulty in accessing the bile duct through fine or bead-like cystic ducts, sometimes requiring dilations to be performed before the cystic duct. When transcystic extraction is not possible, a choledochotomy must be performed and the bile duct explored [33, 36, 39] using balloons or Dormia baskets or through choledochoscopes. All of these techniques are more difficult and dangerous if the bile duct is narrow or if it is affected by inflammatory changes. When exploration of the bile duct has been completed, if a primary suture is not performed —which always poses a risk— drains (a Kher tube) are placed which will prolong the patient's hospital stay. On the whole, the laparoscopic extraction of CBDS has a success rate of 83%-89%, with greater efficiency and lower morbidity for transcystic exploration and extraction of common bile duct stones (68% and 10%, respectively, compared to 31% efficiency with morbidity of 5%-18% for laparoscopic common bile duct exploration) [35, 40]. When its efficiency and costs were compared to the two-stage treatment with preoperative ERCP during a multicentric clinical trial, bile duct cleaning and morbidity had similar success rates, but involved a shorter hospital stay [40]

The difficulties regarding the laparoscopic management of CBDS have been shown in certain algorithms proposed, which show intraoperative or postoperative ERCP as a salvage treatment in the event of failure of the transcystic duct or laparoscopic choledochotomy, [41-42] encouraging joint endoscopic-laparoscopic treatment of CBDS, with which clinical trials have also been performed comparing their results.

The current use of these therapeutic options depends, to a great extent, on the technical skills and experience of the endoscopic and surgical teams [14], which must reach a clearly established and accepted consensus [2, 43].

Postoperative ERCP As a Two-Stage Treatment for CBDS

Postoperative ERCP is an important cost-efficient therapeutic alternative [44], which would be indicated to treat CBDS diagnosed intraoperatively, irrespective of the reason for performing IOC and provided that laparoscopic treatment is unavailable or has failed [30, 35, 39, 41, 43]. One of the pros of postoperative ERCP is that it is available at all equipped hospital centres using the findings from IOC (with high specificity) to establish its indication. However, it also has disadvantages. It requires highly experienced endoscopic support groups with a low ERCP failure rate and the hospital stays arc longer than for single-stage treatments [1, 30, 45]. The possibility that postoperative endoscopic failure could require further surgery should always be taken into account.

Accordingly, the specific circumstances of each hospital centre determine whether or not there is a reluctance to implement the aforementioned technique in clinical practice, although certain studies are available that propose a hopeful wait and see attitude, especially with stones measuring less than 5-6 mm [12, 46-47].

It was also indicated that the possible failure of postoperative ERCP could be avoided by leaving a transcystic catheter in place during surgery or by placing removable biliary stents. However, removing them could lead to an increase in the rate of biliary fistula or biliperitoneum [48].

Intraoperative ERCP As a Single-Stage Treatment for CBDS

There are four main indications for intraoperative ERCP:

a) Patients in which CBDS is highly suspected, with calculi measuring less than 1.5 cm and failed preoperative ERCP
b) Patients at intermediate risk for CBDS in which the MRC/EUS findings and the clinical/analytical data differ
c) CBDS discovered by chance during surgery or if the bile duct clearance using laparoscopic means is unsuccessful
d) patients evidencing CBDS and at high risk for post-ERCP pancreatitis .

A short and successful series of intraoperative ERCP during LC was published in 1993, describing the insertion of a Fogarty balloon catheter into the transcystic duct in order to direct and correctly perform endoscopic papillotomy [49] and a further series of intraoperative ERCP during OC [50]. A transcystic guidewire is inserted laparoscopically and recovered in the duodenum using the endoscope, facilitating selective access to the bile duct and the subsequent sphincterotomy [51-55] (Rendez-vous).

At the beginning Intraoperative ERCP was performed in the theatre immediately after surgery while the patient is still under anaesthesia in order to try to shorten the hospital stay, thereby allowing the endoscopic/surgical treatment to be performed in a single stage. Three different types of catheters or Fogarty balloons [49] or even Dormia basket catheters were initially used which were inserted into the transcystic duct to facilitate insertion of the papillotome in the papilla [56]. However, most endoscopic groups have used and still use a transcystic guidewire. The use of intraoperative ERCP has slowly increased among various endoscopic groups, combining its ease of use with a short learning curve, without the high technical requirements needed by laparoscopic management of the bile duct [22, 57-60].

Very few comparative studies have been made between laparoscopic management with or without intraoperative ERCP [22, 61-64] single-stage treatments, and the two-stage treatment with preoperative ERCP. In fact, five randomised clinical trials have compared preoperative ERCP to intraoperative ERCP, showing that intraoperative ERCP has similar success rates, but has lower morbidity (less post-ERCP pancreatitis), a shorter hospital stay and a lower cost [16, 62] . No differences were observed with regard to conversion to open surgery in either group [16].

Technique

In the rendezvous technique, firstly, a transcystic guidewire (0.025-inch Jagwire; Boston Scientific Inc., Watertown, Massachusetts, USA) is inserted through the cholangiography catheter. Once it emerges from the papilla it should be grasped with a standard snare. It is then withdrawn through the endoscope placed opposite the papilla. A double-lumen sphincterotome is then advanced over the guidewire to facilitate bile duct cannulation and to perform the sphincterotomy, followed by bile duct clearance using a Fogarty balloon or a Dormia basket catheter. Once the sphincterotome is placed inside the papilla reaching the bile duct, the guidewire must be completely retrieved from the cytic duct, pulling it back, in order to avoid the sphincterotome could be wrongly placed in the cystic duct . Then the guidewire must be relocated in the bile duct, with the aid of X-Ray Control in the Operating Theatre, in order to achieve a safety clearance of the bile duct and to avoid liver damage (lacerations of the liver capsule) due to a forceful and uncontrolled insertion of the guidewire.

Finally, the cystic duct is closed and the surgeon proceeds with LC. If the guidewire does not come out through the papilla, the surgeon should try to advance a stiffer Fogarty catheter through the papilla and then a pre-cut sphincterotomy can be performed [22]. If all of these steps fail, intraoperative ERCP must be considered to have failed and postoperative ERCP could be performed using the best technical support available in the Radiology Department or a decision might be made to proceed with OC.

There is another laparoscopic technique to treat CBDS intraoperatively using antegrade sphincterotomy, as described by DePaula et al [65]. The sphincterotome is inserted in an antegrade manner through the cystic duct during the laparoscopy and over the guidewire inserted previously up as far as the papilla and the sphincterotomy is performed using the endoscope. It did not have a significant impact and has also been used by other authors [66] in the management of multiple CBDS.

The Pros and Cons of Intraoperative ERCP

Pros

The main advantage of intraoperative ERCP using the rendezvous technique is the selective cannulation of the bile duct, preventing Wirsung opacification using contrast agents, damage and manipulation of the papilla and the use of risky techniques to access the papilla, such as precut sphincterotomies [58]. This technique results in a lower rate of pancreatitis compared to preoperative ERCP, and of post ERCP acute cholecystitis if the cholecystectomy is delayed [22]. The hospital stay and costs of the process were lower compared to the most used two-stage sequential treatment (preoperative ERCP and laparoscopic surgery) [16, 22, 61-62].

Intraoperative ERCP can be an alternative to the laparoscopic management of CBDS [43, 53, 56], as a salvage treatment during surgery when the bile duct is not adequately cleaned or as an alternative to endoscopic-laparoscopic management in two stages, both with preoperative or postoperative ERCP [41, 57, 67]. Its main advantage is that it is a single-stage treatment and there is no risk of reintervention in the event of intraoperative ERCP failure. It also offers the possibility of salvage for failed preoperative ERCP [64] , attempting to avoid open surgery.

Cons

The main problem is the need to coordinate and synchronise the surgical and endoscopic teams, which must work together. This has caused the most difficulty in generalising its use and this opinion is shared by various authors [59].

Other important concern described was the bowel distention induced by endoscopic insufflation and the possible increase difficulty of the cholecystectomy. However this difficulty has not be found in the different published RC Trials. In order to overcome this possible setback the surgical team has to try to dissect the Calot triangle and the attachment between liver and gallbladder or even almost remove the gallbladder from the liver bed before the endoscopic treatment [61, 68].

Once the endoscopic bile duct cleaning has concluded, the air is endoscopically aspirated with a complete restoration of the surgical field allowing the surgical procedure can be easily concluded.

The endoscopic team must be familiar beforehand with the patient´s surgery programme and be ready to go into theatre once CBDS has been confirmed by IOC. While the endoscopic team is getting ready for theatre, the surgeon passes the guidewire into the duodenum through the IOC catheter. Afterwards, the duodenoscope is introduced in order to grasp the wire. It is important to reduce waiting time as much as possible.

Once the papillotomy has been performed and if the bile duct has not been cleaned completely, a second postoperative ERCP, in the usual radiological environment, is technically easy without the risks associated with the first ERCP.

It is important for the surgical and endoscopic team to agree on the therapeutic options to follow if the rendezvous technique fails. If the guidewire does not emerge through the papilla, an attempt should be made to insert a Fogarty balloon into the transcystic duct, which must always be stiffer than the guidewire, which can prevent it from moving in a retrograde fashion towards the intrahepatic biliary tree. Once the Fogarty balloon emerges from the papilla, a pre-cut papillotomy can be performed using a needle-knife sphincterotome, controlled with the help of the Fogarty balloon catheter. If both manoeuvres fail, the therapeutic options available would be as follows: perform ERCP using a standard technique in surgery immediately after the cholecystectomy has been completed [2, 67, 69-70], postpone the ERCP to the postoperative stage depending on the patient´s evolution or convert the LC to open surgery. The option to take will vary depending on the anatomical characteristics (intradiverticular papilla) and the difficulties envisaged in the standard ERCP of that patient, the quality of the surgical equipment available in theatre and the size of the CBDS.

Special mention should be made of intraoperative ERCP treatment for patients with common bile duct stones measuring more than 15-20 mm detected intraoperatively, or when multiple stones are found. In these cases, although intraoperative ERCP may not be as definitive and conclusive as when it is performed in our usual radiological environment, at the same time, it can prolong the length of surgery unnecessarily. However, it allows and guarantees that intraoperative papillotomy can be performed with lower morbidity than conventional ERCP, helping in particular if the bile duct has not been fully cleaned, during a second stage with postoperative ERCP, with or without dilation of the papilla or with the use of mechanical lithotripsy systems.

Conclusion

During the preoperative study of cholelithiasis pending surgery, it is clear that the risk of associated CBDS must be assessed. There is a consensus to perform preoperative ERCP if the patient can be classified as high risk for CBDS following the 2010 ASGE guidelines. There is also complete agreement not to perform any other diagnostic or therapeutic radiological or endoscopic studies if the patient has a low risk of CBDS. The ASGE suggests that the preoperative study should be completed using MRC or EUS in patients with intermediate risk or in an intraoperative manner using intraoperative ultrasound or IOC11. However, not every hospital in the world is equipped with these facilities nor have they easy or timely access to them. Nevertheless, we will still find patients in whom clinical/analytical/radiological discordance makes it advisable to perform a new radiological study, such as IOC, to establish the most appropriate surgical treatment, or patients in which CBDS appears as a casual finding in IOC. The three possible therapeutic options for these intermediate risk patients are the single-stage treatment, total laparoscopic treatment with intraoperative ERCP or the two-stage treatment with postoperative ERCP. The three types of treatment are correct and their choice will depend on the particular circumstances and on the experience of the different endoscopic and surgical teams at each centre. However, randomised clinical trials have compared preoperative ERCP and intraoperative ERCP (rendez-vous) showing that intraoperative ERCP has similar success rates, but has lower morbidity (post-ERCP pancreatitis), a shorter hospital stay [16, 62] and lower costs [22]. Moreover, intraoperative ERCP has an easy learning curve.

Postoperative ERCP is a good choice which has the same drawbacks as preoperative ERCP (ERCP complications). Also, in the event of ERCP failure, further surgical intervention might be needed. The laparoscopic management of CBDS is a single–stage treatment needs a highly-skilled and experienced surgical team, and in order to acquire this expertise a long learning curve is required.

Intraoperative ERCP could also be a perfect salvage treatment for failed preoperative ERCP [64] in the event of failure of total laparoscopic management, in order to avoid open surgery. It maintains a high success rate with very low morbidity and mortality. It also has some drawbacks such as the need for good coordination between surgical and endoscopic teams and cholecystectomy should be virtually completed before the ERCP is performed.

Therefore, in coming years, we may witness an increase in the use of intraoperative ERCP, not to compete with the indications of preoperative ERCP in general, but rather to prevent the improper use of preoperative ERCP in patients at intermediate risk for CBDS, and to provide a diagnostic and therapeutic alternative to sophisticated techniques that are not always available in all societies and countries throughout the world.

References

[1] Martin, D.J., D.R. Vernon, and J. Toouli, Surgical versus endoscopic treatment of bile duct stones. *Cochrane Database Syst Rev*, 2006(2): p. CD003327.

[2] Memon, M.A., H. Hassaballa, and M.I. Memon, Laparoscopic common bile duct exploration: the past, the present, and the future. *Am J Surg*, 2000. 179(4): p. 309-15.

[3] Prat, F., et al., Early EUS of the bile duct before endoscopic sphincterotomy for acute biliary pancreatitis. *Gastrointest Endosc*, 2001. 54(6): p. 724-9.

[4] Palazzo, L., et al., Value of endoscopic ultrasonography in the diagnosis of common bile duct stones: comparison with surgical exploration and ERCP. *Gastrointest Endosc*, 1995. 42(3): p. 225-31.

[5] Bosch, F., et al., Laparoscopic or open conventional cholecystectomy: clinical and economic considerations. *Eur J Surg*, 2002. 168(5): p. 270-7.

[6] Cronan, J.J., US diagnosis of choledocholithiasis: a reappraisal. *Radiology*, 1986. 161(1): p. 133-4.

[7] Verma, D., et al., EUS vs MRCP for detection of choledocholithiasis. *Gastrointest Endosc*, 2006. 64(2): p. 248-54.

[8] Tse, F., et al., EUS: a meta-analysis of test performance in suspected choledocholithiasis. *Gastrointest Endosc*, 2008. 67(2): p. 235-44.

[9] Garrow, D., et al., Endoscopic ultrasound: a meta-analysis of test performance in suspected biliary obstruction. *Clin Gastroenterol Hepatol*, 2007. 5(5): p. 616-23.

[10] Srinivasa, S., et al., Selective use of magnetic resonance cholangiopancreatography in clinical practice may miss choledocholithiasis in gallstone pancreatitis. *Can J Surg*, 2010. 53(6): p. 403-7.

[11] Tham, T.C., et al., Role of endoscopic retrograde cholangiopancreatography for suspected choledocholithiasis in patients undergoing laparoscopic cholecystectomy. *Gastrointest Endosc*, 1998. 47(1): p. 50-6.

[12] Graham, S.M., et al., Laparoscopic cholecystectomy and common bile duct stones. The utility of planned perioperative endoscopic retrograde cholangiography and sphincterotomy: experience with 63 patients. *Ann Surg*, 1993. 218(1): p. 61-7.

[13] Maple, J.T., et al., The role of endoscopy in the evaluation of suspected choledocholithiasis. *Gastrointest Endosc*, 2010. 71(1): p. 1-9.

[14] Clayton, E.S., et al., Meta-analysis of endoscopy and surgery versus surgery alone for common bile duct stones with the gallbladder in situ. *Br J Surg*, 2006. 93(10): p. 1185-91.

[15] Girard, R.M. and M. Morin, Open cholecystectomy: its morbidity and mortality as a reference standard. *Can J Surg*, 1993. 36(1): p. 75-80.

[16] Gurusamy, K., et al., Systematic review and meta-analysis of intraoperative versus preoperative endoscopic sphincterotomy in patients with gallbladder and suspected common bile duct stones. *Br J Surg*, 2011. 98(7): p. 908-16.

[17] Freeman, M.L., et al., Complications of endoscopic biliary sphincterotomy. *N Engl J Med,* 1996. 335(13): p. 909-18.

[18] Sackmann, M., et al., Extracorporeal shock wave lithotripsy for clearance of bile duct stones resistant to endoscopic extraction. *Gastrointest Endosc,* 2001. 53(1): p. 27-32.

[19] Choudhary, A., et al., Pancreatic stents for prophylaxis against post-ERCP pancreatitis: a meta-analysis and systematic review. *Gastrointest Endosc,* 2011. 73(2): p. 275-82.

[20] Williams, E.J., et al., Guidelines on the management of common bile duct stones (CBDS). *Gut,* 2008. 57(7): p. 1004-21.

[21] Carr-Locke, D.L., Therapeutic role of ERCP in the management of suspected common bile duct stones. *Gastrointest Endosc,* 2002. 56(6 Suppl): p. S170-4.

[22] Rabago, L.R., et al., Two-stage treatment with preoperative endoscopic retrograde cholangiopancreatography (ERCP) compared with single-stage treatment with intraoperative ERCP for patients with symptomatic cholelithiasis with possible choledocholithiasis. *Endoscopy,* 2006. 38(8): p. 779-86.

[23] Siegel, J.H., et al., Duodenoscopic sphincterotomy in patients with gallbladders in situ: report of a series of 1272 patients. *Am J Gastroenterol,* 1988. 83(11): p. 1255-8.

[24] Hendolin, H.I., et al., Laparoscopic or open cholecystectomy: a prospective randomised trial to compare postoperative pain, pulmonary function, and stress response. *Eur J Surg,* 2000. 166(5): p. 394-9.

[25] Sarli, L., D.R. Iusco, and L. Roncoroni, Preoperative endoscopic sphincterotomy and laparoscopic cholecystectomy for the management of cholecystocholedocholithiasis: 10-year experience. *World J Surg,* 2003. 27(2): p. 180-6.

[26] Poon, R.T., et al., Management of gallstone cholangitis in the era of laparoscopic cholecystectomy. *Arch Surg,* 2001. 136(1): p. 11-6.

[27] Ishizaki, Y., et al., Conversion of elective laparoscopic to open cholecystectomy between 1993 and 2004. Br J Surg, 2006. 93(8): p. 987-91.

[28] Bagnato, J., Laparoscopic common bile duct exploration. *J Miss State Med Assoc,* 1990. 31(11): p. 361-2.

[29] Lezoche, E., et al., Laparoscopic treatment of gallbladder and common bile duct stones: a prospective study. *World J Surg,* 1996. 20(5): p. 535-41; discussion 542.

[30] Rhodes, M., et al., Randomised trial of laparoscopic exploration of common bile duct versus postoperative endoscopic retrograde cholangiography for common bile duct stones. *Lancet,* 1998. 351(9097): p. 159-61.

[31] Millat, B., et al., Prospective evaluation in 121 consecutive unselected patients undergoing laparoscopic treatment of choledocholithiasis. *Br J Surg,* 1995. 82(9): p. 1266-9.

[32] Chander, J., et al., Laparoscopic management of CBD stones: an Indian experience. *Surg Endosc,* 2011. 25(1): p. 172-81.

[33] Tinoco, R., et al., Laparoscopic common bile duct exploration. *Ann Surg,* 2008. 247(4): p. 674-9.

[34] Bingener, J. and W.H. Schwesinger, Management of common bile duct stones in a rural area of the United States: results of a survey. *Surg Endosc,* 2006. 20(4): p. 577-9.

[35] Millat, B., F. Borie, and G. Decker, Treatment of choledocholithiasis: therapeutic ERCP versus peroperative extraction during laparoscopic cholecystectomy. *Acta Gastroenterol Belg,* 2000. 63(3): p. 301-3.

[36]   Ponsky, J.L., B.T. Heniford, and K. Gersin, Choledocholithiasis: evolving intraoperative strategies. *Am Surg*, 2000. 66(3): p. 262-8.

[37]   Sgourakis, G. and K. Karaliotas, Laparoscopic common bile duct exploration and cholecystectomy versus endoscopic stone extraction and laparoscopic cholecystectomy for choledocholithiasis. A prospective randomized study. *Minerva Chir*, 2002. 57(4): p. 467-74.

[38]   Tokumura, H., et al., Laparoscopic management of common bile duct stones: transcystic approach and choledochotomy. *J Hepatobiliary Pancreat Surg*, 2002. 9(2): p. 206-12.

[39]   Nathanson, L.K., et al., Postoperative ERCP versus laparoscopic choledochotomy for clearance of selected bile duct calculi: a randomized trial. *Ann Surg*, 2005. 242(2): p. 188-92.

[40]   Cuschieri, A., et al., E.A.E.S. multicenter prospective randomized trial comparing two-stage vs single-stage management of patients with gallstone disease and ductal calculi. *Surg Endosc*, 1999. 13(10): p. 952-7.

[41]   Phillips, E.H., et al., Laparoscopic trans-cystic-duct common-bile-duct exploration. Surg Endosc, 1994. 8(12): p. 1389-93; discussion 1393-4.

[42]   Berci, G., Laparoscopic management of common bile duct stones. *Surg Endosc*, 1994. 8(12): p. 1452-3.

[43]   Lilly, M.C. and M.E. Arregui, A balanced approach to choledocholithiasis. *Surg Endosc*, 2001. 15(5): p. 467-72.

[44]   Waye, J.D., et al., Endoscopic sphincterotomy: 2002. Gastrointest Endosc, 2002. 55(1): p. 139-40.

[45]   Schroeppel, T.J., et al., An economic analysis of hospital charges for choledocholithiasis by different treatment strategies. *Am Surg*, 2007. 73(5): p. 472-7.

[46]   Collins, C., et al., A prospective study of common bile duct calculi in patients undergoing laparoscopic cholecystectomy: natural history of choledocholithiasis revisited. *Ann Surg*, 2004. 239(1): p. 28-33.

[47]   Kondylis, P.D., et al., Abnormal intraoperative cholangiography. Treatment options and long-term follow-up. *Arch Surg*, 1997. 132(4): p. 347-50.

[48]   Arregui, M.E., et al., Laparoscopic cholecystectomy combined with endoscopic sphincterotomy and stone extraction or laparoscopic choledochoscopy and electrohydraulic lithotripsy for management of cholelithiasis with choledocholithiasis. *Surg Endosc*, 1992. 6(1): p. 10-5.

[49]   Deslandres, E., et al., Intraoperative endoscopic sphincterotomy for common bile duct stones during laparoscopic cholecystectomy. *Gastrointest Endosc*, 1993. 39(1): p. 54-8.

[50]   Mayrhofer, T., R. Schmiederer, and P. Razek, Intraoperative endoscopic papillotomy and stone removal. *Endosc Surg Allied Technol*, 1993. 1(3): p. 144-9.

[51]   Cavina, E., et al., Laparo-endoscopic "rendezvous": a new technique in the choledocholithiasis treatment. *Hepatogastroenterology*, 1998. 45(23): p. 1430-5.

[52]   Basso, N., et al., Laparoscopic cholecystectomy and intraoperative endoscopic sphincterotomy in the treatment of cholecysto-choledocholithiasis. *Gastrointest Endosc*, 1999. 50(4): p. 532-5.

[53]   Tricarico, A., et al., Digestive hemorrhages of obscure origin. *Surg Endosc*, 2002. 16(4): p. 711-3.

[54] Nakajima, H., et al., Intraoperative endoscopic sphincterotomy during laparoscopic cholecystectomy. *Endoscopy*, 1996. 28(2): p. 264.

[55] Miscusi, G., et al., [Endolaparoscopic "Rendez-vous" in the treatment of cholecysto-choledochal calculosis]. *G Chir*, 1997. 18(10): p. 655-7.

[56] Montori, A., et al., Endoscopic and surgical integration in the approach to biliary tract disease. *J Clin Gastroenterol*, 1999. 28(3): p. 198-201.

[57] Wright, B.E., et al., Current management of common bile duct stones: is there a role for laparoscopic cholecystectomy and intraoperative endoscopic retrograde cholangiopancreatography as a single-stage procedure? *Surgery*, 2002. 132(4): p. 729-35; discussion 735-7.

[58] La Greca, G., et al., Laparo-endoscopic "Rendezvous" to treat cholecysto-choledocolithiasis: Effective, safe and simplifies the endoscopist's work. *World J Gastroenterol*, 2008. 14(18): p. 2844-50.

[59] La Greca, G., et al., Simultaneous laparoendoscopic rendezvous for the treatment of cholecystocholedocholithiasis. *Surg Endosc*, 2009.

[60] Ghazal, A.H., et al., Single-step treatment of gall bladder and bile duct stones: a combined endoscopic-laparoscopic technique. *Int J Surg*, 2009. 7(4): p. 338-46.

[61] Morino, M., et al., Preoperative endoscopic sphincterotomy versus laparoendoscopic rendezvous in patients with gallbladder and bile duct stones. *Ann Surg*, 2006. 244(6): p. 889-93; discussion 893-6.

[62] ElGeidie, A.A., G.K. ElEbidy, and Y.M. Naeem, Preoperative versus intraoperative endoscopic sphincterotomy for management of common bile duct stones. *Surg Endosc*, 2011. 25(4): p. 1230-7.

[63] Lella, F., et al., Use of the laparoscopic-endoscopic approach, the so-called "rendezvous" technique, in cholecystocholedocholithiasis: a valid method in cases with patient-related risk factors for post-ERCP pancreatitis. *Surg Endosc*, 2006. 20(3): p. 419-23.

[64] Tzovaras, G., et al., Laparoendoscopic rendezvous versus preoperative ERCP and laparoscopic cholecystectomy for the management of cholecysto-choledocholithiasis: interim analysis of a controlled randomized trial. *Ann Surg*, 2012. 255(3): p. 435-9.

[65] DePaula, A.L., et al., Laparoscopic antegrade sphincterotomy. *Surg Laparosc Endosc*, 1993. 3(3): p. 157-60.

[66] Curet, M.J., et al., Laparoscopic antegrade sphincterotomy. A new technique for the management of complex choledocholithiasis. *Ann Surg*, 1995. 221(2): p. 149-55.

[67] Cemachovic, I., et al., Intraoperative endoscopic sphincterotomy is a reasonable option for complete single-stage minimally invasive biliary stones treatment: short-term experience with 57 patients. *Endoscopy*, 2000. 32(12): p. 956-62.

[68] Berggren, U., et al., Laparoscopic versus open cholecystectomy: hospitalization, sick leave, analgesia and trauma responses. *Br J Surg*, 1994. 81(9): p. 1362-5.

[69] Siddiqui, M.N., et al., Per-operative endoscopic retrograde cholangio-pancreatography for common bile duct stones. *Gastrointest Endosc*, 1994. 40(3): p. 348-50.

[70] Cox, M.R., T.G. Wilson, and J. Toouli, Peroperative endoscopic sphincterotomy during laparoscopic cholecystectomy for choledocholithiasis. *Br J Surg*, 1995. 82(2): p. 257-9.

In: Cholecystectomies
Editors: Miyu Akiyama and Satomi Kunomasu

ISBN: 978-1-62257-890-0
© 2013 Nova Science Publishers, Inc.

Chapter VI

Difficult Cholecystectomies: Procedures, Prognosis and Potential Complications

*Edwin O. Onkendi and Juliane Bingener**
Department of Surgery, Mayo Clinic,
Rochester, MN, US

Abstract

Background: Complications from gallstone disease continue to cause patient morbidity and mortality, although less frequently now. Complications of gallstone disease are more likely to result in difficult cholecystectomies. A difficult cholecystectomy refers to a case in which exposure of the critical anatomy necessary to conduct a safe procedure is challenging as a result of acute inflammation, dense scarring, gallstone impaction, bleeding, liver pathology or hepatobiliary anatomy. These difficult laparoscopic cholecystectomies demand advanced strategies to ensure safe operative approaches.

Aim: To review the evidence-based advanced operative procedures for difficult laparoscopic cholecystectomies, and outcomes of these approaches for difficult gall bladder problems.

Methods: A review of literature databases of PubMed, MEDLINE, EMBASE, and SCOPUS was performed. Advanced operative approaches for difficult laparoscopic cholecystectomy and their outcomes in patients with gangrenous cholecystitis, inflamed mega-gall bladder, perforated gall bladder, a short or large cystic duct, Mirizzi syndrome and cholecystectomy in liver cirrhosis and portal hypertension are reviewed. Factors influencing the decision to convert to open cholecystectomy are discussed.

Results: From a review of 100 studies including 2 meta-analyses, 12 randomized controlled trials (RCTs), and 86 prospective and retrospective studies, several different operative approaches for a difficult cholecystectomy were identified. They include fundus-first/dome down approach, ultrasonic dissection with or without fundus first or

---

* Corresponding Author: Juliane Bingener, M.D. Department of Surgery, 200 First Street SW, Rochester, MN 55905, Ph (507) 293-0767, Fax (507) 284-5196, Email: Bingenercasey.juliane@mayo.edu

half-dome approach and subtotal/partial cholecystectomy. Another approach, the half dome down approach, is also discussed. From the existing literature, the fundus-first approach, ultrasonic dissection and subtotal cholecystectomy have been found to reduce the rate of conversion of a laparoscopic to open cholecystectomy with no associated increase in the risk of injury to the liver, duodenum, colon or the biliary tree. They have been found to lower the complication rates.

Ultrasonic dissection has been demonstrated to be safe and very valuable for bloodless dissection especially in acute cholecystitis, but a learning curve exists. There is also a risk of thermal injury from instrument misuse. With these techniques, outcomes similar to standard retrograde cholecystectomy for uncomplicated and acute cholecystitis can be reached.

Conclusion: Advanced operative approaches for difficult laparoscopic cholecystectomy should be considered prior to converting to open cholecystectomy. In situation where it is still difficult to perform a safe laparoscopic cholecystectomy or the surgeon is inexperienced, conversion to open cholecystectomy should be considered or the patient referred to an experienced center.

Introduction

Symptomatic gallstone disease leads to more than 500,000 cholecystectomies per year in the United States. Since the early 1990s, laparoscopic cholecystectomy has been considered the standard treatment for gallbladder pathology.

This procedure can often be accomplished with little difficulty in experienced hands, thus the American Board of Surgery currently considers laparoscopic cholecystectomy a basic laparoscopy procedure. In the United States, patients expect to undergo an outpatient surgical procedure with the entire stay not lasting much longer than 6 to 8 hours. However, some patients experience a different course than expected, sometimes due to other medical conditions, sometimes due to complicated gallbladder disease. In this chapter, we review these difficult gallbladder scenarios.

We examine how a change from the routine may be predicted and what alternative approaches are available to deal with the difficult scenarios.

Preoperative Considerations

Difficult situations may present if the patient has pre-existing disease such as heart and lung conditions, liver cirrhosis, super morbid obesity, or multiple previous surgical procedures.

These conditions render the perioperative anesthesia more challenging and limit some technical aspects of the planned procedure. Technical aspects are also involved for patients with a severely inflamed or even gangrenous gallbladder, a perforated gallbladder or situations where gallstones have migrated into adjacent ducts or organs.

It would be advantageous for the patient and the surgical team to know in advance if a change in course is to be expected.

How to Predict Difficulties Due to Pre-Existing Disease

The tools available to assess the risk of a "difficult gallbladder" are a detailed history and physical examination, preoperative laboratory and imaging studies. Factors that have been correlated with a "difficult cholecystectomy" are repeat or prolonged attacks of acute cholecystitis or prior severe pancreatitis, both leading to inflammation and swelling. Multiple previous upper abdominal operations and a very large body habitus may result in dense adhesions or distorted anatomy surrounding the liver and gallbladder. Male patients and patient of advanced age often present with longstanding undiagnosed disease in advanced stages of inflammation. However, it is not always easy to predict this. Presence of ultrasound features of acute cholecystitis (gallbladder wall thickening of >4 mm and pericholecystic fluid), or contracted gallbladder may indicate significant acute inflammation or scarring, respectively, which may make dissection difficult. Below we briefly review the "routine scenario" and then examine different predictive factors and possible adjustment strategies.

Routine Laparoscopic Cholecystectomy

After anesthesia induction, the patient is prepared and trocars are placed. Pneumoperitoneum is established to provide operative space. Adhesions around the gallbladder and hepatocystic triangle are removed to provide unobstructed view of the gallbladder. The gallbladder is then lifted up over the liver to expose the neck of the gallbladder (Hartman's pouch). Beginning with dissection at the lateral aspect of the gallbladder with opening of the peritoneum has the least chance of encountering aberrant anatomy. Subsequently, the medial peritoneum can be opened and stripped back to expose Calot's triangle. Calot's triangle dissection starts by caudad and lateral retraction of the Hartmann pouch, a strategy helpful to avoid common bile duct injuries. Blunt dissection around the cystic artery and duct will usually lead to the critical view of safety. The critical view of safety consists of three requirements: Calot's triangle must be cleared of connective tissue, the caudal part of the gallbladder and its infundibulum must be separated from the cystic plate and only 2 structures should be entering the gallbladder. The surgeon should be able to see the liver surface behind these 2 structures [1] (Figure 1). Once the critical view is obtained, the cystic artery and duct are clipped and divided and the gallbladder dissected off the liver.

Helpful Anatomic Landmark: Rouviere Sulcus/Fissure of Gans

The fissure of Ganz also known as the sulcus of Rouviere is a 2-5 cm sulcus consistently located to the right of the hepatic hilum and anterior to the caudate lobe (Figures 1 and 2). It is found in approximately 70-80% of livers and is a helpful landmark to locate the right posterior sectoral pedicle [2, 3]

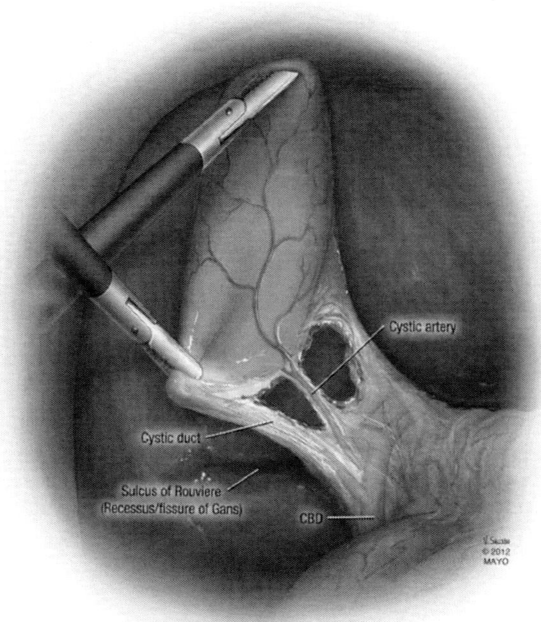

Figure 1. Critical view of safety obtained. The Calot's triangle has been cleared of fat, adhesions and fibrous tissue and 2 structures are seen entering the gall bladder. The liver surface can be seen behind these 2 structures. By permission of Mayo Foundation for Medical Education and Research. All rights reserved.

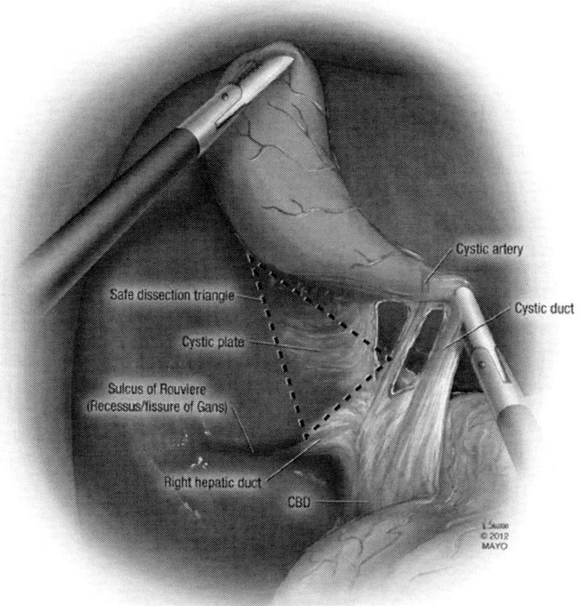

Figure 2. Exposed Rouviere's sulcus with the triangle of safety on the lateral aspect of the gallbladder. Beginning dissection here with opening of the peritoneum has the least chance of encountering aberrant anatomy. By permission of Mayo Foundation for Medical Education and Research. All rights reserved.

It typically contains the right portal triad or its branches. In difficult cholecystectomy cases due to edema, scarring and adhesions where delineation of the gallbladder-cystic duct junction is difficult, the fissure of Gans reliably indicates the plane of the common bile duct. Dissection posterior to this plane should be avoided.

Dissection of the peritoneum immediately ventral to a line through the sulcus and within the triangle bounded by liver surface, gallbladder neck and the plane of the sulcus decreases the chance of encountering aberrant anatomy [3]. Anterior dissection is then performed using the posterior landmarks, eventually connecting the two areas of dissection.

Prediction and Intraoperative Classification of Difficult Cholecystectomy

In more than half of the cases of difficult laparoscopic cholecystectomies that require conversion to laparotomy, the reason for conversion is difficult dissection or inability to identify the anatomy [4].

Table 1. Predictive factors of laparoscopic cholecystectomy surgery risk and possibility of conversion

History and physical exam	Prior upper abdominal surgery
	Repeated or prolonged attacks of acute cholecystitis or pancreatitis
	RUQ focal peritonitis
	Male gender
	History of advanced liver cirrhosis
Ultrasound features	Gallbladder wall thickness >4-5 mm
	Pericholecystic fluid
	Shrunken/contracted gallbladder
Laboratory findings	Leukocytosis > 10×10^9/L

The remaining cases are due to the need for open common bile duct exploration, an intraoperative complication, unsuspected findings, misdiagnosis, or bleeding [4, 5]. When caring for a patient with complicated gallbladder disease, it is critical to anticipate difficulties and carry out the appropriate preoperative surgical planning. Therefore, predictive factors and scores for a difficult laparoscopic cholecystectomy have been developed.

Several preoperative predictive factors have been studied in literature and have been used to model and score the likelihood for a likely difficult cholecystectomy. These factors include history of prior upper abdominal surgery, focal peritonitis in the right upper quadrant, leucocytosis, sonographic features of acute cholecystitis, Mirizzi syndrome or contracted gallbladder, male gender age over 60 years and advanced liver cirrhosis [5-8] (Table 1). Most of these factors point to the presence of acute cholecystitis as indicated by suggestive history, presence of clinical and/or sonographic Murphy's sign, leucocytosis and ultrasound findings of gallbladder wall thickening >3 mm and presence of pericholecystic fluid. Prior abdominal surgeries increase the complexity of a laparoscopic cholecystectomy by presence of adhesions in the right upper abdomen. Studies have shown that, compared to female patients, male patients are more likely to have adhesions, five times higher conversion rates to open cholecystectomy, and thicker gallbladder walls (>3 mm) during acute cholecystitis [9-12].

Even though several preoperative predictive models and scoring systems for difficult cholecystectomy have been developed using these factors, none of them has been shown to be reliable enough to accurately predict intraoperative difficulty of cholecystectomy. However, Bouarfa et al found that the complexity of intraoperative findings for patients undergoing laparoscopic cholecystectomy can be predicted preoperatively using four preoperative features i.e. inflammation, gallbladder wall thickness, sex and BMI with an accuracy of 83% using the linear discriminant classifier and independent of the subjective opinions of surgeons regarding complexity [9]. In this study, they found that gallbladder inflammation was the most important predictive feature followed by gallbladder wall thickening, male gender and high BMI. It has been suggested that the triad of obesity, upper abdominal surgery and acute cholecystitis is associated with longer operative times, higher morbidity and higher conversion rates to open cholecystectomy [12, 13].

In order to compare studies among different populations, an intraoperative classification of inflammation was proposed by Nassar [14]. The classification is based on the visibility of the cystic pedicle, the appearance of the gallbladder, and the presence of adhesions around the gallbladder, liver, duodenum and hepatic flexure of the colon. Grade I was defined as intraoperative findings of a soft gallbladder wall with a free thin cystic pedicle and simple adhesions involving the infundibulum or Hartmann's pouch. Grade II comprised of impacted gallbladder stones or mucocele, with simple adhesions involving the gallbladder body and the cystic pedicle covered by fat. Grade III was defined as presence of acute cholecystitis, compressed or intrahepatic gallbladder or a fibrous Hartmann's pouch adhering to the biliary tree associated with cystic pedicle anatomical irregularities or a short, dilated or obscured cystic duct or the presence of dense adhesions involving the gallbladder bed, duodenum or hepatic flexure [14]. Grade IV had a completely hidden gallbladder, or gangrenous gallbladder, empyema, gallbladder perforation with a completely obscured cystic pedicle, or dense, fibrous adhesions completely the gallbladder that are difficult to separate from the surrounding structures [14]. Higher grades suggest increased difficulty with cholecystectomy.

Difficult Cholecystectomy Scenarios

1. Perforated Gallbladder

Gallbladder perforation occurs in 3-15% of cases of acute calculous cholecystitis. It is rarer in acute acalculous cholecystitis. It is associated with increased morbidity and mortality. The most common site of perforation is the gallbladder fundus or body. According to a classification by Niemeier, gallbladder perforation can be acute with generalized biliary peritonitis (type 1), subacute with localized peritonitis, pericholecystic abscess or fluid collection or perforation into the liver (type 2) or chronic with chronic inflammation, scarring and internal or external fistulae to the duodenum, colon or CBD (type 3) [15]. Early identification and intervention is warranted to reduce morbidity, mortality and hospital costs. Laparoscopic cholecystectomy in cases of gallbladder perforation is difficult and is associated with a high rate of conversion to cholecystectomy due to marked inflammation, bleeding and scarring. Early cholecystectomy within 24 hours is associated with few complications and shorter hospital stay [16]. However, preoperative identification is a significant challenge and most cases are not diagnosed preoperatively. When a perforated gangrenous or inflamed gallbladder is identified intraoperatively, a subtotal laparoscopic cholecystectomy may be considered if feasible, as described below. A complete cholecystectomy may be a challenge but may still be accomplished in the standard retrograde manner.

2. Large Dilated Cystic Duct

During a laparoscopic cholecystectomy, a large dilated cystic duct (>1.0 cm in diameter) requires alternative approaches other than the standard laparoscopic endo clips to control it. This is because the endo clips may not cover the entire cystic duct and therefore may result in a cystic duct stump leak. In case of a large edematous and inflamed cystic duct, the clips may fall off once the duct edema and inflammation resolves. Other approaches to controlling a large cystic duct include an Endo-GIA stapling, Endoloop, intracorporeal or extracorporeal suture ligature of the cystic duct. Endo-GIA stapling has been shown to be safe and feasible in selected patients with difficult laparoscopic cholecystectomies with large cystic ducts. Prior to application of the EndoGIA, the cystic duct should be completely skeletonized and the critical view obtained. One should ensure that the cystic duct in of adequate length to accommodate the EndoGIA without catching the CBD/CHD side wall. Due to ease of application, the EndoGIA may be the preferred method to control a large dilated cystic duct. Its main drawback is that it is expensive.

Use of an Endoloop often requires dividing the cystic duct prior applying the Endoloop, unless the fundus-first or subtotal cholecystectomy approach is performed first, in which case gallbladder may be passed through the Endoloop to allow ligation of the cystic duct without prior division. Prior division of the cystic duct prior to application of the Endoloop may retraction of the divided cystic duct stump due to loss of traction on the CBD.

Similar to open cholecystectomy, a laparoscopic suture ligature may be used to control a large or dilated cystic duct. Its main drawback is that it is time consuming and requires expertise. Other methods that have been described include ultrasonic coagulating shears, or electrothermal bipolar sealer.

3. Laparoscopic Cholecystectomy in Liver Cirrhosis

The frequency of gallstone disease in more than twice that in noncirrhotic patients presumably due to increased intravascular hemolysis with a reduction in gallbladder emptying and motility, hypersplenism and increased levels of estrogen [17, 18]. Majority of these are asymptomatic. Management of symptomatic gallstone disease in patients with cirrhosis may be associated with higher mortality bases on the MELD score. LC in cirrhotic portal hypertension patients is more complicated with associated excessive bleeding, postoperative hepatic failure and sepsis. Animal studies have demonstrated that ischemia-reperfusion injury due to pneumoperitoneum may play an important in liver impairment. This injury is positively correlated with the pressure of pneumoperitoneum. Use of pneumoperitoneum with a lower flow of CO2, maintaining the intra-abdominal pressure at about 10 mmHg, and gradually relieving the pneumoperitoneum after LC has been suggested to minimize liver ischemic injury. Randomized studies have shown that laparoscopic cholecystectomy by itself and specifically with the use of Harmonic scalpel is safe and feasible in patients with Child A and B cirrhosis associated with shorter operative and anesthesia time, lesser intraoperative bleeding and a lower rate of gallbladder perforation compared to standard cholecystectomy with clipping[19, 20].

4. Mirizzi Syndrome

Mirizzi syndrome is characterized by common hepatic duct obstruction owing to extrinsic mechanical compression and surrounding inflammation by a gallstone impacted at the gallbladder neck or cystic duct. It is classified into two types: Mirizzi type I, limited to external compression of the common hepatic duct by a stone impacted in the cystic duct or Hartmann pouch, and Mirizzi type II, associated with a fistula between the gallbladder and the common duct from inflammation and erosion of the impacted stone (Figure 3). In a series from Mayo Clinic, laparoscopic cholecystectomy in Mirizzi syndrome was associated with a 67% conversion rate to open cholecystectomy due to intense inflammation and peribiliary adhesions [21]. Laparoscopic cholecystectomy was successfully completed in 15% of patients all of whom had Mirizzi type 1 syndrome.

The authors concluded that laparoscopic cholecystectomy is feasible Mirizzi syndrome especially type I if the critical view can be demonstrated [21]. In these patients, handling of the Hartmann pouch or infundibulum with the impacted stone for adequate retraction for exposure is the challenging part. A fundus-first of half-dome down approaches will solve this problem. Following dissection of the fundus and body of the gallbladder, the area of gallbladder with the impacted can then be adequately assessed. Also attempts to dislodge the stone into the gallbladder fundus can be tried. Dissection then leads to identification of the critical view.

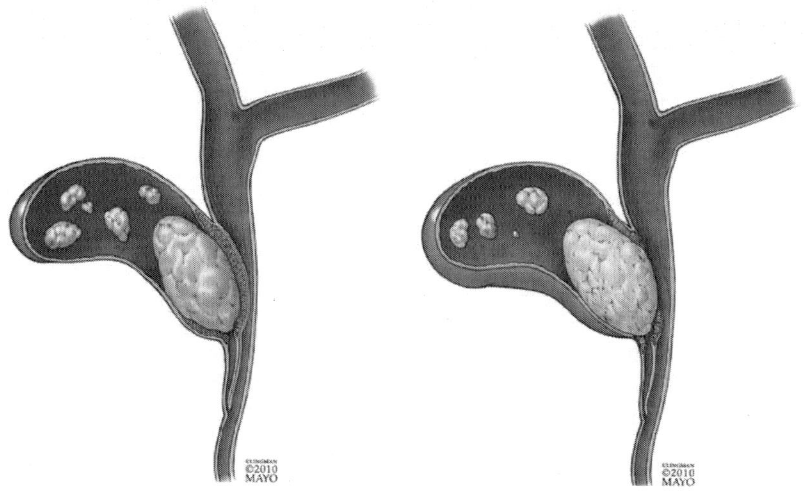

Figure 3. McSherry Classification of Mirizzi syndrome. By permission of Mayo Foundation Medical Education and Research. All rights reserved.

Different approaches can be used to control the cystic duct depending on the degree of inflammation and size of the cystic duct. These include clip application to those described discussed below for handling a large cystic duct. Evaluation of the site of compression of the common duct should be done to identify any coexisting cystoenteric fistula. In Mirizzi type 2, dealing with the fistula becomes the major issue. If it is a small fistula, simple closure over T-tube choledochostomy. If local conditions like inflammation and scarring do not allow for simple closure over a T-tube, a Roux-en-Y jejunal serosal patch can be performed for duct closure. If this is not feasible, a Roux-en-Y hepaticojejunostomy or choledochojejunostomy may be performed. Whether these can be completed laparoscopically depends on the skills of the surgeon.

5. Xanthogranulomatous Cholecystitis

Xanthogranulomatous cholecystitis (XGC) is a rare intense chronic inflammatory process that causes asymmetrical thickening of the gallbladder wall with formation of nodules. It results in a tendency of the inflamed gallbladder tissue to adhere or fistulize into neighboring organs like the duodenum or colon [22]. This intraoperative finding can mimic gallbladder cancer and result in unnecessary extensive resection. It occurs in 1-13% of cases of cholecystitis. The clinical presentation is similar to that of acute or chronic cholecystitis, and cholecystectomy is often difficult.

Typical ultrasound findings are focal and diffuse gallbladder thickening ranging from 5-9 mm with presence of cholelithiasis in up to 80% of cases. Laparoscopy cholecystectomy in XGC cases can be associated with a high conversion rate to open procedure (up to 80%) due to the marked thickening and fibrosis as well as adherence to neighboring organs that make dissection very challenging [22, 23].

Partial cholecystectomy often becomes the safest and appropriate alternative approach in these cases. The gallbladder tissue should be excised as much as is possible, leaving the part of the gallbladder wall adherent to the hepatic bed, part of the Hartmann pouch, or the gallbladder neck.

The residual gallbladder mucosa should be fulgurated with electrocautery. Guzma′n-Valdivia reported a postoperative complication rate of 11% with partial cholecystectomy and 3% following complete cholecystectomy in XGC including controlled bile fistula, surgical site infection, biliary peritonitis and hemoperitoneum.[22]. Given the resemblance of XGC to gall bladder carcinoma, intraoperative frozen section histologic evaluation is recommended if available.

Intraoperative Difficulties

Some of the challenges that may be encountered intraoperatively may range from difficulties with peritoneal access with trocar placement due to the patient's body habitus or pregnancy, limited access sites due to prior abdominal operations, difficulties with tolerating pneumoperitoneum due to the patient's comorbidities or challenges encountered during hepatobiliary dissection due to the gallbladder pathology. These may be approached as described below.

A. Difficult Trocar Placement

I. Super morbid obesity

A large pannus in morbidly obese patients will pull the umbilicus down further thereby altering the usual anatomical landmarks and access points. The altered geometry of the abdominal wall may require adjustments of the access technique. A careful Veress needle access and optical access trocar can be considered as the Hasson trocar placement may be difficult to accomplish due to thick abdominal wall. A hybrid technique involves an incision into the subcutaneous fatty tissue, dissection to the fascial level, elevation the fascia securely with small hook retractors, and subsequent access with a Veress needle and optical access trocar. For super morbidly obese patients, extra long trocars may be required. At times, a fifth trocar will assist in retraction of large fatty liver or copious amounts of omentum.

II. Prior abdominal operations

With multiple previous upper abdominal operations, the choice of access point is sometimes difficult. If the operations were performed a long time ago, the possibility of a traditional Hasson trocar placement exists. Alternatives are Veress needle access in the right or left upper quadrant or cut-down trocar placement at more distant sites. Hasson technique has been shown to have fewer complications that Veress needle in these patients [24]. Yu et al suggested that the use of Hasson technique with prior adhesiolysis before placement of the epigastric port and a fundus first technique was associated with fewer complications in patients who have had prior upper abdominal operations [25].

B. Difficulty of Establishing Pneumoperitoneum

The establishment of pneumoperitoneum is the first step in laparoscopic cholecystectomy after trocar access into the abdomen. Establishing a pneumoperitoneum may be a challenge in pregnancy or patients with significant cardiopulmonary disease due to hemodynamic compromise.

In a patient with pre-existing cardiopulmonary disease, the pressure may have to be kept between 8 and 10 cm H2O. Pre-existing bradycardia or hypotension will lead to a lower rate of insufflation.

Surgeons performing laparoscopic bariatric procedures will often have to resort to higher pressures than 15 cm H2O.

C. Dissection in Inflamed Tissues

Significant inflammation will lead to omental, colonic and duodenal adhesions obscuring the view of the gallbladder on initial entry. Therefore, blunt and sharp dissection without much energy can be helpful in identifying the gallbladder and retracting it. Below we discuss some techniques that may aide in the safe conduct of the laparoscopic cholecystectomy in inflamed tissue.

Techniques for Dealing with Inflamed Gallbladders

1. Aspiration
2. Dome-down dissection
3. Half dome-down dissection
4. Subtotal/Partial cholecystectomy
5. Alternative instrumentation: role of ultrasonic dissection
6. Cholecystostomy tube

In some patients, routine LC technique proves difficult to carry out either due to gall bladder pathologies or patient factors that make it challenging to obtain the critical view of safety during laparoscopic cholecystectomy. These difficult situations may be encountered in patients with gangrenous cholecystitis, inflamed distended gallbladder, perforated gallbladder, large cystic duct, Mirizzi syndrome and cholecystectomy in liver cirrhosis and portal hypertension. Alternative approaches to standard retrograde LC may be necessary to complete the procedure laparoscopically. These are described below.

1. Aspiration

During laparoscopic cholecystectomy in acute cholecystitis, the inflamed and distended gallbladder is sometimes difficult to grasp for adequate retraction for exposure of Calot's triangle. In these cases, prior aspiration of the gallbladder contents with a 14 or 16 gauge needle inserted into the gallbladder fundus and suctioned out with the suction aspirator or aspiration with a large syringe may be helpful.

2. Fundus-First/Dome-Down/Top-Down Approach

Laparoscopic fundus-first/dome-down/top-down approach mimics the open cholecystectomy technique which is now rarely performed as a primary procedure. The fundus first approach has been shown to be safe for difficult cholecystectomies and to decrease conversion rates to open cholecystectomy [26, 27]. The principle steps of a dome down approach are as follows: the gallbladder fundus is gently grasped and retracted caudad and the overlying edge of the liver is gently retracted cephalad with a blunt grasping forceps. If a tense, markedly distended gallbladder is difficult to grasp, prior gallbladder aspiration can be performed to decompress it.

A diathermy L-hook is used to dissect the plane between the gallbladder fundus and the liver. Liver retraction is often difficult with this approach. Leaving a rim of peritoneum on the edge of the liver if it is thick enough to be grasped may be used for liver retraction [27]. Otherwise a blunt instrument is used to gently push the liver cephalad with ongoing dissection. A liver retractor may be used instead of the blunt grasper for liver retraction. The plane may be very bloody in these cases.

Every effort should be made to maintain hemostasis. The most critical moment of the fundus down approach is when the Hartmann's pouch is reached because proximity to the cystic, main hepatic and aberrant hepatic ducts may result in their injury. Care should therefore be taken when approaching the Calot's triangle with this approach to avoid bile duct injury. Medial rotation of the gallbladder neck is the next step with right side blunt dissection of the cystic duct off the common hepatic duct and the infundibulum off the cystic plate. No sharp dissection or diathermy hook dissection should be performed in the area to avoid damage to the cystic or hepatic ducts. If a gallstone is impacted in the Hartmann's pouch, it can be removed by opening the Hartmann's pouch if attempts to push it back into the gallbladder body fail [27].

Previous authors have recommended mandatory intraoperative cholangiogram in these cases to confirm the anatomy and due to a high incidence of CBD stones in the difficult gallbladder pathologies and the increased likelihood of stones entering the CBD with a dome down approach.

The main drawbacks of a dome down approach are that liver retraction during the dissection may be challenging and bleeding may interfere with visualization of the plane of dissection since the cystic artery remains intact until the end of the dome down dissection. Gallstones may also find their way into the common bile duct during the dissection.

3. Half-Dome Down Approach

The gall bladder is retracted cephalad and laterally in the usual manner. Beginning with dissection at the lateral aspect of the gallbladder with opening of the peritoneum has the least chance of encountering aberrant anatomy. Dissection therefore starts on the lateral side of the gallbladder by separating the gallbladder off the cystic plate starting just above the level of the lymph node of Calot and proceeding cephalad to the body of the gallbladder. The cystic plate is the fibrous surface of the liver to which the non-peritonealized portion of the gall bladder is attached.

The same dissection is carried out on the medial side at the same level as the lateral side and the two sides are connected behind the gall bladder. Retrocystic dissection may be carried out bluntly with Maryland dissector or the laparoscopic swab (Kittner)/peanut swab dissector or suction irrigator dissection. Once the two ends are connected, dissection can cautiously proceed proximally towards Calot's triangle taking care to avoid injury of any anomalous bile ducts especially an anomalous posterior sectoral duct draining into the cystic duct. A posterior sectoral duct, if present, is usually below the level of Calot's node. If Hartmann's pouch or cystic duct is adherent to the common hepatic duct or the common bile duct, only blunt swab dissection should be performed to avoid injuring these structures. The critical view of safety is then confirmed prior to clipping the cystic artery and cystic duct. Intraoperative cholangiography may be performed to confirm the anatomy. The main advantage of this approach is that retraction of the liver is not lost since the fundus of the gall bladder remains attached to the liver and can be used to provide adequate exposure by the cephalad hepatic retraction throughout the procedure.

The half-dome approach is best for cases with dense scarring of the hepatocystic triangle, or when it is difficult to dissect out and identify the anatomy of the hepatocystic triangle despite adequate cephalad retraction of the gall bladder.

4. Partial/Subtotal Cholecystectomy

Subtotal laparoscopic cholecystectomy (LSC) may sometimes be the safest option in a difficult laparoscopic cholecystectomy [12, 28]. This is especially so if the cystic pedicle area is obscured by dense adhesions or inflammation that precludes a safe dissection to obtain a critical view without causing injury to the CBD or surrounding structures. LSC has been shown to prevent bile duct injuries and significantly lowers the rate of conversion to open in severe cholecystitis and hence offers the patient the benefits of minimally invasive cholecystectomy [29-31]. LSC may be a safe alternative for cases of gangrenous cholecystitis, perforated gall bladder, dense adhesions at the cystic triangle ("frozen Calot's triangle), markedly inflamed hepatocystic triangle and Mirizzi syndrome. The procedure is started as a standard cholecystectomy. The gallbladder is aspirated through the body/fundus and opened through an incision at the Hartmann's pouch leaving enough stump for subsequent closure. Any stones extracted into an endo bag exercising care to prevent loss of stones. This can be achieved by ensuring that prior to opening the gallbladder, the body of the gallbladder or Hartmann's pouch are ligated circumferentially distal to the site where the incision will be made on the Hartmann's pouch following posterolateral dissection of the gallbladder off the cystic plate [12, 29]. If posterolateral dissection off the cystic plate and circumferential ligature of the gallbladder cannot be achieved, other maneuvers to prevent spillage of gallbladder contents should be employed. The incision through the Hartmann pouch is then completed circumferentially and retrograde gall bladder dissection is completed in the usual manner. In cases of severe inflammation with difficulty identifying the dissection plane or associated hemorrhage, a strip of posterior wall of the GB may be left in situ adhered to the liver and the remnant GB mucosa fulgurated with diathermy [28, 29]. The Hartmann pouch or cystic stump may be closed with an Endo loop, stapler, intracorporeal or extra-corporeal sutures. Drainage may be used in select cases. Alternatively, LSC may be accomplished by through a fundus-first /half-dome down dissection, with the gall bladder being transected at the neck following Endoloop ligation or intra/extra-corporeal suture ligation. Other techniques of performing a subtotal cholecystectomy have been described. One of these is the endovesicular (inside approach of the gallbladder) approach described by Hubert et al [32]. Briefly, a longitudinal incision is made on the gallbladder from the fundus to Hartmann's pouch and the gallbladder dissected off the liver bed from the inside and outside and is completed by performing a subtotal cholecystectomy while avoiding dissection in the Calot's triangle. Closure of the cystic duct was done from the inside by intracorporeal suture. The residual gallbladder mucosa was destroyed by argon beam coagulation [32]. Combined fundus-down dissection first then subtotal cholecystectomy may be another option.

The main drawbacks of LSC include the risk of cystic duct stump leak, retained common bile duct stones and future recurrent cholecystitis of the remnant gallbladder mucosa. Some cases of adhesive small bowel obstruction related to the remnant gallbladder wall have been described [28].

5. Cholecystostomy Tube

Percutaneous cholecystostomy has been considered as a safe treatment alternative for critically ill or elderly patients with medical comorbidities who develop acute cholecystitis and are not good candidates for cholecystectomy. In these patients, tube cholecystostomy allows for resolution of acute cholecystitis with associated sepsis and elective cholecystectomy in controlled settings. Another potential indication for a cholecystostomy tube is presence of severe inflammation in complicated acute cholecystitis that makes performing a safe dissection of the hepatocystic structures difficult. Studies have, however, shown that cholecystostomy tube is associated with a higher complication rates, prolonged ICU stays and higher readmission rate compared to patients who undergo cholecystectomy.

6. Role of Ultrasonic (Harmonic) and Kittner dissection

Ultrasound dissection involves the application of harmonic frequency range ultrasound to tissues to simultaneously achieve coagulation, coaptation, cavitation and cutting with very minimal lateral spread of energy and hence lower risk of collateral tissue injury [33-35]. Ultrasonic dissection has been shown to be safe in the vicinity of biliary structures and to have an incidence of bile duct injury comparable to open cholecystectomy. Its main advantage is low-risk dissection in the proximity of biliary structures, ability to carry out several functions i.e. simultaneous dissection, coagulation, hemostasis, coaptation and cutting which increase efficiency and safety by avoiding distraction from repeated instrument change. Ultrasonic dissection also results in a bloodless dissection that enables easy anatomic delineation.

A significant drawback is the cost of the instrumentation. Control of the cystic duct requires two applications of the ultrasonic shears initially achieving simple sealing of the cystic duct, then dividing the duct without applying too much tension [33]. Reinforcement with an Endoloop may be necessary if the cystic duct is very inflamed or large [33]. A learning curve exists and is associated with a potential risk of thermal injury with instrument misuse.

References

[1]   Strasberg SM, Brunt LM (2010) Rationale and use of the critical view of safety in laparoscopic cholecystectomy. *J. Am. Coll Surg.*, 211:132-138.

[2]   Liau KH, Blumgart LH, DeMatteo RP (2004) Segment-oriented approach to liver resection. *The Surgical clinics of North America*, 84:543-561.

[3]   Hugh TB, Kelly MD, Mekisic A (1997) Rouviere's sulcus: a useful landmark in laparoscopic cholecystectomy. *The British journal of surgery*, 84:1253-1254.

[4]   Bingener-Casey J, Richards ML, Strodel WE, Schwesinger WH, Sirinek KR (2002) Reasons for conversion from laparoscopic to open cholecystectomy: a 10-year review. J. Gastrointest Surg., 6:800-805.

[5]   Kama NA, Kologlu M, Doganay M, Reis E, Atli M, Dolapci M (2001) A risk score for conversion from laparoscopic to open cholecystectomy. *Am. J. Surg.*, 181:520-525.

[6]   Schrenk P, Woisetschlager R, Rieger R, Wayand WU (1998) A diagnostic score to predict the difficulty of a laparoscopic cholecystectomy from preoperative variables. *Surg. Endosc.*, 12:148-150.

[7]   Rosen M, Brody F, Ponsky J (2002) Predictive factors for conversion of laparoscopic cholecystectomy. *Am. J. Surg.*, 184:254-258.

[8]   Kologlu M, Tutuncu T, Yuksek YN, Gozalan U, Daglar G, Kama NA (2004) Using a risk score for conversion from laparoscopic to open cholecystectomy in resident training. *Surgery*, 135:282-287.

[9]   Bouarfa L, Schneider A, Feussner H, Navab N, Lemke HU, Jonker PP, Dankelman J (2011) Prediction of intraoperative complexity from preoperative patient data for laparoscopic cholecystectomy. *Artif. Intell. Med.*, 52:169-176.

[10]   Gabriel R, Kumar S, Shrestha A (2009) Evaluation of predictive factors for conversion of laparoscopic cholecystectomy. Kathmandu Univ. Med. *J.*, *(KUMJ)* 7:26-30.

[11]   Zisman A, Gold-Deutch R, Zisman E, Negri M, Halpern Z, Lin G, Halevy A (1996) Is male gender a risk factor for conversion of laparoscopic into open cholecystectomy? *Surg. Endosc.*, 10:892-894.

[12]   Hussain A (2011) Difficult laparoscopic cholecystectomy: current evidence and strategies of management. *Surg. Laparosc. Endosc. Percutan. Tech.*, 21:211-217.

[13]   Simopoulos C, Botaitis S, Karayiannakis AJ, Tripsianis G, Pitiakoudis M, Polychronidis A (2007) The contribution of acute cholecystitis, obesity, and previous abdominal surgery on the outcome of laparoscopic cholecystectomy. *Am. Surg.*, 73:371-376.

[14]   Nassar AHM, Ashkar KA, Mohamed AY, Hafiz AA (1995) Is Laparoscopic Cholecystectomy Possible without Video Technology. *Minimal Invasiv Ther.*, 4:63-65.

[15]   Niemeier OW (1934) Acute Free Perforation of the Gall-Bladder. *Ann. Surg.*, 99:922-924.

[16]   Stefanidis D, Sirinek KR, Bingener J (2006) Gallbladder perforation: risk factors and outcome. The Journal of surgical research 131:204-208.

[17]   Poggio JL, Rowland CM, Gores GJ, Nagorney DM, Donohue JH (2000) A comparison of laparoscopic and open cholecystectomy in patients with compensated cirrhosis and symptomatic gallstone disease. *Surgery*, 127:405-411.

[18]   Morino M, Cavuoti G, Miglietta C, Giraudo G, Simone P (2000) Laparoscopic cholecystectomy in cirrhosis: contraindication or privileged indication? *Surg. Laparosc. Endosc. Percutan. Tech.*, 10:360-363.

[19]   El Nakeeb A, Askar W, El Lithy R, Farid M (2010) Clipless laparoscopic cholecystectomy using the Harmonic scalpel for cirrhotic patients: a prospective randomized study. *Surg. Endosc.*, 24:2536-2541.

[20]   El-Awadi S, El-Nakeeb A, Youssef T, Fikry A, Abd El-Hamed TM, Ghazy H, Foda E, Farid M (2009) Laparoscopic versus open cholecystectomy in cirrhotic patients: a prospective randomized study. *Int. J. Surg.*, 7:66-69.

[21]   Erben Y, Benavente-Chenhalls LA, Donohue JM, Que FG, Kendrick ML, Reid-Lombardo KM, Farnell MB, Nagorney DM (2011) Diagnosis and treatment of Mirizzi syndrome: 23-year Mayo Clinic experience. J *Am. Coll Surg.*, 213:114-119; discussion 120-111.

[22]   Guzman-Valdivia G (2004) Xanthogranulomatous cholecystitis: 15 years' experience. *World J. Surg.*, 28:254-257.

[23]   Kim JH, Jeong IH, Yoo BM, Kim MW, Kim WH (2009) Is xanthogranulomatous cholecystitis the most difficult for laparoscopic cholecystectomy? *Hepatogastroenterology*, 56:597-601.

[24] Yerdel MA, Karayalcin K, Koyuncu A, Akin B, Koksoy C, Turkcapar AG, Erverdi N, Alacayir I, Bumin C, Aras N (1999) Direct trocar insertion versus Veress needle insertion in laparoscopic cholecystectomy. *Am. J. Surg.*, 177:247-249.

[25] Yu SC, Chen SC, Wang SM, Wei TC (1994) Is previous abdominal surgery a contraindication to laparoscopic cholecystectomy? *J. Laparoendosc Surg.*, 4:31-35.

[26] Gupta A, Agarwal PN, Kant R, Malik V (2004) Evaluation of fundus-first laparoscopic cholecystectomy. JSLS : Journal of the Society of Laparoendoscopic Surgeons / *Society of Laparoendoscopic Surgeons*, 8:255-258.

[27] Mahmud S, Masaud M, Canna K, Nassar AH (2002) Fundus-first laparoscopic cholecystectomy. *Surg. Endosc.*, 16:581-584.

[28] Bornman PC, Terblanche J (1985) Subtotal cholecystectomy: for the difficult gallbladder in portal hypertension and cholecystitis. *Surgery*, 98:1-6.

[29] Singhal T, Balakrishnan S, Hussain A, Nicholls J, Grandy-Smith S, El-Hasani S (2009) Laparoscopic subtotal cholecystectomy: initial experience with laparoscopic management of difficult cholecystitis. *Surgeon*, 7:263-268.

[30] Beldi G, Glattli A (2003) Laparoscopic subtotal cholecystectomy for severe cholecystitis. *Surg. Endosc.*, 17:1437-1439.

[31] Ji W, Li LT, Li JS (2006) Role of laparoscopic subtotal cholecystectomy in the treatment of complicated cholecystitis. *Hepatobiliary Pancreat. Dis. Int.*, 5:584-589.

[32] Hubert C, Annet L, van Beers BE, Gigot JF (2010) The "inside approach of the gallbladder" is an alternative to the classic Calot's triangle dissection for a safe operation in severe cholecystitis. *Surg. Endosc.*, 24:2626-2632.

[33] Huscher CG, Lirici MM, Di Paola M, Crafa F, Napolitano C, Mereu A, Recher A, Corradi A, Amini M (2003) Laparoscopic cholecystectomy by ultrasonic dissection without cystic duct and artery ligature. *Surg. Endosc.*, 17:442-451.

[34] Emam TA, Cuschieri A (2003) How safe is high-power ultrasonic dissection? *Ann. Surg.*, 237:186-191.

[35] Sasi W (2010) The outcome of laparoscopic cholecystectomy by ultrasonic dissection. *Surg. Technol. Int.*, 19:70-78.

In: Cholecystectomies
Editors: Miyu Akiyama and Satomi Kunomasu

ISBN: 978-1-62257-890-0
© 2013 Nova Science Publishers, Inc.

Chapter VII

Cholecystectomy for Acute Cholecystitis in the Elderly

Takahisa Fujikawa[*], Seiichiro Tada and Akira Tanaka*
Department of Surgery, Kokura Memorial Hospital, Kitakyushu,
Fukuoka, Japan

Abstract

Background: Acute cholecystitis in the elderly is a serious condition with high operative mortality and morbidity. Both acute cholecystitis and high age are significant risk factors for mortality and prolonged hospital stay after cholecystectomy.

Methods: A review of the English language literature listed on Medline database, concerning cholecystectomy for acute cholecystitis in the elderly, was performed.

Results: It is generally accepted that early cholecystectomy is the preferred approach for most patients with acute cholecystitis, and laparoscopic cholecystectomy is increasingly advocated for experienced surgeons. Several randomized controlled trials that compared early surgery with delayed one found that early surgery had the advantages of shorter operation time, less blood loss, and less length of hospital stay. Results of randomized controlled trials comparing early and delayed laparoscopic cholecystectomy have also shown that early laparoscopic surgery is superior to delayed surgery in terms of the conversion rate to open surgery, complication rate, and total hospital stay. On the other hand, recent reports still showed that acute cholecystitis in the elderly may be associated with higher morbidity and mortality. Some encouraging papers demonstrated early laparoscopic cholecystectomy in the elderly patients suffering from acute cholecystitis is feasible and effective if an appropriate surgery candidate is selected.

Conclusion: The elderly patients with acute cholecystitis still represent a challenging group and need to be carefully managed. Early laparoscopic cholecystectomy is a safe, effective treatment option for acute cholecystitis if an appropriate selection for candidate is secured.

[*] Corresponding Author. MD, PhD, FACS, Department of Surgery, 3-2-1 Asano, Kokurakita-ku, Kitakyushu, Fukuoka 802-8555, JAPAN. Tel: 81-93-511-2000, fax: 81-93-511-3240; e-mail: fujikawa-t@kokurakinen.or.jp.

Keywords: Acute cholecystitis, elderly patients, early laparoscopic cholecystectomy, surgical risks

Introduction

Gallstone disease is one of the most common digestive diseases. In the United States, approximately 20 million people have gallstones and more than 700,000 annual operative procedures [1, 2]. The prevalence of gallstones increases sharply with age. About 20% of people have gallstones by age 70, and this increases to 30% by age 90 [3, 4]. Annually, 1% to 4% of patients with gallstones will develop complications including acute cholecystitis (AC) and common bile duct (CBD) stones [5-7]. Cholecystectomy is the only definitive therapy for gallstone-related complications.

AC is a common cause of inflammatory acute abdomen. Although laparoscopic cholecystectomy (LC) is initially contraindicated in AC, LC is shown to be a feasible, safe and effective treatment of AC with laparoscopic experience accumulated, and is currently considered as the standard treatment option [8-10]. LC for AC has the advantages of less pain, shorter hospital stay, early return to work, and minimal invasiveness compared with open cholecystectomy [11-14].

AC in the elderly is a serious condition with high operative mortality and morbidity [14-18]. Both AC and high age are significant risk factors for mortality and prolonged hospital stay after cholecystectomy [9, 16, 19, 20]. The main goal of managing AC in the elderly is to provide them the best surgical treatment concomitant with possible quality of life. Recently, some studies have confirmed that early LC (within 24-72 hours of diagnosis) is feasible and reduces total length of hospital stay as compared to delayed LC [15, 21, 22]. Therefore, it is requisite to investigate the impact of early LC on the elderly patients with AC. The aim of this paper is to discuss trends and feasibility of LC in elderly patients suffering from AC, with reference to its technical aspects and perioperative management.

Analytical Methods

A review of the English language literature listed on Medline database, concerning cholecystectomy for AC in the elderly, was performed. We specially focused on indication of early LC to AC in the elderly, and data of Medline database, as well as our personal surgical experience, were comprehensively investigated.

Diagnosis of Acute Cholecystitis

Diagnosis is the starting point of the management of AC, and prompt and timely diagnosis should lead to early treatment and lower mortality and morbidity [23]. Specific diagnostic criteria are necessary to accurately diagnose AC. Tokyo Guidelines [23] propose diagnostic criteria for AC which included (A) local signs of inflammation such as Murphy's sign and right upper quadrant mass/pain/tenderness, (B) systemic signs of inflammation such as fever, elevated WBC count, and elevated C-reactive protein (CRP), and (C) Imaging findings characteristic of AC (by ultrasonography, computed tomography, or magnetic resonance imaging). Definite diagnosis is made when (1) one item in (A) and one item in (B) are positive, or (2) C confirms the diagnosis when AC is clinically suspected.

Severity and Management of Acute Cholecystitis

Patients with AC may present with a spectrum of disease stages ranging from a mild, self-limited illness to a fulminant, potentially life-threatening illness. According to Tokyo Guidelines [24], the severity of AC is classified into the following three categories: "mild (grade I)", "moderate (grade II)", and "severe (grade III)". Usually, the vast majority of patients present with less severe forms of the disease.

"Mild (grade I)" AC is defined as AC without having a severity index that meets the criteria for "severe" or "moderate" cholecystitis. Mild AC can also be defined as AC in a healthy patient with no organ dysfunction and only mild inflammatory changes in the gallbladder, making cholecystectomy a safe and low-risk operative procedure.

"Moderate (grade II)" AC is accompanied by any one of the following conditions: (1) elevated WBC count (>18 000/mm3), (2) palpable tender mass in the right upper abdominal quadrant, (3) duration of complaints >72 hours, or (4) marked local inflammation (biliary peritonitis, pericholecystic abscess, hepatic abscess, gangrenous cholecystitis, emphysematous cholecystitis). In moderate AC, the degree of acute inflammation is likely to be associated with increased operative difficulty to perform a cholecystectomy [25-30].

"Severe (grade III)" AC is accompanied by dysfunctions in any one of the following organs/systems: (1) cardiovascular dysfunction (hypotension requiring treatment with dopamine 5μg/kg per min, or any dose of dobutamine), (2) neurological dysfunction (decreased level of consciousness), (3) respiratory dysfunction (PaO2/FiO2 ratio <300), (4) renal dysfunction (oliguria, creatinine >2.0 mg/dl), (5) hepatic dysfunction (PT-INR >1.5), and (6) hematological dysfunction (platelet count <100 000/mm3). Severe AC is associated with organ dysfunction. This type requires intensive care and urgent treatment (operation and/or drainage) to save the patient's life.

In AC patients, the major practical question regarding management is whether it is advisable to perform cholecystectomy at the time of presentation in the acute phase or whether other strategies of management should be chosen during the acute phase, followed by an interval cholecystectomy.

The treatment of AC should be guided by the grade of severity of the disease and concomitant surgical risk factors. Assessing preoperative surgical risk factors is also an important step for the management of AC.

Surgical risk factors include severe organ failure (cardiopulmonary and/or renal failure) presented, performance status level 2 or more, those with acute cholangitis and/or CBD stones, and patients under anti-thrombotics (anticoagulation or antiplatelet agents). With increasing age, all of the risk factors mentioned above are likely to be more frequently met in patient with AC. Especially, patients who receive anti-thrombotics have a risk of both thromboembolic and bleeding complications.

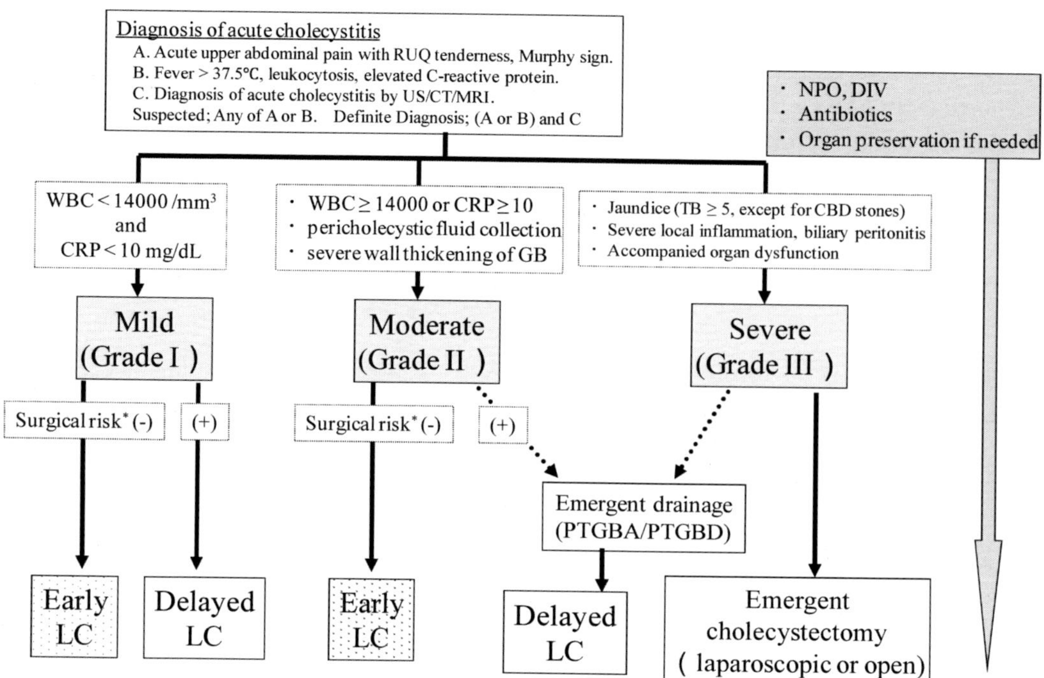

Figure 1. A flowchart for the management of acute cholecystitis proposed by Fujikawa *et al.* Early cholecystectomy, especially early laparoscopic approach if possible, is recommended for most patients. If surgical risks were presented, conservative management (intravenous antibiotics and fluids), with percutaneous gallbladder drainage if needed, and subsequent delayed LC were an alternative therapy for those patients.

Figure 1 demonstrates a flowchart for the management of acute cholecystitis in our institute. Considering the grade of severity of AC and preexisting surgical risks, appropriate management can be selected using this flowchart. Early cholecystectomy, especially early LC if possible, is recommended for most patients in Grade I or II. If grade of AC is "severe" or surgical risks are present, conservative management (definitive organ support with intravenous antibiotics and fluids), with percutaneous gallbladder drainage if needed, and subsequent delayed LC is an alternative therapy.

Early LC for Acute Cholecystitis

About 10-15% of all cholecystectomies performed are for AC [31]. Although both laparoscopic and open cholecystectomy have been shown to be safe in the setting of AC [21, 32-38], LC has currently become the preferred approach in patients with AC [10, 31, 37-43] with conversion rates to an open procedure of 6-35% [44-50]. Furthermore, additional gallstone-related complications occur in 20% to 30% of patients after an initial episode of AC if definitive therapy is not performed [33, 51-54]. Since early cholecystectomy (within 24-72 hours of diagnosis) for AC has been studied and shown to be safe in recent papers, early cholecystectomy is increasingly advocated for patients who can tolerate the procedure. A Cochrane group comprehensive review of randomized controlled trials (1998 to 2003) evaluating cholecystectomy during initial hospitalization versus delayed laparoscopic cholecystectomy for acute cholecystitis concluded that laparoscopic cholecystectomy during initial hospitalization was associated with reduced hospital stays and no difference in rates of conversion to open cholecystectomy, complications, or mortality [55]. Results of several other randomized controlled trials comparing early and delayed laparoscopic cholecystectomy have also shown that early laparoscopic cholecystectomy had the advantages of shorter operation time, less blood loss, and less length of hospital stay. It can be performed without increased rates of conversion to an open procedure, and without an increased risk of complications, including bile duct injury [22, 43-45, 48, 49, 55-59].

Technical Aspects of LC for Acute Cholecystitis

In addition to appropriate preoperative assessment of biliary anatomy and patients' medical condition, it is generally accepted that some basic and important techniques are needed to avoid major complications like bile duct injuries [60-63]. Figure 2 demonstrated operative view of early laparoscopic cholecystectomy for AC.

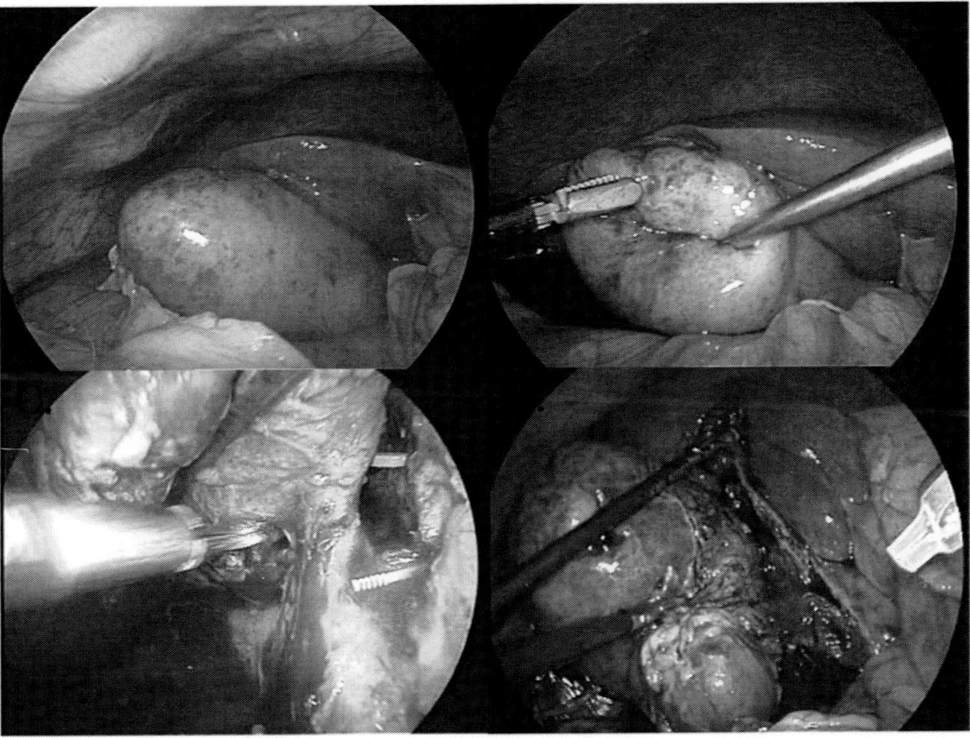

Figure 2. Operative view of early laparoscopic cholecystectomy for acute cholecystitis in the elderly. (A) After the first port is inserted through umbilicus, initial intraabdominal view was obtained showing badly inflamed and distended gallbladder. (B) Due to significant distention of the gallbladder, a needle is used to drain some bile so that grasper clamps can be applied for dissection and manipulation. (C) The Hartmann's pouch is retracted laterally and upward to expose Calot's triangle, then both cystic duct and cystic artery was recognized and dissected. (D) After clipping and dividing the cystic artery and duct, the gallbladder is dissected off the liver bed. Remember that we should care for exposing the layer between the inner and outer layers of the subserosal tissue.

After the first port is inserted through umbilicus, initial intraabdominal view was obtained to determine whether a laparoscopic approach is possible or not. In case of significant distention of the gallbladder, a needle is used to drain some bile so that grasper clamps can be applied for dissection and manipulation (Figure 2B). Inability to identify the structures in Calot's triangle led us to conversion to open surgery. The Hartmann's pouch is retracted laterally and upward to sufficiently expose Calot's triangle (gaining the "critical view of safety"), then both cystic duct and cystic artery are recognized and dissected (Figure 2C). Retrograde dissection of the gallbladder from the fundus was attempted in case of severe inflammation and anatomical difficulty of the pericystic space. After clipping and dividing the cystic artery and duct, the gallbladder is dissected off the liver bed (Figure 2D). Remember that we should care for exposing the layer between the inner and outer layers of the subserosal tissue recommended by Honda *et al.* [64] A plastic bag was used for gallbladder removal from the abdomen for prevention of wound infection and falling of stones.

The "critical view of safety" has been accepted as the most important concept to gain a sufficient view of Calot's triangle before transecting the cystic duct [61]. However, in cases of highly inflamed gallbladders, it is often hard to achieve a critical view of safety, because Calot's triangle is likely to be solid and cannot be expanded. Some landmarks including cystic lymph node, gall bladder neck, Hartman's pouch, and Rouviere's sulcus have been advocated for identifying the cystic duct and safe dissection [65]. Although it may be distorted and is carefully identified in patients with atrophic cholecystitis or adhesions around cystic duct, Hartman's pouch is often used as a landmark as it is easily visualized and connects gallbladder to cystic duct [66]. Hugh *et al.* recommends identifying Rouviere's sulcus as a fixed extra-biliary point ventral to the right portal pedicle, and dissection ventral to this sulcus and extending this dissection as far as possible up the gallbladder fossa both posteriorly and anteriorly allows the hepatobiliary triangle to open out [67]. Strasberg *et al.* suggested that misidentification of the CBD as cystic duct can be attributed to the direction of traction on the gallbladder in superior direction rather than laterally bringing the cystic duct and CBD into alignment, thus it is essential to retract the gallbladder in lateral direction when clipping or dividing the cystic duct [62]. Honda *et al.* recommended exposing the inner layer of the subserosal layer (ss-i) to achieve the "critical view of safety" in case of severe acute cholecystitis [64].

LC for Acute Cholecystitis in the Elderly

Recently, since the proportion of the elderly population continues to increase worldwide each year, cholecystitis in the elderly is becoming a serious and often a critical problem. Management of complicated gallstones presents a unique set of challenges in the elderly population such as delayed presentation, significant comorbid illness, or increased postoperative morbidity [3, 4, 54].

After the introduction and popularization of LC, its superiority has been reported in an increasing number of studies, and currently the indication of LC is extended to more challenging patient population. Although initial reports showed that LC in the elderly may be associated with higher morbidity and mortality [16, 68, 69], recent papers showed that LC performed for AC in the elderly 75 years and over requires a shorter time of operation and a shorter length of hospitalization, and reduces the number of patients who need rehabilitation and the mortality rate, as compared with open cholecystectomy [18, 70]. The mortality rate of LC is the same as that of open cholecystectomy [71]. The morbidity rate of open cholecystectomy is about seven times higher than that of LC, and the elderly and high risk patients in higher American Society of Anesthesiology (ASA) Physical Class System classes should undergo LC [14]. LC performed in the elderly 75 years and over reduces the morbidity rate and shortens the duration of hospitalization, and thus reduces medical costs [72].

On the other hand, there is a report that LC for elderly patients 75 years and over is not very beneficial, because many of the elderly need to undergo open cholecystectomy later and to stay in hospital for the same length of time as those with open cholecystectomy [73]. There is an opinion that LC is preferable, similarly to delayed surgery, for patients without complications, whereas for elderly patients with complications, early conversion to open cholecystectomy or the performance of open cholecystectomy is recommended [74].

Early vs Delayed LC for Acute Cholecystitis in the Elderly

Recently, some studies have confirmed that early LC is feasible and reduces total length of hospital stay as compared to delayed LC [15, 21, 22], but the data about the impact of early LC on the outcome of elderly patients with AC are limited and its effect and feasibility remains controversial.

The U.S. population-based study by Riall *et al.* concerning the rate of AC in the elderly reported that early cholecystectomy during initial hospitalization for AC is appropriate and safe, with low rates of further gallstone-related problems and low gallstone-related readmission rates [3]. The conversion and open cholecystectomy rate for elderly patients with AC was 71%, which is similar to that reported in previous single institution studies [3, 71, 74-76]. The 2.1% in-hospital mortality rate for AC is consistent with the 0.5% to 2.5% rate reported for elective cholecystectomy in elderly patients [18, 75] and actually much lower than a 1980's report of 10% to 19% mortality for emergency cholecystectomy in elderly patients [3, 75, 76]. Cui *et al.* also demonstrated the retrospective review of 4048 patients (among them 18% is the elderly) receiving early LC for AC and reported that the elderly patients had higher rate of ASA score III or IV (18% vs 3%) and higher co-morbidity rates (62% vs 21%) than younger patients, but there was no difference in operative time, intraoperative complications, hospital stay, and mortality between the groups, and concluded that early LC for elderly patients with AC is safe and practical [15].

On the other hand, Moyson *et al.* retrospectively examined 100 patients aged 75 years and older who underwent cholecystectomy for AC, in which 55% of patients received emergent operation with higher conversion or open surgery rate (86.7%) and high morbidity (33%) and mortality (14.5%) rate, and suggested that elective LC for elderly patients with AC is recommended due to high morbidity and mortality risks after emergent cholecystectomy [17]. Kirshtein *et al.* also reported that among 225 patients undergoing attempted LC for AC (19% of which is the elderly), elderly patients had higher rate of ASA score III or IV (21% vs 4% in the younger), high postoperative complication rate (31% vs 15%), and high mortality rate (4.8% vs 0.5%), although mean operative time and conversion rate to open surgery were similar between the elderly and the younger [69]. They concluded that LC in elderly patients suffering from AC is feasible and effective, but stronger selection of elderly patients for surgery is recommended due to their high rate of mortality and morbidity unrelated to the surgical site. Fujikawa *et al.* reported their strategy for the management of acute cholecystitis, which included selection system of AC patients according to the severity of AC and preoperative risk factors [77] (Figure 1). When severity of AC, presence of preoperative surgical risks, feasibility of early LC done, and outcome of early and delayed LC were compared between 49 elderly patients and 62 younger patients, the severity of AC were similar, but the elderly patients had higher occurrence of preoperative surgical risk (53%, vs 24% in the younger), including high rate of antithrombotic use (35%). Since the rate of early LC (55% vs 47%), conversion rate (4% vs 5%), and duration of surgery (120 min vs 125 min) were all similar between the groups, and there was neither operative death nor bile duct injury in both groups, it is concluded that early LC is a safe and effective treatment for AC even in the elderly if an appropriate patient selection is performed [77].

Thus, controversy over the timing of LC in elderly patients suffering from AC still exists. However, early LC by experienced surgeons is feasible and safely applied even for this challenging patient population, and an appropriate preoperative assessment and patient selection under a standardized managing protocol is of paramount importance.

Conclusion

It is generally accepted that early cholecystectomy is the preferred approach for most patients with acute cholecystitis. Appropriate patient selection for early or delayed cholecystectomy according to the severity of acute cholecystitis and preexisting surgical risks is of paramount importance. During operation, basic and important techniques to avoid major complications like bile duct injuries should be carefully applied. The elderly patients with acute cholecystitis still represent a challenging group and need to be carefully managed. Indication of laparoscopic cholecystectomy to elderly patients is increasingly advocated for experienced surgeons. If an appropriate selection for candidate is secured, early laparoscopic cholecystectomy can be a safe and effective treatment option for acute cholecystitis even in the elderly.

References

[1] Steiner CA, Bass EB, Talamini MA, Pitt HA, Steinberg EP. Surgical rates and operative mortality for open and laparoscopic cholecystectomy in Maryland. *N Engl J Med.* 1994;330(6):403-408.

[2] Gallstones and laparoscopic cholecystectomy. *NIH Consensus Statement.* 1992.

[3] Riall TS, Zhang D, Townsend CM, Jr., Kuo YF, Goodwin JS. Failure to perform cholecystectomy for acute cholecystitis in elderly patients is associated with increased morbidity, mortality, and cost. *J Am Coll Surg.* 2010;210(5):668-677, 677-669.

[4]   Khang K, Wargo J. Gallstone disease in the elderly. In: Rosenthal RA, Zenilman ME, Katlic MR, editors. *Principles and Practice of Geriatric Surgery*. Verlag: Springer; 2001. pp. 690–710.

[5]   Chiang W, Lee F, Santen S. *Cholelithiasis* [EMedicine web site] 2008 [Accessed 07/28/09]; Available at: http://emedicine.medscape.com/ article/774352-overview.

[6]   Gracie WA, Ransohoff DF. The natural history of silent gallstones: the innocent gallstone is not a myth. *N Engl J Med.* 1982;307(13):798-800.

[7]   McSherry CK, Ferstenberg H, Calhoun WF, Lahman E, Virshup M. The natural history of diagnosed gallstone disease in symptomatic and asymptomatic patients. *Ann Surg.* 1985;202(1):59-63.

[8]   Garber SM, Korman J, Cosgrove JM, Cohen JR. Early laparoscopic cholecystectomy for acute cholecystitis. *Surg Endosc.* 1997;11(4):347-350.

[9]   Kiviluoto T, Siren J, Luukkonen P, Kivilaakso E. Randomised trial of laparoscopic versus open cholecystectomy for acute and gangrenous cholecystitis. *Lancet.* 1998;351(9099):321-325.

[10]   Lam CM, Yuen AW, Chik B, Wai AC, Fan ST. Variation in the use of laparoscopic cholecystectomy for acute cholecystitis: a population-based study. *Arch Surg.* 2005;140(11):1084-1088.

[11]   Eldar S, Sabo E, Nash E, Abrahamson J, Matter I. Laparoscopic versus open cholecystectomy in acute cholecystitis. *Surg Laparosc Endosc.* 1997;7(5):407-414.

[12]   Golden WE, Cleves MA, Johnston JC. Laparoscopic cholecystectomy in the geriatric population. *J Am Geriatr Soc.* 1996;44(11):1380-1383.

[13]   Kanaan SA, Murayama KM, Merriam LT, Dawes LG, Prystowsky JB, Rege RV, et al. Risk factors for conversion of laparoscopic to open cholecystectomy. *J Surg Res.* 2002;106(1):20-24.

[14]   Massie MT, Massie LB, Marrangoni AG, D'Amico FJ, Sell HW, Jr. Advantages of laparoscopic cholecystectomy in the elderly and in patients with high ASA classifications. *J Laparoendosc Surg.* 1993;3(5):467-476.

[15]   Cui W, Zhang RY, Sun DQ, Gong RH, Han TQ. Early laparoscopic *cholecystectomy for acute gallbladder disease in Chinese elderly. Hepatogastroenterology.* 2010;57(99-100):409-413.

[16]   do Amaral PC, Azaro Filho Ede M, Galvao TD, Ettinger JE, Silva Reis JM, Lima M, et al. Laparoscopic cholecystectomy for acute cholecystitis in elderly patients. *JSLS.* 2006;10(4):479-483.

[17]   Moyson J, Thill V, Simoens C, Smets D, Debergh N, Mendes da Costa P. Laparoscopic cholecystectomy for acute cholecystitis in the elderly: a retrospective study of 100 patients. *Hepatogastroenterology.* 2008;55(88):1975-1980.

[18]   Pessaux P, Tuech JJ, Derouet N, Rouge C, Regenet N, Arnaud JP. Laparoscopic cholecystectomy in the elderly: a prospective study. *Surg Endosc.* 2000;14(11):1067-1069.

[19]   Bingener J, Richards ML, Schwesinger WH, Strodel WE, Sirinck KR. Laparoscopic cholecystectomy for elderly patients: gold standard for golden years? *Arch Surg.* 2003;138(5):531-535; discussion 535-536.

[20]   Hazzan D, Geron N, Golijanin D, Reissman P, Shiloni E. Laparoscopic cholecystectomy in octogenarians. *Surg Endosc.* 2003;17(5):773-776.

[21] Chandler CF, Lane JS, Ferguson P, Thompson JE, Ashley SW. Prospective evaluation of early versus delayed laparoscopic cholecystectomy for treatment of acute cholecystitis. *Am Surg.* 2000;66(9):896-900.

[22] Lau H, Lo CY, Patil NG, Yuen WK. Early versus delayed-interval laparoscopic cholecystectomy for acute cholecystitis: a metaanalysis. *Surg Endosc.* 2006;20(1): 82-87.

[23] Hirota M, Takada T, Kawarada Y, Nimura Y, Miura F, Hirata K, et al. Diagnostic criteria and severity assessment of acute cholecystitis: Tokyo Guidelines. *J Hepatobiliary Pancreat Surg.* 2007;14(1):78-82.

[24] Miura F, Takada T, Kawarada Y, Nimura Y, Wada K, Hirota M, et al. Flowcharts for the diagnosis and treatment of acute cholangitis and cholecystitis: Tokyo Guidelines. *J Hepatobiliary Pancreat Surg.* 2007;14(1):27-34.

[25] Chopra S, Dodd GD, 3rd, Mumbower AL, Chintapalli KN, Schwesinger WH, Sirinek KR, et al. Treatment of acute cholecystitis in non-critically ill patients at high surgical risk: comparison of clinical outcomes after gallbladder aspiration and after percutaneous cholecystostomy. *AJR Am J Roentgenol.* 2001;176(4):1025-1031.

[26] Kendall JL, Shimp RJ. Performance and interpretation of focused right upper quadrant ultrasound by emergency physicians. *J Emerg Med.* 2001;21(1):7-13.

[27] Ralls PW, Halls J, Lapin SA, Quinn MF, Morris UL, Boswell W. Prospective evaluation of the sonographic Murphy sign in suspected acute cholecystitis. *J Clin Ultrasound.* 1982;10(3):113-115.

[28] Rosen CL, Brown DF, Chang Y, Moore C, Averill NJ, Arkoff LJ, et al. Ultrasonography by emergency physicians in patients with suspected cholecystitis. *Am J Emerg Med.* 2001;19(1):32-36.

[29] Soyer P, Brouland JP, Boudiaf M, Kardache M, Pelage JP, Panis Y, et al. Color velocity imaging and power Doppler sonography of the gallbladder wall: a new look at sonographic diagnosis of acute cholecystitis. *AJR Am J Roentgenol.* 1998;171(1):183-188.

[30] Sugiyama M, Tokuhara M, Atomi Y. Is percutaneous cholecystostomy the optimal treatment for acute cholecystitis in the very elderly? *World J Surg.* 1998;22(5): 459-463.

[31] Ainsworth AP, Adamsen S, Rosenberg J. Surgery for acute cholecystitis in Denmark. *Scand J Gastroenterol.* 2007;42(5):648-651.

[32] Hunter JG. Acute cholecystitis revisited: get it while it's hot. *Ann Surg.* 1998;227(4):468-469.

[33] Jarvinen HJ, Hastbacka J. Early cholecystectomy for acute cholecystitis: a prospective randomized study. *Ann Surg.* 1980;191(4):501-505.

[34] Johansson M, Thune A, Blomqvist A, Nelvin L, Lundell L. Management of acute cholecystitis in the laparoscopic era: results of a prospective, randomized clinical trial. *J Gastrointest Surg.* 2003;7(5):642-645.

[35] Lai PB, Kwong KH, Leung KL, Kwok SP, Chan AC, Chung SC, et al. Randomized trial of early versus delayed laparoscopic cholecystectomy for acute cholecystitis. *Br J Surg.* 1998;85(6):764-767.

[36] Lo CM, Liu CL, Fan ST, Lai EC, Wong J. Prospective randomized study of early versus delayed laparoscopic cholecystectomy for acute cholecystitis. *Ann Surg.* 1998;227(4):461-467.

[37] Shikata S, Noguchi Y, Fukui T. Early versus delayed cholecystectomy for acute cholecystitis: a meta-analysis of randomized controlled trials. *Surg Today.* 2005;35(7):553-560.

[38] Siddiqui T, MacDonald A, Chong PS, Jenkins JT. Early versus delayed laparoscopic cholecystectomy for acute cholecystitis: a meta-analysis of randomized clinical trials. *Am J Surg.* 2008;195(1):40-47.

[39] Campbell EJ, Montgomery DA, MacKay CJ. A survey of current surgical treatment of acute gallstone disease in the west of Scotland. *Scott Med J.* 2007;52(4):15-19.

[40] Campbell EJ, Montgomery DA, Mackay CJ. A national survey of current surgical treatment of acute gallstone disease. *Surg Laparosc Endosc Percutan Tech.* 2008;18(3):242-247.

[41] Csikesz NG, Tseng JF, Shah SA. Trends in surgical management for acute cholecystitis. *Surgery.* 2008;144(2):283-289.

[42] Yamashita Y, Takada T, Hirata K. A survey of the timing and approach to the surgical management of patients with acute cholecystitis in Japanese hospitals. *J Hepatobiliary Pancreat Surg.* 2006;13(5):409-415.

[43] Yamashita Y, Takada T, Kawarada Y, Nimura Y, Hirota M, Miura F, et al. Surgical treatment of patients with acute cholecystitis: Tokyo Guidelines. *J Hepatobiliary Pancreat Surg.* 2007;14(1):91-97.

[44] Johansson M, Thune A, Nelvin L, Stiernstam M, Westman B, Lundell L. Randomized clinical trial of open versus laparoscopic cholecystectomy in the treatment of acute cholecystitis. *Br J Surg.* 2005;92(1):44-49.

[45] Kolla SB, Aggarwal S, Kumar A, Kumar R, Chumber S, Parshad R, et al. Early versus delayed laparoscopic cholecystectomy for acute cholecystitis: a prospective randomized trial. *Surg Endosc.* 2004;18(9):1323-1327.

[46] Simopoulos C, Botaitis S, Polychronidis A, Tripsianis G, Karayiannakis AJ. Risk factors for conversion of laparoscopic cholecystectomy to open cholecystectomy. *Surg Endosc.* 2005;19(7):905-909.

[47] Soffer D, Blackbourne LH, Schulman CI, Goldman M, Habib F, Benjamin R, et al. Is there an optimal time for laparoscopic cholecystectomy in acute cholecystitis? *Surg Endosc.* 2007;21(5):805-809.

[48] Stevens KA, Chi A, Lucas LC, Porter JM, Williams MD. Immediate laparoscopic cholecystectomy for acute cholecystitis: no need to wait. *Am J Surg.* 2006;192(6): 756-761.

[49] Tzovaras G, Zacharoulis D, Liakou P, Theodoropoulos T, Paroutoglou G, Hatzitheofilou C. Timing of laparoscopic cholecystectomy for acute cholecystitis: a prospective non randomized study. *World J Gastroenterol.* 2006;12(34):5528-5531.

[50] Wang YC, Yang HR, Chung PK, Jeng LB, Chen RJ. Urgent laparoscopic cholecystectomy in the management of acute cholecystitis: timing does not influence conversion rate. *Surg Endosc.* 2006;20(5):806-808.

[51] Cheruvu CV, Eyre-Brook IA. Consequences of prolonged wait before gallbladder surgery. *Ann R Coll Surg Engl.* 2002;84(1):20-22.

[52] Lahtinen J, Alhava EM, Aukee S. Acute cholecystitis treated by early and delayed surgery. A controlled clinical trial. *Scand J Gastroenterol.* 1978;13(6):673-678.

[53] McArthur P, Cuschieri A, Shields R, Sells RA. Controlled clinical trial comparing early with interval cholecystectomy for acute cholecystitis. *Proc R Soc Med.* 1975;68(11):676-678.

[54] Siegel JH, Kasmin FE. Biliary tract diseases in the elderly: management and outcomes. Gut. 1997;41(4):433-435.

[55] Gurusamy K, Samraj K. Early versus delayed laparoscopic cholecystectomy for acute cholecystitis. *Cochran Database of Systematic Reviews.* 2009 Article number: CD005440.(4).

[56] Casillas RA, Yegiyants S, Collins JC. Early laparoscopic cholecystectomy is the preferred management of acute cholecystitis. *Arch Surg.* 2008;143(6):533-537.

[57] Daniak CN, Peretz D, Fine JM, Wang Y, Meinke AK, Hale WB. Factors associated with time to laparoscopic cholecystectomy for acute cholecystitis. *World J Gastroenterol.* 2008;14(7):1084-1090.

[58] Hadad SM, Vaidya JS, Baker L, Koh HC, Heron TP, Hussain K, et al. Delay from symptom onset increases the conversion rate in laparoscopic cholecystectomy for acute cholecystitis. *World J Surg.* 2007;31(6):1298-1201; discussion 1302-1293.

[59] Lee AY, Carter JJ, Hochberg MS, Stone AM, Cohen SL, Pachter HL. The timing of surgery for cholecystitis: a review of 202 consecutive patients at a large municipal hospital. *Am J Surg.* 2008;195(4):467-470.

[60] Hunter JG. Avoidance of bile duct injury during laparoscopic cholecystectomy. *Am J Surg.* 1991;162(1):71-76.

[61] Strasberg SM. Avoidance of biliary injury during laparoscopic cholecystectomy. J Hepatobiliary Pancreat Surg. 2002;9(5):543-547.

[62] Strasberg SM, Hertl M, Soper NJ. An analysis of the problem of biliary injury during laparoscopic cholecystectomy. *J Am Coll Surg.* 1995;180(1):101-125.

[63] Troidl H. Disasters of endoscopic surgery and how to avoid them: error analysis. *World J Surg.* 1999;23(8):846-855.

[64] Honda G, Iwanaga T, Kurata M, Watanabe F, Satoh H, Iwasaki K. The critical view of safety in laparoscopic cholecystectomy is optimized by exposing the inner layer of the subserosal layer. *J Hepatobiliary Pancreat Surg.* 2009;16(4):445-449.

[65] Singh K, Ohri A. Anatomic landmarks: their usefulness in safe laparoscopic cholecystectomy. *Surg Endosc.* 2006;20(11):1754-1758.

[66] van Eijck FC, van Veen RN, Kleinrensink GJ, Lange JF. Hartmann's gallbladder pouch revisited 60 years later. *Surg Endosc.* 2007;21(7):1122-1125.

[67] Hugh TB. New strategies to prevent laparoscopic bile duct injury--surgeons can learn from pilots. *Surgery.* 2002;132(5):826-835.

[68] Kauvar DS, Brown BD, Braswell AW, Harnisch M. Laparoscopic cholecystectomy in the elderly: increased operative complications and conversions to laparotomy. *J Laparoendosc Adv Surg Tech A.* 2005;15(4):379-382.

[69] Kirshtein B, Bayme M, Bolotin A, Mizrahi S, Lantsberg L. Laparoscopic cholecystectomy for acute cholecystitis in the elderly: is it safe? *Surg Laparosc Endosc Percutan Tech.* 2008;18(4):334-339.

[70] Yasuda H, Takada T, Kawarada Y, Nimura Y, Hirata K, Kimura Y, et al. Unusual cases of acute cholecystitis and cholangitis: Tokyo Guidelines. J Hepatobiliary *Pancreat Surg.* 2007;14(1):98-113.

[71] Feldman MG, Russell JC, Lynch JT, Mattie A. Comparison of mortality rates for open and closed cholecystectomy in the elderly: Connecticut statewide survey. *J Laparoendosc Surg.* 1994;4(3):165-172.

[72] Chau CH, Tang CN, Siu WT, Ha JP, Li MK. Laparoscopic cholecystectomy versus open cholecystectomy in elderly patients with acute cholecystitis: retrospective study. *Hong Kong Med J.* 2002;8(6):394-399.

[73] Uecker J, Adams M, Skipper K, Dunn E. Cholecystitis in the octogenarian: is laparoscopic cholecystectomy the best approach? *Am Surg.* 2001;67(7):637-640.

[74] Magnuson TH, Ratner LE, Zenilman ME, Bender JS. Laparoscopic cholecystectomy: applicability in the geriatric population. *Am Surg.* 1997;63(1):91-96.

[75] Houghton PW, Jenkinson LR, Donaldson LA. Cholecystectomy in the elderly: a prospective study. *Br J Surg.* 1985;72(3):220-222.

[76] Margiotta SJ, Jr., Horwitz JR, Willis IH, Wallack MK. Cholecystectomy in the elderly. *Am J Surg.* 1988;156(6):509-512.

[77] Fujikawa T, Tanaka A, Abe T, Yoshimoto Y, Tada S, Maekawa H. Is early laparoscopic cholecystectomy feasible for acute cholecystitis in the elderly? *J Gastroenterol Hepatol Res* (in press).

In: Cholecystectomies
Editors: Miyu Akiyama and Satomi Kunomasu

ISBN: 978-1-62257-890-0
© 2013 Nova Science Publishers, Inc.

Chapter VIII

Optimal Surgical Strategy for Gallbladder Carcinoma According to Clinical and Pathological Background

Keita Kai[1,], Kohji Miyazaki[2], Naohiko Kohya[2], Kenji Kitahara[2], Takao Ide[2], Atsushi Miyoshi[2], Hirokazu Noshiro[2] and Osamu Tokunaga[1]*

Departments of [1]Pathology and Microbiology and [2]Surgery,
Faculty of Medicine, Saga University, Saga, Japan

Abstract

The surgical strategy for gallbladder carcinoma (GBC) depends on the extent of disease, especially the T-stage in TNM classification. Our institution has developed an original surgical strategy for GBC based on the accumulation of clinical and pathological studies. The previous study about the efficacy of extended surgical resection, such as hepatectomy, extrahepatic bile duct resection (BDR) or pancreatoduodenectomy (PD) in T2 and T3 GBC revealed that S4a+5 hepatectomy combined with BDR and regional lymphadenectomy is recommendable for the treatment of T2 or T3 GBC. An original scoring system, the "subserosal cancer invasion score (ss score)" was developed to discriminate favorable cases in T2 GBC. The score divides the lesion into three categories: ss minimum (ss min), ss medium (ss med), and ss massive (ss mas) and our previous study indicated the survival of an ss min GBC patient would be satisfactory with simple cholecystectomy. We focused on the phenomena of dedifferentiation (DD) and tumor budding (BD), which have been reported as markers predictive of poor prognosis in other malignancies, particularly in colorectal cancer and analyzed 80 consecutive patients with GBC exceeding stage T1b. This study revealed both BD and DD correlated significantly with survival in patients with T2 tumor whereas no prognostic impact was evident in patients with other T-stage of tumor. Our accumulated experience and studies

---

[*] Correspondence to: Keita Kai. Department of Pathology & Microbiology, Faculty of Medicine, Saga University; 5-1-1 Nabesima, Saga City, Saga 849-8501, Japan. Tel.: +81-952-34-2234; Fax: +81-952-34-2055; E-mail: kaikeit@cc.saga-u.ac.jp.

enable us to select meticulous surgical strategies for individual patients. However, practical use of these strategies in clinical settings requires close cooperation between surgeons and pathologists.

Introduction

The surgical strategy for gallbladder carcinoma (GBC) depends on the extent of the disease, particularly the T-stage from the TNM classification [1]. Our institution has developed an original surgical strategy for GBC based on the accumulation of clinical and pathological studies. This chapter introduces our strategies and the clinical and pathological backgrounds with a review of the literature.

Survival and General Strategies According to T-stage

The prognosis after surgery for GBC differs strikingly according to T-stage. The Kaplan-Meier curve of disease-specific survival according to T-stage in our institution is demonstrated in Figure 1.

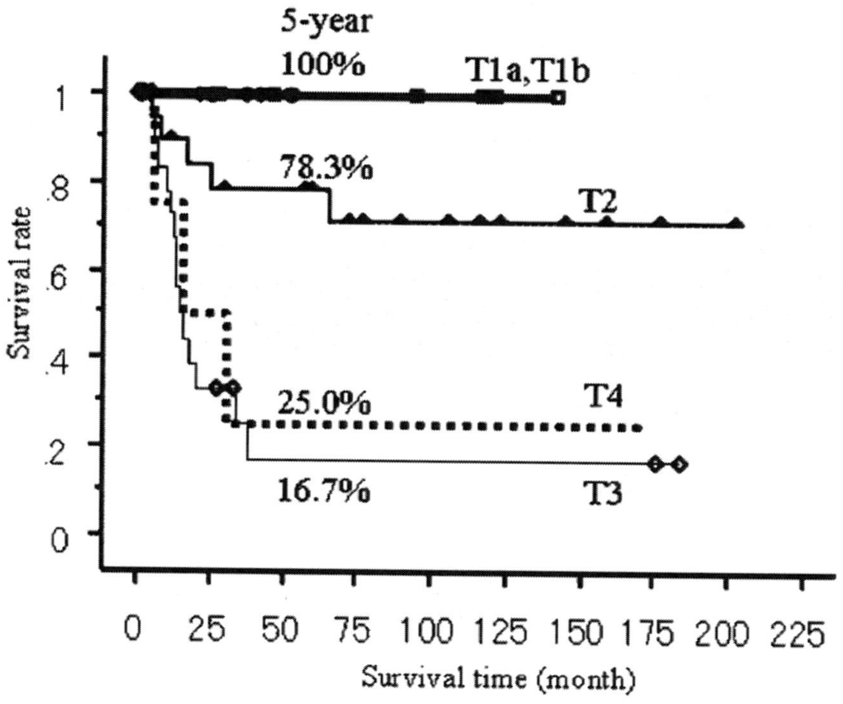

Figure 1. Kaplan-Meier survival analysis for the T-factor component of TNM staging in gallbladder carcinoma. Five-year survival rates for T1, T2, T3, and T4 were 100%, 78.3%, 16.7%, and 25.0%, respectively.

Five-year survival rates for T1, T2, T3, and T4 stage were 100%, 78.3%, 16.7%, and 25.0%, respectively [2]. These survival rates from our series were consistent with findings from previous reports [3-6]. Survival of patients with T1a lesions (invasion restricted to the lamina propria) is particularly good and lymph node metastasis is extremely rare. Simple cholecystectomy with or without lymphadenectomy is thus widely accepted as sufficient for T1a lesions [3, 7, 8]. Areas requiring attention in cholecystectomy for such cases are intraoperative perforation of the gallbladder and surgical margins around the cystic duct, as important prognostic factors in surgery for early GBC [9].

Survival and strategies for T1b (invasion to the muscle layer) remain somewhat controversial. Although our T1b series showed favorable prognosis without lymph node (LN) metastasis, several studies have reported LN metastasis in up to 20% of cases, with recurrence rates of 30-60% following simple cholecystectomy [10-16]. In addition, distinguishing T1b lesions from T2 lesions pre- or intraoperatively is usually difficult. Performing cholecystectomy combined with lymphadenectomy with or without liver resection in patients with pre- or intraoperative presumption of T1b GBC thus seems reasonable. However, T1b GBC is often discovered after laparoscopic cholecystectomy for presumed benign disease. Our experience is that lymph vessel invasion is extremely rare and no LN metastases or recurrences were observed in our T1b series, so additional lymphadenectomy does not always seem necessary in patients with T1b lesion diagnosed after routine cholecystectomy. However, caution is required in that the pathological work for resected specimens must be performed intensively with sections of the whole specimen, to minimize the possibility that a more invasive site or findings of residual lesion remained present in the resected specimen.

The prognosis for T2 (invasion to the subserosal layer) lesions varies widely, showing 5-year survival rates of approximately 20-70% after simple cholecystectomy, compared to 60-100% after radical surgery [8, 17-20]. The surgical strategy for T2 lesion thus remains controversial. However, the conventional opinion is that patients with T2 lesions should be treated using radical cholecystectomy, including en bloc resection of the adjacent liver as well as regional lymphadenectomy with or without extrahepatic bile duct resection (BDR) [3, 21]. Pathologists should take care that T1a tumor invading the Rokitansky-Aschoff sinuses (RAS) is not misdiagnosed as T2 tumor with invasion of the subserosal layer.

Prognosis is poor for most patients with T3 tumor, which shows perforation of the serosa and/or direct invasion of the liver and/or one other adjacent organ or structure). Surgery for T3 lesions is only appropriate if there is potential to achieve a curative resection. T3 lesions require hepatic resection with regional lymphadenectomy at a minimum. This can include major hepatectomy if there is extensive extension into the liver or major vascular structures. In addition, if direct invasion into an adjacent organ (duodenum, pancreas, stomach or colon) is suspected, en bloc resection would be required for curative resection. Because of the high degree of surgical stress involved, the utility of aggressive surgery with extended resection for T3 lesions is often debated in clinical practice and case-by-case selection is required with consideration of patient performance status, complications, and age.

Chemotherapy or palliation is typically appropriate for T4 disease (tumor invading into the main portal vein or two or more extrahepatic organs or structures), except in rare cases where en bloc resection of multiple organs is possible. This is because of the unfortunate prognosis and difficulty of achieving curative resection. Unresectablility discovered at the time of laparotomy may be treated with bypass surgery to relieve symptoms related to biliary obstruction. Cases identified preoperatively as unresectable may be considered for percutaneous biliary drainage or endoscopic stenting to address biliary obstruction.

Radical Surgery for T2 and T3 Tumors

As mentioned above, T2 and T3 tumors are indications for radical surgery. However, the substance of radical surgery is obscure. Although regional lymphadenectomy is widely accepted as necessary at a minimum, the efficacy of extended resection, such as hepatectomy, extrahepatic bile duct resection (BDR) or pancreatoduodenectomy (PD) remains controversial. The necessity of BDR is supported by biliary infiltration associated with perineural invasion and complete lymphadenectomy and eradication of the connective tissue around the common bile duct [22-25]. In terms of hepatectomy for GBC, the resection may vary from a small wedge resection near the gallbladder fossa to an extended right hepatectomy.

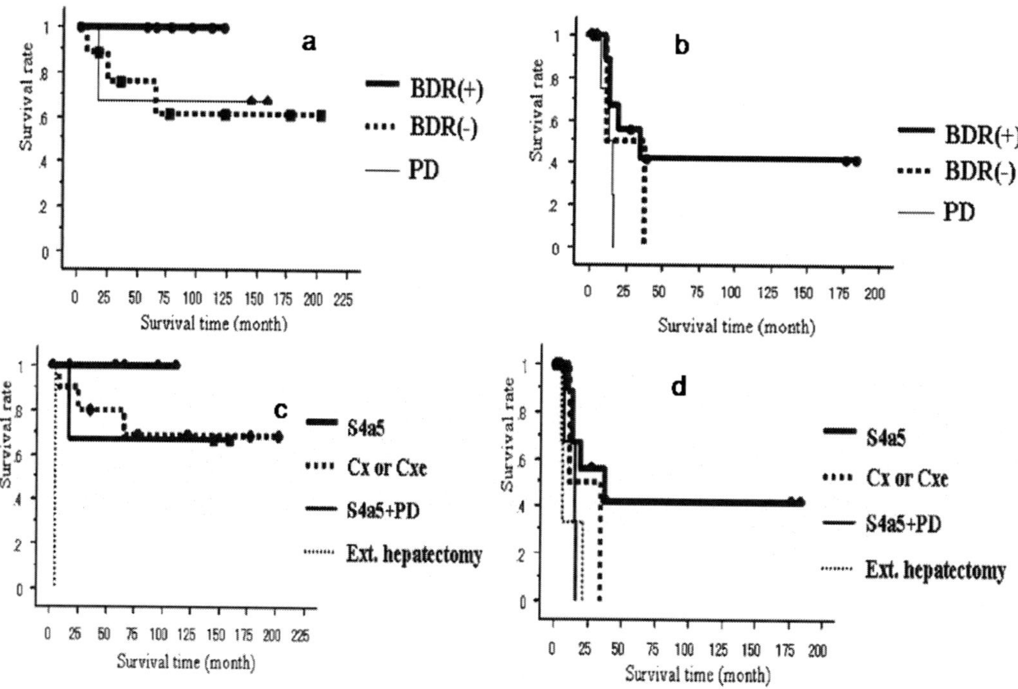

Figure 2. Kaplan-Meier survival analysis by operation procedures in T2 and T3 gallbladder carcinoma. a, b) Kaplan-Meier survival analysis by operation procedures for evaluating the importance of extrahepatic bile duct resection in T2 (a) and T3 (b) gallbladder carcinoma. BDR(+), group with extrahepatic bile duct resection; BDR(-), group without extrahepatic bile duct resection; PD, group with pancreatoduodenectomy or pylorus-preserving pancreatoduodenectomy. c, d) Kaplan-Meier survival analysis by operation procedures for evaluating the importance of liver resection in T2 (c) and T3 (d) gallbladder carcinoma. S4a5, S4a5 hepatectomy; Cx, simple cholecystectomy; Cxe, Cx with liver bed resection; S4a5+PD, S4a5 hepatectomy combined with PD; Ext. hepatectomy, including extended right hepatectomy and right trisegmentectomy.

The reasonability of segment 4a+5 (S4a+5) hepatectomy for advanced GBC is supported by the drainage of the cystic vein into anatomic Couinaud's segments IVa and V and the frequency of liver metastases in this anatomical area [26]. We have previously investigated the efficacy of extended resection, hepatectomy, BDR, and PD in a consecutive surgical series of 23 cases of T2 GBC and 29 cases of T3 GBC [2]. Indications for PD in these cases were obvious duodenal or pancreatic invasion, or infiltrating LN metastases at the retro-pancreatic head portion. Survival curves for evaluating the efficacy of BDR in T2 GBC (Figure 2a) revealed significantly better survival in the BDR(+) group compared to the BDR(-) group. Survival curves according to the status of BDR in T3 GBC (Figure 2b) showed that the BDR(+) group included few long-term survivors. Survival curves for evaluating the efficacy of hepatectomy in T2 GBC (Figure 2c) revealed significantly favorable survival of the S4a+5 hepatectomy group, with a 5-year survival rate of 100%. Survival curves according to the status of hepatectomy in T3 GBC (Figure 2d) revealed the S4a+5 hepatectomy group as the only group with long-term survivors. Furthermore, both uni- and multivariate analyses using Cox proportional hazards models identified the strong efficacy of S4a+5 hepatectomy combined with BDR (P=0.0006 in univariate analysis, P=0.012 in multivariate analysis; relative risk, 0.035; 95% confidence interval, 0.005-0.271). We therefore concluded that S4a+5 hepatectomy combined with BDR and regional lymphadenectomy is recommendable for the treatment of T2 or T3 GBC. On the other hand, additional PD showed no significant difference in survival for both T2 and T3 GBC. Further extension of the operation, such as the addition of PD or extended hepatectomy, should thus be carefully modified for each individual according to the extent of the cancer.

Table 1. Extent of tumor spread by ss score

Vertical invasion	<1/3 in depth	score 1
	≥1/3 and <2/3	score 2
	≥2/3	score 3
Horizontal invasion	<5mm	score1
	≥5mm and <10mm	score2
	≥10mm	score3

The sum total of ss score was calculated. ss minimum (ss min): 2; ss medium (ss med): 3-4; ss massive (ss mas): 5-6.

Attempts to Discriminate Favorable Cases in T2 GBC

T2 GBC shows a wide variety of tumor spread. Some T2 tumors show none of the histological invasive factors of LN metastasis, lymphatic or venous invasion. However, others show prominent LN metastases, along with venous, lymphatic, or perineural invasion, resulting in poor prognosis. This indicates that patients with T2 GBC can allocated to a favorable prognosis group or a poor prognosis group. Although we have documented that S4a+5 hepatectomy combined with BDR and regional lymphadenectomy is the recommended surgery for the treatment of T2 GBC, could the ability to discriminate patients with favorable prognosis even following limited surgery for stage T2 GBC would free these patients from the need for extended radical surgery. To identify cases with a favorable prognosis, an original scoring system, the "subserosal cancer invasion score (ss score)" was developed. The ss score was histologically determined by measuring vertical and horizontal tumor spread in the subserosal layer. Each score was divided according to tumor invasion as follows: vertical invasion <1/3, score 1; ≥1/3 but <2/3, score 2; ≥2/3, score 3; horizontal invasion <5 mm, score 1; ≥5 mm but <10 mm, score 2; and ≥10 mm, score 3. The sum of horizontal and vertical scores was identified as the ss score. Finally, patients were divided into three groups according to the ss score: ss minimum (ss min), ss score 2; ss medium (ss med), ss score 3-4; or ss massive (ss mas), ss score 5-6 (Table 1).

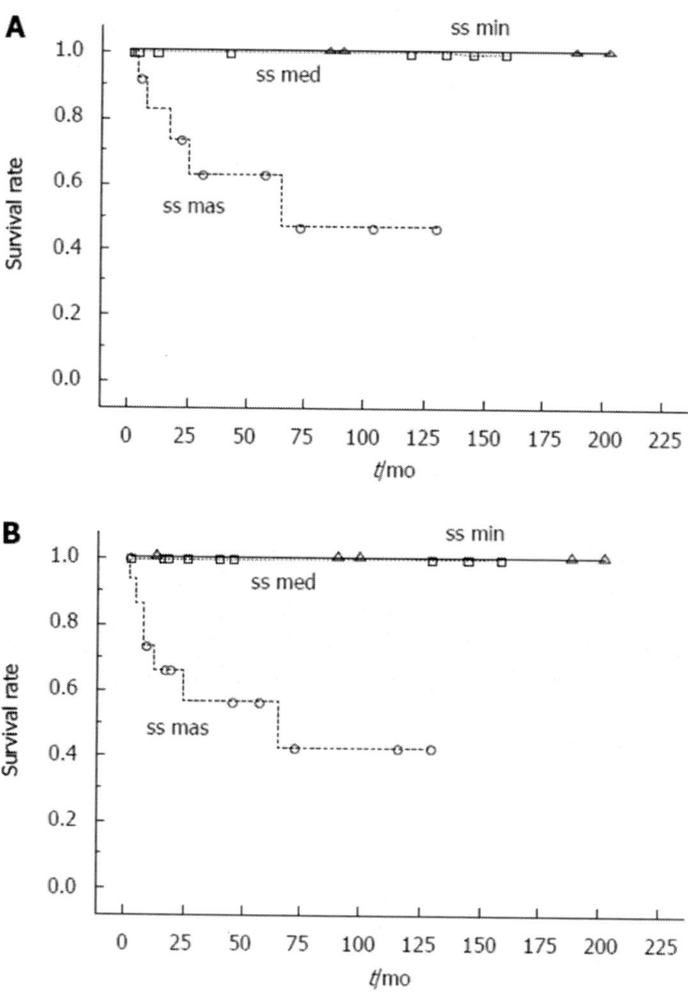

Figure 3. Kaplan-Meier survival analysis of patients with T2 gallbladder carcinoma by ss score. a) Disease-specific survival; the 5-year survival rate for ss min and ss med was 100%. In ss mas gallbladder carcinoma, the 5-year survival rate was 59.7%. b) Disease-free survival; the 5-year survival rate for ss min and ss med was 100%. In ss mas gallbladder carcinoma, the 5-year survival rate was 56.6%.

We have previously reported analyses using ss scores from 30 consecutive cases of T2 GBC [27]. Table 2 describes the relationship between classification of ss score and pathological factors such as hepatic infiltration (h-inf), bile duct invasion (b-inf), lymphatic invasion (ly), venous invasion (v), perineural invasion (pn), and lymph node metastasis (n). The ss min group showed no positive pathological factors. In the ss med group, pathological factors of h-inf, ly, pn, and n were positive in 50%, 60%, 10%, and 30% of patients, respectively. All pathological factors showed high rates of positivity in the ss mas group. Figure 3A shows the disease-specific survival curve for patients with T2 GBC by ss score. All patients with ss min and ss med survived until the end of the follow-up period and 5-year survival rates were 100% in the ss min and ss med groups. In the ss mas group, survival was significantly worse than for the ss min and ss med groups, and the 5-year survival rate was 59.7%. Figure 3B shows the disease-free survival curve. Five-year survival rates in the ss min and ss med groups were 100%. In ss mas GBC, disease-free 5-year survival rate was 56.6%. Seven patients with cancer recurrence were included in the ss mas group. The pattern of recurrence was lymph node recurrence in 3 patients, local recurrence in 2, liver metastasis in 1, and peritoneal dissemination in 1. To evaluate the appropriate surgical procedure for ss mas GBC, survival was analyzed according to the surgical procedures. In ss mas GBC, the cholecystectomy + BDR + regional lymphadenectomy and S4a+5 hepatectomy + BDR + regional lymphadenectomy groups showed significantly better survival than the other groups (Figure 4). The 5-year survival following the cholecystectomy + regional lymphadenectomy without BDR group was 33.3%, worse than for the cholecystectomy + BDR + regional lymphadenectomy group. Other extended operations, including PD and extended hepatectomy, showed dismal outcomes. Surgery in these patients revealed massive lymph node metastasis intraoperatively. These findings by ss score indicate that ss min GBC shows no pathological factors suggestive of a need for radical surgery. While ss med GBC is considered an indication for radical surgery, the lack of recurrence suggests that adjuvant therapy is unwarranted, while radical surgery and adjuvant therapy remain necessary for ss mas GBC. The current algorithm applied in determining the therapeutic strategy for T2 GBC is based on ss score, as shown in Figure 5.

We consider that ss min GBC patients can be treated satisfactorily with simple cholecystectomy. Patients with ss med or ss mas GBC should undergo cholecystectomy with BDR plus regional lymphadenectomy, while these patients and those with or without S4a+5 hepatectomy and ss mas GBC patients should undergo adjuvant therapy.

Table 2. The ss score and clinicopathological factors, n (%)

	ss min (n = 4)	ss med (n = 10)	ss mas (n = 16)
h-inf (+)	0	5 (50.0)	2 (12.5)
b-inf (+)	0	0	1 (6.3)
ly (+)	0	6 (60.0)	15 (93.8)
v (+)	0	0	5 (35.7)
pn (+)	0	1 (10.0)	6 (37.5)
n (+)	0	3 (30.0)	4 (25.0)

h-inf: Hepatic invasion; b-inf: Bile duct invasion; ly: Lymphatic invasion; v: Venous invasion; pn: Peri-neural invasion; n: Lymph node metastasis.

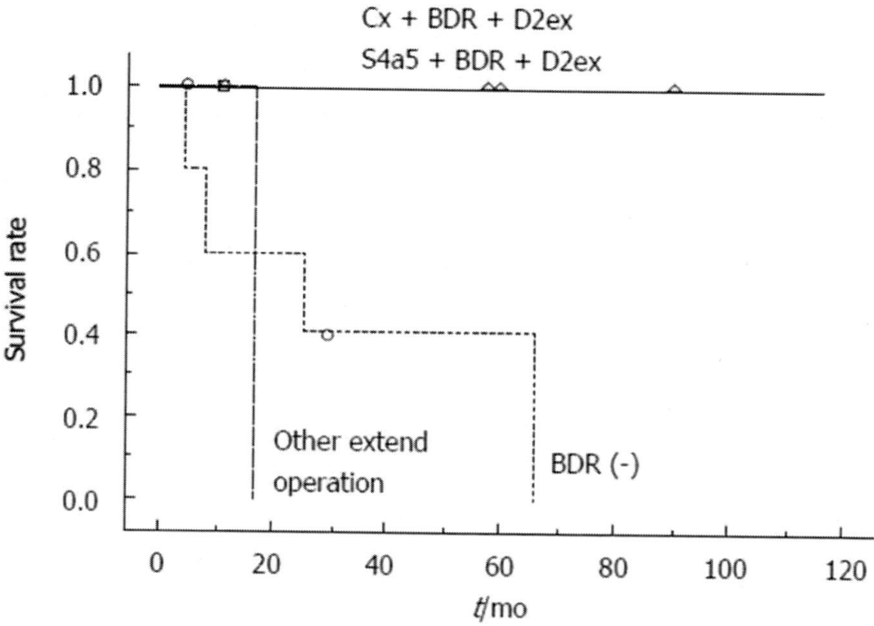

Figure 4. Kaplan-Meier survival analysis by surgical procedure for T2 gallbladder carcinoma. BDR, with extrahepatic BDR; BDR(-), without extrahepatic BDR; S4a5, S4a5 hepatectomy; Cx, simple cholecystectomy; D2ex, D2 lymph node dissection with para-aortic lymph node sampling; BDR, bile duct resection.

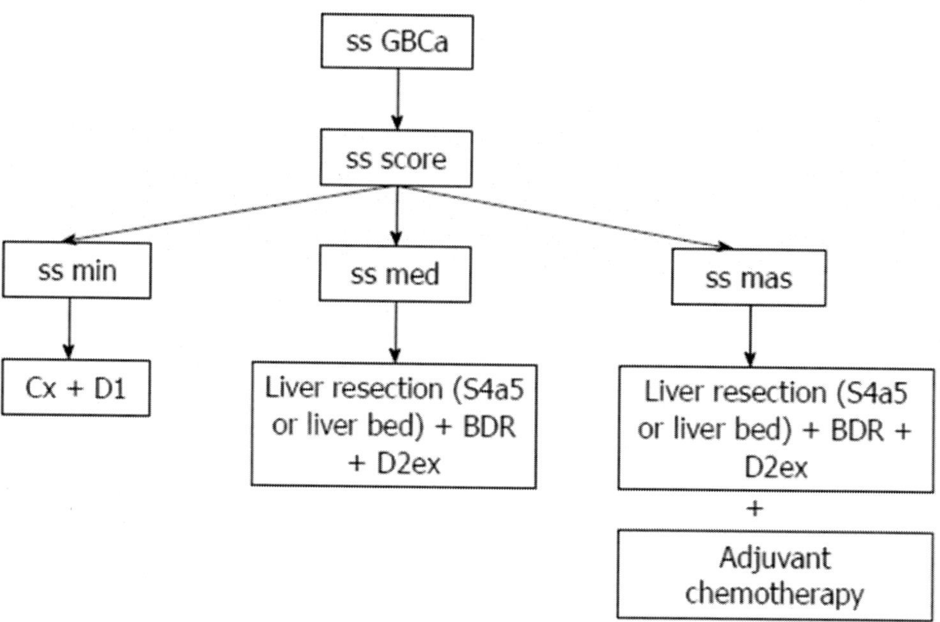

Figure 5. Algorithm of therapeutic strategy for T2 gallbladder carcinoma by ss score. Cx, simple cholecystectomy; BDR, with extrahepatic BDR; S4a5, S4a5 hepatectomy; D2ex, D2 lymph node dissection with para-aortic lymph node sampling.

Histological Approach to Discriminating Favorable Cases of T2 GBC

Under pathological examination of GBC, well-differentiated adenocarcinoma in the mucosal layer is often seen to dedifferentiate into poorly or moderately differentiated adenocarcinoma on the invading side. We focused on the phenomena of dedifferentiation (DD, Figure 6) and tumor budding (BD, Figure 7), which have been reported as markers predictive of poor prognosis in other malignancies, particularly in colorectal cancer [28-34]. We therefore analyzed 80 consecutive patients with GBC exceeding stage T1b [35]. In this study, DD was histopathologically evaluated as tumor in which the histological grade of the invasive front was higher than the histological grade at the surface. BD was defined as an isolated single cancer cell or cluster of fewer than five cancer cells at the invasive front. Among the 80 patients, 47 (58.8%) were positive for BD and 33 (41.2%) were positive for DD. Both BD and DD correlated significantly with disease-specific survival in univariate analysis ($P<0.0001$, $P=0.0013$, respectively). In univariate analysis according to T stage, both BD and DD correlated significantly with survival in patients with T2 tumor (n=32) ($P=0.0011$ and $P=0.0018$, respectively), whereas no prognostic impact was evident in patients with T1b (n=8), T3 (n=34) or T4 (n=6) tumor. The status of BD and DD thus correlates with the prognosis of T2 GBC, suggesting BD and DD as useful markers to discriminate favorable cases in T2 GBC.

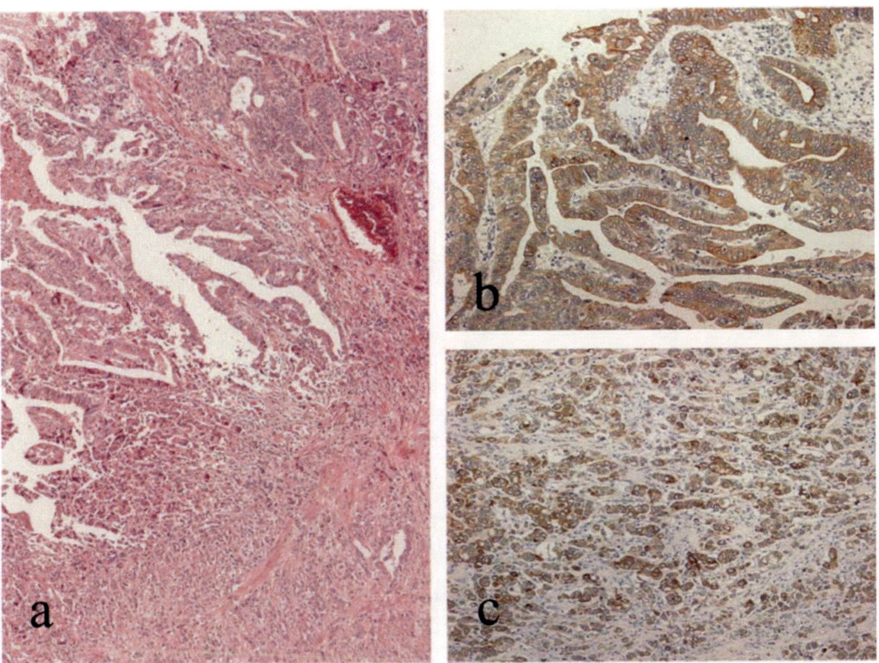

Figure 6. A representative case of dedifferentiation. a) Well-differentiated adenocarcinoma showing dedifferentiation into poorly differentiated adenocarcinoma at the subserosal layer (hematoxylin and eosin, original magnification ×40). b) Immunohistochemical staining of cytokeratin at the tumor surface. The tubular structure of the tumor was highlighted (original magnification ×100). c) Immunohistochemical staining for cytokeratin at the invasive front of the tumor. The dedifferentiated structure of the tumor is highlighted (original magnification ×100).

Table 3. Population of ss score, BD and DD

	ss min (n=6, CD;0, LMN;0)	ss med (n=9, CD;1, LMN;3)	ss mas (n=17, CD;8, LNM;7)
BD positive (n=14)	0	3 (CD;1, LNM;1)	11 (CD;7, LNM;6)
BD negative (n=18)	6	6 (LNM;2)	6 (CD;1, LNM;1)
DD positive (n=15)	0	3 (CD;1, LNM;2)	12 (CD;7, LNM;6)
DD negative (n=15)	6	6 (LNM;1)	5 (CD;1, LNM;1)
Both BD and DD positive (n= 11)	0	2 (CD;1, LNM;1)	9 (CD;4, LNM;5)
Both BD and DD negative (n=14)	6	5	3 (LNM;1)

BD; budding, DD; dedifferentiation, CD;cancer related death, LNM; lymph node metastasis,

Table 4. Details of ss score, and interaction of BD and DD with cancer-related death and LN metastasis in T2 GBC

	ss min (n=6, CD;0, LMN;0)	ss med (n=9, CD;1, LMN;3)	ss mas (n=17, CD;8, LNM;7)
BD positive (n=14)	0	3 (CD;1, LNM;1)	11 (CD;7, LNM;6)
BD negative (n=18)	6	6 (LNM;2)	6 (CD;1, LNM;1)
DD positive (n=15)	0	3 (CD;1, LNM;2)	12 (CD;7, LNM;6)
DD negative (n=15)	6	6 (LNM;1)	5 (CD;1, LNM;1)
Both BD and DD positive (n= 11)	0	2 (CD;1, LNM;1)	9 (CD;4, LNM;5)
Both BD and DD negative (n=14)	6	5	3 (LNM;1)

BD; budding, DD; dedifferentiation, LN; lymph node, CD; cancer related death, LNM; lymph node metastasis.

Table 3 shows the correlation of BD and DD with LN metastasis in T2 GBC patients. A significant correlation with LN metastasis was observed for DD (P=0.0209), but not for BD (P=0.0623). Significant differences were observed in the comparison of LN metastasis between patients showing BD and DD double-positive results and patients with either BD- or DD-negative results (P=0.0396). More marked differences were observed between patients with BD and DD double-negative results and patients with either BD- or DD-positive findings (P=0.0059). As DD status or the combination of BD and DD status show significant correlations with LN metastasis, assessment of BD and DD could provide an indicator of the need for extended resection or lymphadenectomy. The interactions of BD, DD, and ss score and relationships with cancer-related deaths and LN metastasis were examined (Table 4). A notable finding was that no LN metastases and no cancer-related deaths were observed in ss med cases negative for both BD and DD. This suggests that simple cholecystectomy would suffice for ss med patients with negative results for both BD and DD. Furthermore, only 1 patient with LN metastasis and no cancer-related deaths were observed among ss mas patients, so DD and BD status appears to have the potential to discriminate favorable cases even among patients with ss mas T2 GBC.

Pathological Examination for Optimal Surgery

Preoperative diagnosis using an imaging study is very important for selecting the optimal surgery according to T-stage. However, preoperative diagnosis of T-stage in T1 or T2 GBC is not easy, despite advances in medical imaging. As a result, stage T1 or T2 GBC is often discovered incidentally after routine cholecystectomy. In such cases, the entire series of tumor sections and pathological evaluations of ss score, BD, and DD could be available for determining the need for additional extended radical surgery. Intraoperative histological examination is usually performed during surgery for lesions preoperatively diagnosed as "suspected GBC" or "possible T1 or T2 GBC". In such cases, the resected specimen from cholecystectomy with or without en bloc liver resection (S4a5 or liver bed) is submitted for intraoperative histological examination. Diagnosis of the depth of invasion from frozen sections of GBC is not a common pathological work. The actual procedure and pitfalls in intraoperative histological examination of GBC from our experience proceeds as follows. First, observe the entire gallbladder and recognize the cut end of the cystic duct and the presence or absence of combined liver resection. Next, open the resected gallbladder and drain the bile juices, then identify the presence or absence of gallstones and gross features of adenomyomatosis. Examine the gross features with care and take photographs of both the mucosal and serosal sides (Figure 8a).

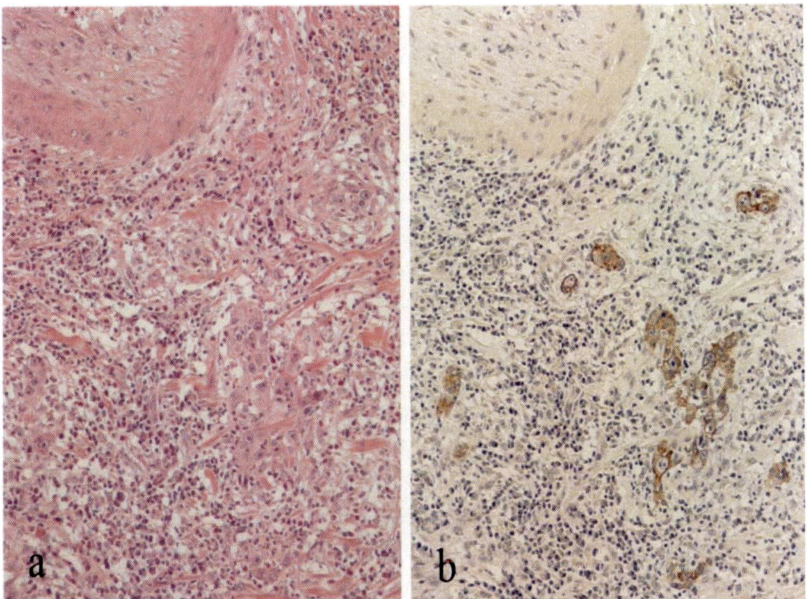

Figure 7. A representative case of budding with inflammation. a) Invasive front of the gallbladder carcinoma. The dense inflammation masks a small cluster of tumor cells (hematoxylin and eosin, original magnification ×100). b) Clusters of tumor cells are highlighted by immunohistochemical staining of cytokeratin (original magnification ×100).

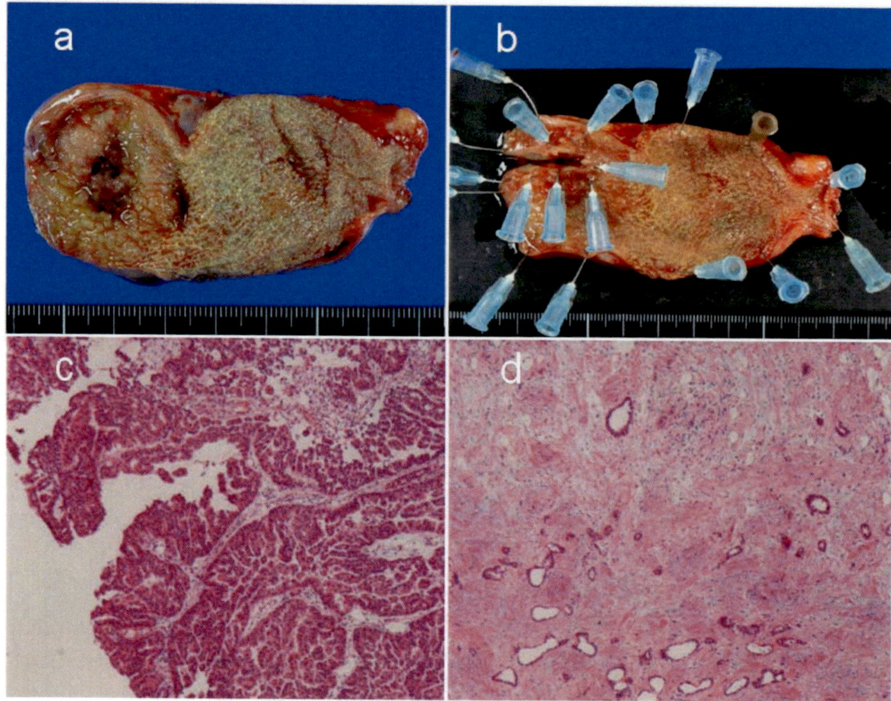

Figure 8. Case presentation for a 66-year-old woman. Wall thickening on the fundal side of the gallbladder with segmental-type adenomyomatosis was identified in an imaging study following complaints of right hypochondrial discomfort. Under a presumed diagnosis of gallbladder cancer, cholecystectomy combined with liver bed resection was performed and the resected specimen was submitted for intraoperative histological examination. a) Gross appearance. Papillary tumor was found on the fundal side of segmental-type adenomyomatosis. b) The gallbladder was fixed on the rubber board by pins and a specimen for the frozen section was cut out. The surface of the tumor showed well-differentiated tubular adenocarcinoma (c), whereas the invasive site showed dedifferentiation of the moderately differentiated tubular adenocarcinoma (d). The intraoperative diagnosis was ss mas gallbladder cancer with dedifferentiation. Additional regional lymphadenectomy and bile duct resection were therefore performed. The intraoperative diagnosis was confirmed following examination of the formalin-fixed samples and lymph node metastases were identified (#12c and #13a). The patient remains alive without recurrence as of 2 years postoperatively.

After taking photographs, fix the gallbladder on the rubber board using pins. Identify the most invasive site from gross examination to make the most informative frozen sections (1 or 2) for diagnosis. The subserosal and muscle layers of the fresh gallbladder easily slide and become disordered from the original arrangement. Frozen sections thus need to be made carefully under fixation by pins to allow the creation of informative and effective frozen sections (Figure 8b). When embedding fresh tissues in the optimal cutting temperature compound, it is important to retain the natural arrangement, and not to wrench or bend tissues, particularly for the subserosal layer. When diagnosing the depth of invasion for a tentative ss score on frozen sections sliced using a microtome-cryostat, it is important to recognize that subserosal tissue is often lacking after preparation with a microtome-cryostat. The presence of an inflammatory reaction means that the assessment of BD on the frozen section is often difficult. Conversely, assessment of DD is easily performed even on frozen examination (Figure 8c, d). Gross features of adenomyomatosis are sometimes present in gallbladders resected under a diagnosis of gallbladder carcinoma [36].

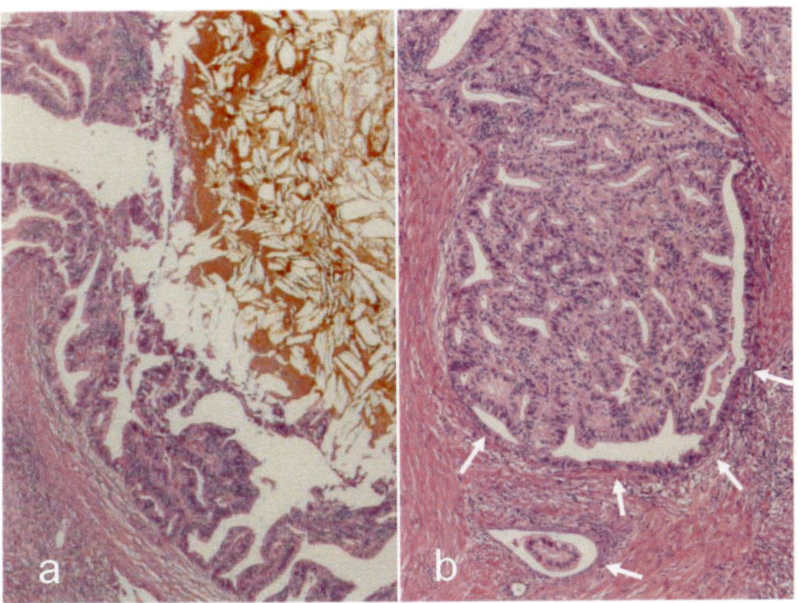

Figure 9. Cancer invading into Rokitansky-Aschoff sinuses (RAS). Discriminating between tumor invading into the RAS and tumor invading into the subserosal layer is very important, but sometimes difficult. The presence of intramural bile stones (a) and lining of epithelial cells or tumor cells replacing lining epithelial cells (b, arrow) in cystic lesions and surrounding smooth muscle bundles are important findings suggesting tumor invading into the RAS.

In such cases, cautioned is needed to avoid taking cancer invading into Rokitansky-Aschoff sinuses as invasion into the subserosal layer (Figure 9). When the tumor lesion is small, care must be taken to avoid obstructing the pathological diagnosis of formalin-fixed specimens. In our institution, the pathologist who treats the fresh specimen and makes the intraoperative histological diagnosis from frozen sections also takes charge of pathological diagnosis of the formalin-fixed specimens.

Conclusion

This chapter has documented the surgical strategies for GBC based on clinical and pathological data from previous studies. Our accumulated experience and studies enable us to select meticulous surgical strategies for individual patients. However, practical use of these strategies in clinical settings requires close cooperation between surgeons and pathologists.

References

[1]   Sobin L, Gospodarowicz M, Wittekind C, editor. *TNM Classification of malignant tumors.* 7th ed. 2009. John Wiley & Sons, Inc., Hoboken, NJ

[2]   Kohya N, Miyazaki K. Hepatectomy of segment 4a and 5 combined with extra-hepatic bile duct resection for T2 and T3 gallbladder carcinoma. *J Surg Oncol.* 2008;97(6):498-502.

[3]   Pilgrim C, Usatoff V, Evans PM. A review of the surgical strategies for the management of gallbladder carcinoma based on T stage and growth type of the tumour. *Eur J Surg Oncol.* 2009;35(9):903-7..

[4]   Bartlett DL, Fong Y, Fortner JG, Brennan MF, Blumgart LH. Longterm results after resection for gallbladder cancer. Implications for staging and management. *Ann Surg* 1996;224(5):639–46.

[5]   Kai M, Chijiiwa K, Ohuchida J, Nagano M, Hiyoshi M, Kondo K. A curative resection improves the postoperative survival rate even in patients with advanced gallbladder carcinoma. *J Gastrointest Surg* 2007; 11(8):1025–32.

[6]   Misra S, Chaturvedi A, Misra NC, Sharma ID. Carcinoma of the gallbladder. *Lancet Oncol* 2003;4(3):167–76.

[7]   Mekeel KL, Hemming AW. Surgical management of gallbladder carcinoma: a review. *J Gastrointest Surg* 2007;11(9):1188–93.

[8]   Wakai T, Shirai Y, Yokoyama N, Nagakura S, Watanabe H, Hatakeyama K. Early gallbladder carcinoma does not warrant radical resection. *Br J Surg* 2001;88(5):675–8.

[9]   Eguchi H, Ishikawa O, Ohigashi H, et al. Surgical significance of superficial cancer spread in early gallbladder cancer. *Jpn J Clin Oncol* 2005;35(3):134–8

[10]   Yildirim E, Celen O, Gulben K, Berberoglu U. The surgical management of incidental gallbladder carcinoma. *Eur J Surg Oncol* 2005;31(1):45–52.

[11]   de Aretxabala X, Roa I, Burgos L, et al. Gallbladder cancer in Chile. A report on 54 potentially resectable tumors. *Cancer* 1992;69(1):60–5.

[12]   Ogura Y, Mizumoto R, Isaji S, Kusuda T, Matsuda S, Tabata M. Radical operations for carcinoma of the gallbladder: present status in Japan. *World J Surg* 1991;15(3):337–43.

[13]   Cucinotta E, Lorenzini C, Melita G, Iapichino G, Curro G. Incidental gall bladder carcinoma: does the surgical approach influence the outcome? *ANZ J Surg* 2005;75(9):795–8.

[14]   Wagholikar GD, Behari A, Krishnani N, et al. Early gallbladder cancer. *J Am Coll Surg* 2002; 194(2):137–41.

[15]   Ouchi K, Suzuki M, Tominaga T, Saijo S, Matsuno S. Survival after surgery for cancer of the gallbladder. *Br J Surg* 1994;81(11):1655–7.

[16]   Matsumoto Y, Fujii H, Aoyama H, Yamamoto M, Sugahara K, Suda K. Surgical treatment of primary carcinoma of the gallbladder based on the histologic analysis of 48 surgical specimens. *Am J Surg* 1992; 163(2):239–45

[17]   Shirai Y, Yoshida K, Tsukada K, Muto T, Watanabe H. Early carcinoma of the gallbladder. *Eur J Surg* 1992;158(10):545–8.

[18]   Fong Y, Brennan MF, Turnbull A, Colt DG, Blumgart LH. Gallbladder cancer discovered during laparoscopic surgery. Potential for iatrogenic tumor dissemination. *Arch Surg* 1993;128(9):1054–6.

[19]   Chijiiwa K, Kai M, Nagano M, Hiyoshi M, Ohuchida J, Kondo K. Outcome of radical surgery for stage IV gallbladder carcinoma. *J Hepatobiliary Pancreat Surg* 2007;14(4):345–50.

[20]   Principe A, Del Gaudio M, Ercolani G, Golfieri R, Cucchetti A, Pinna AD. Radical surgery for gallbladder carcinoma: possibilities of survival. *Hepatogastroenterology* 2006;53(71):660–4.

[21]   Miller G, Jarnagin WR (2008) Gallbladder carcinoma. *Eur J Surg Oncol* 34:306-312.

[22] Kaneoka Y, Yamaguchi A, Isogai M, Harada T, Suzuki M. Hepatoduodenal ligament invasion by gallbladder carcinoma: Histologic patterns and surgical recommendation. *World J Surg.* 2003;27(3):260-5.

[23] Shimizu Y, Ohtsuka M, Ito H, Kimura F, Shimizu H, Togawa A, Yoshidome H, Kato A, Miyazaki M.. Should the extrahepatic bile duct be resected for locally advanced gallbladder cancer? *Surgery.* 2004;136(5):1012-7

[24] Kosuge T, Sano K, Shimada K, Yamamoto J, Yamasaki S, Makuuchi M. Should the bile duct be preserved or removed in radical surgery for gallbladder cancer? *Hepatogastroenterology* 1999;46(28):2133-7.

[25] Burdiles P, Csendes A, Diaz JC, Maluenda F, Avila S, Jorquera P, Aldunate M. Factors affecting mortality in patients over 70 years of age submitted to surgery for gallbladder or common bile duct stones. *Hepatogastroenterology* 1989;36(3):136-9.

[26] Araida T, Higuchi R, Hamano M, Kodera Y, Takeshita N, Ota T, Yoshikawa T, Yamamoto M, Takasaki K. Hepatic resection in 485 R0 pT2 and pT3 cases of advanced carcinoma of the gallbladder: results of a Japanese Society of Biliary Surgery survey--a multicenter study. *J Hepatobiliary Pancreat Surg.* 2009;16(2):204-15

[27] Kohya N, Kitahara K, Miyazaki K. Rational therapeutic strategy for T2 gallbladder carcinoma based on tumor spread. *World J Gastroenterol.* 2010;16(28):3567-72.

[28] Prall F. Tumour budding in colorectal carcinoma. *Histopathology.* 2007;50(1):151-62.

[29] Morodomi T, Isomoto H, Shirouzu K, Kakegawa K, Irie K, Morimatsu M An index for estimating the probability of lymph node metastasis in rectal cancers. Lymph node metastasis and the histopathology of actively invasive regions of cancer. *Cancer.* 1989;63(3):539-43.

[30] Okuyama T, Oya M, Ishikawa H. Budding as a risk factor for lymph node metastasis in pT1 or pT2 well-differentiated colorectal adenocarcinoma. *Dis Colon Rectum.* 2002;45(5):628-34.

[31] Ueno H, Mochizuki H, Shinto E, Hashiguchi Y, Hase K, Talbot IC. Histological indices in biopsy specimens for estimating the probability of extended local spread in rectal cancer. *Cancer.* 2002;94(11):2882-91.

[32] Hase K, Shatney C, Johnson D, Trollope M, Vierra M. Prognostic value of "tumour budding" in patients with colorectal cancer. *Dis Colon Rectum.* 1993;36(7):627-35.

[33] Ueno H, Mochizuki H, Hatsuse K, Hase K, Yamamoto T .Indicators for treatment strategies of colorectal liver metastases. *Ann Surg.* 2000;231(1):59-66.

[34] Ueno H, Murphy J, Jass JR, Mochizuki H, Talbot IC. Tumour "budding" as an index to estimate the potential of aggressiveness in rectal cancer. *Histopathology.* 2002;40(2):127-32.

[35] Kai K, Kohya N, Kitahara K, Masuda M, Miyoshi A, Ide T, Tokunaga O, Miyazaki K, Noshiro H. Tumor budding and dedifferentiation in gallbladder carcinoma: potential for the prognostic factors in T2 lesions. *Virchows Arch.* 2011;459(4):449-56.

[36] Kai K, Ide T, Masuda M, Kitahara K, Miyoshi A, Miyazaki K, Noshiro H, Tokunaga O. Clinicopathologic features of advanced gallbladder cancer associated with adenomyomatosis. *Virchows Arch.* 2011; 459(6):573-80.

ISBN: 978-1-62257-890-0
© 2013 Nova Science Publishers, Inc.

Chapter IX

Mininvasive Laparoscopic Cholecystectomy: From three-port to New Laparoendoscopic Single Site (Less) Access. Evaluating a New Technology

A. Puzziello, G. Orlando, R. Gervasi and M. A. Lerose*
Endocrine Sugery Unit, University Magna Graecia of Catanzaro,
Catanzaro, Italy

Abstract

Laparoscopic cholecystectomy is the gold standard for the treatment of gallbladder stone disease. The advantages of this procedure compared with the open approach include less postoperative pain, shorter recovery time and better cosmetic results. In recent years, many surgeons have attempted to reduce the number and size of ports to decrease parietal trauma and improve cosmetic results. The first step was to remove the fourth trocar that is used to grasp the fundus of the gallbladder, pulling upward and outward to expose Calot's triangle or to retract the liver. A recent meta-analysis of randomized clinical trials confirms that three port technique has similar operating time, success rate, analgesia requirement and postoperative hospital stay.

In the past three years laparoendoscopic single-site surgery (LESS) has also gained greater interest and diffusion as a less invasive laparoscopic cholecystectomy. The cosmetic outcomes of LESS are expected to be better when the operation is performed through the umbilicus because the surgical wound is hidden within the umbilicus, leaving no visible abdominal scars, virtually "scarless" surgery.

The best procedure to evaluate a new technology and/or an innovative surgical technique is a prospective trial comparing the new technique with the gold standard.

---

* Corresponding author: Alessandro Puzziello MD, Chief of Endocrine Surgery Unit, Surgical &Medical Sciences Dept., School of Medicine, University Magna Graecia of Catanzaro, Viale Europa 1, 88100 Catanzaro, Italy. Private address: Alessandro Puzziello, via G. Bonito 32 – 80129 Napoli, Italia.

Otherwise a literature review of the best available evidence is necessary to make the best choice. This critical review aims to evaluate the feasibility and safety of LESS cholecystectomy versus the three-port technique through a comparative analysis of five parameters: mean operative time, intraoperative and postoperative complications, conversion to open, conversion to the four-trocar technique and postoperative hospital stay. Although LESS cholecystectomy is a fashionable technique there are few data available for an evidence-based determination as to the real benefits of this technique. Well-designed comparative studies are suggested to validate the clinical benefits, missing the cosmetic outcome, and ensure that there are no new complications or added costs associated with the new technique.

Laparoscopic cholecystectomy (LC) is the gold standard for the treatment of gallbladder stone disease [1]. The advantages of this procedure compared with the open approach include less postoperative pain, shorter recovery time and better cosmetic results.

History of Laparoscopic Surgery and Standard Cholecystectomy

The development of "closed-cavity" endoscopy, of which laparoscopy is one form, followed the establishment of open-cavity endoscopic procedures such as esophagoscopy, proctoscopy, and laryngoscopy. The first laparoscopy was carried out using a cystoscope (a rigid telescopic endoscope) with distal light illumination. The development of laparoscopic surgery can be described by three main eras: diagnostic laparoscopy (1901-1933), therapeutic laparoscopy (1933-1987), and the modern era using computer chips and television monitors. In the 1933 Fervers performed laparoscopic adhesiolysis with biopsy instruments and cauterization of intraabdominal adhesions and in 1987 Mouret performed the first laparoscopic cholecystectomy.

Until 1987 laparoscopic visualization of the abdominal cavity was restricted to the individual directing the operative procedure, and participation by other members of the surgical team was limited. Therefore complicated operative procedures proved to be tedious because of the inability of the assistant(s) to effectively interact with the surgeon. Although articulated attachments containing a series of mirrors could split the laparoscopic image, they proved to be cumbersome and ineffective. In 1986 this problem was solved with the development of a computer chip television camera attached to the laparoscope, and so began the era of video-guided surgery in which laparoscopic surgical techniques could be used for more complicated gastrointestinal procedures. Video-imaging has also facilitated the education of other surgeons and house staff. In addition, videos can now be used to document the diagnostic or operative procedure. Rapid developments in the area of video-imaging have resulted in higher resolution video monitors that afford greater clarity and definition as well as improved magnification of the operative field, making fine dissection of the tissue plane easier. [2]

In 1987 Mouret, in France, removed a diseased gallbladder from a patient by exposing the porta hepatis by forceful cephalad retraction of the gallbladder fundus. This started the modern era of laparoscopy.

From then on various operative procedures have been performed by the new laparoscopic approach, but the cholecystectomy is still the most performed in surgical units. [3]

According to the standard technique four trocars are used: two 10 mm trocars and two 5 mm trocars. The consolidated experience and cultural push towards a less invasive surgery have stimulated some authors to develop different mini-invasive solutions. Therefore in recent years many surgeons have further attempted to reduce the number and/or size of ports in LC to decrease parietal trauma and improve cosmetic results. The first step was to remove the fourth trocar that is used to grasp the fundus of the gallbladder, pulling upward and outward to expose Calot's triangle, or to retract the liver. A recent meta-analysis of randomized clinical trials confirms that three port technique has similar operating time, success rate, analgesia requirement and postoperative hospital stay. [4] Another way has been a reduction of trocar size (minilaparoscopic cholecystectomy) [5]

In the last three years, laparoendoscopic single-site surgery (LESS) has gained greater interest and diffusion. The cosmetic outcomes of LESS are expected to be better when the operation is performed through the umbilicus because the surgical wound is hidden within the umbilicus, leaving no visible abdominal scars, virtually ''scarless'' surgery.

The recent interest for this new technique is attributable to several factors:

- the consolidated experience in the standard four-trocar technique;
- the availability of different devices that make easier the insertion of trocars with a reduction of umbilical incision;
- the development of new instruments for LESS and related marketing strategies;
- an easier, although controversial, patients' choice of innovative techniques assuring a "scarless" surgery.

Diffusion of a new technique in surgery, as LESS in these years, requires a careful scientific evaluation of the available evidence. Nowadays the best procedure to evaluate a new technology and/or an innovative surgical technique is a prospective trial comparing the new technique with the gold standard. Otherwise a literature review of the best available evidence is necessary to make the best choice.

LESS Cholecystectomy: Evaluating a New Technique

This chapter shows how to review the literature and in this case the object is to evaluate feasibility and safety of LESS cholecystectomy versus three-port technique (TPT), through a comparative analysis of five parameters: mean operative time, intraoperative and postoperative complications, conversion to open, conversion to standard four-trocar technique (FTT), and postoperative hospital stay.

According to PICO model (Problem, Intervention, Comparison and Outcome) you have to keep in your mind the clinical scenario and to indentify the key concepts. In this case we wanted to know if there is an evidence to support LESS for the cholecystectomy rather than a conventional intervention as three trocars technique. The first step was a systematic search of the medical literature, identifying all published work on the topic of single-incision and three-port cholecystectomy in the peer-reviewed literature, as demonstrated in Figures 1 and 2.

Original published studies on laparoscopic surgery performed through a single-incision or the 3-port technique were identified through a search of PubMed and Ovid EMBASE. Inclusion criteria were:

- publication date between January 1, 2005, and December 31, 2010;
- English and Italian language;
- human subjects;
- series of twenty operations or more.

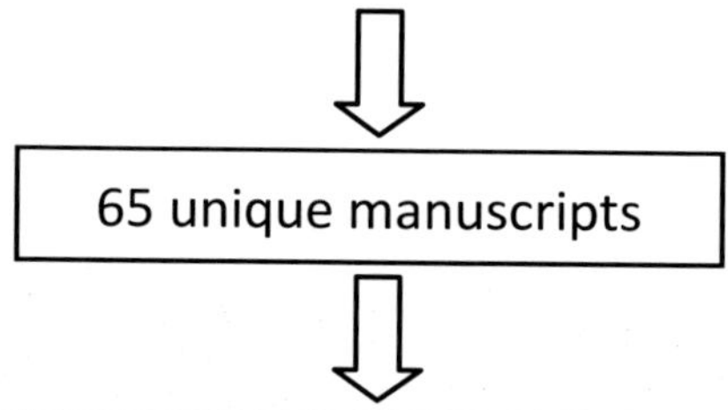

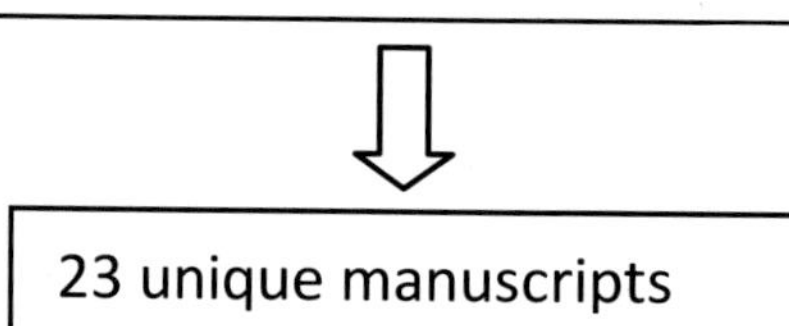

Figure 1. Flowchart for single-incision literature search.

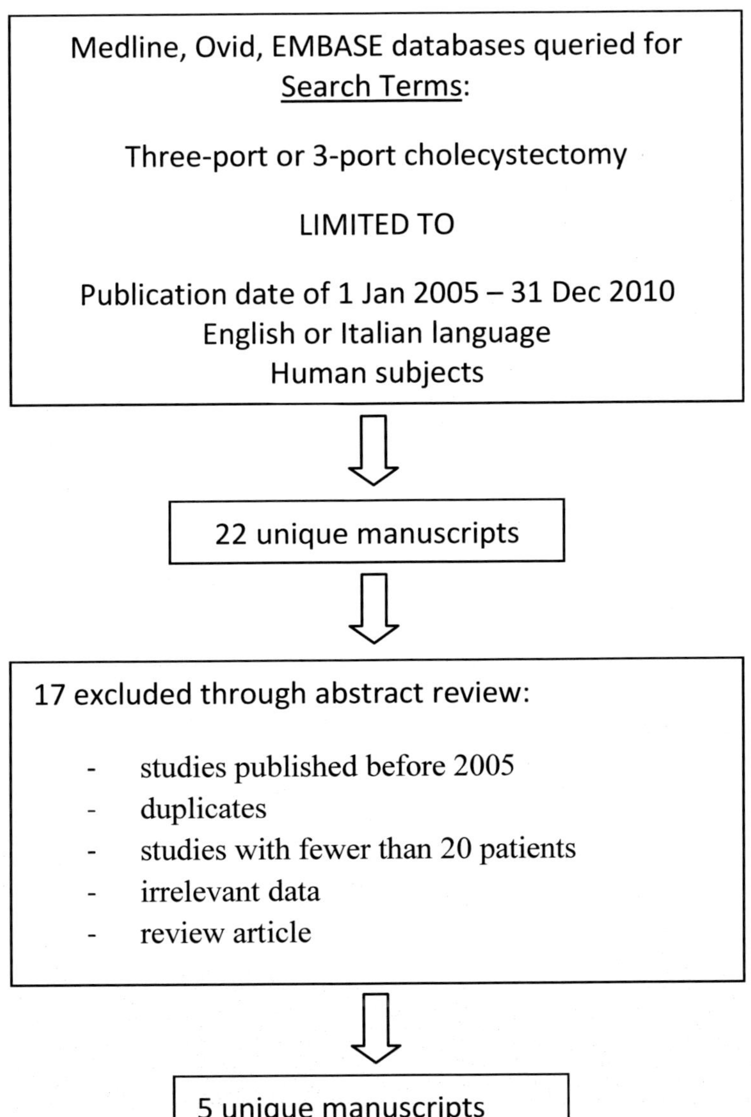

Figure 1. Flowchart for three-port technique literature search.

Reviews, letters to the editor and commentaries were excluded a priori. Then the revision of the bibliography of each selected paper was also performed.

All complete manuscripts were carefully reviewed and data on LESS and TPT were separately recorded in an electronic spreadsheet (Excel; Microsoft®). Data collected included year of publication, procedures performed, number of patients, description of ports used and rate of patients with cholecystitis or pancreatitis. Outcomes data included mean operative time, complications, conversions to open, conversion to standard four-trocar technique (FTT), and postoperative hospital stay.

The data were processed to obtain the weighted average of operative time and length of stay. With regard to the other three parameters, the incidence was calculated on the total number of patients enrolled in each of the two clusters of studies (LESS and TPT).

Results

There were 5 manuscripts meeting the inclusion criteria for TPT and 23 for LESS. This represented 2640 and 1448 operations, respectively. Only one prospective randomized controlled trial comparing TPT and LESS was identified in our review [6].

Operative time is significantly longer in the single-incision group. Also, the rate of complications and conversions to standard four-port technique is higher in LESS. Tables 2 and 3 show complications in detail. They are mostly minimal. In addition, 3.8% of LESS operations were noted to have been converted into a two- or three-trocar technique. In LESS the use of one or more additional trocars in a different site from the umbilical is 8.2%. Postoperative hospital stay is the same in the two groups. Rate of conversion to open is higher in TPT (Table 1). It's notable that the length of incision in TPT ranges from 5 mm to 10 mm depending on the trocar's dimension. In LESS the use of new devices requires an incision from 10 to 30 mm with an average lenght of 18 mm. Furthermore some surgeons performed a single incision through the skin and the abdominal fascia to introduce a device [7]. Others performed a single skin incision and inserted trocars through separate fascial incisions (swiss cheese technique) [8].

In LESS the longer operative time and the higher conversion rate to classic FTT is certainly due not only to the learning curve but also to the technique. The position of instruments compared with the surgical field and the target makes exposure of Calot's triangle more difficult, especially in the presence of adhesions or particular anatomical features as "floppy gallbladder" and Hartmann's pouch stretched by the gallstone. Furthermore, the closeness of instruments and optic caused their clash. For this reason, some authors suggest the use of new curved or flexible-tip instruments [9].

Table 1. LESS vs TPT: comparative data

PARAMETER	THREE-PORT	Patients n (%)[1]	LESS	Patients n (%)[1]
Average operative time (minutes)	45.78	2536 (96%)	64.57	1366 (94%)
Rate of complications (%)	2.0	2536 (96%)	5.9	1110 (77%)
Rate of conversion to open (%)	2.8	2640 (100%)	0.8	1060 (73%)
Rate of conversion to FTT (%)	3.7	2357 (89%)	4.4 (8.2)°	1305 (90%)
Average length of stay (day)	1	2490 (94%)	1.1	1056 (73%)

[1] n is the number of patients from which the entry shown in bold has been computed. In brackets, the rate on the total number of patients of the two clusters of studies (n/2640 and n/1448).

° Rate of cases turned to the standard four-trocar technique. The rate rises to 8.2% if we consider the cases in which one or more trocar is put in a different site from the umbilical, essentially transforming the LESS into a two- or three-trocar technique.

The higher incidence of complications in the LESS could be a bias. It had been explained as a greater attention of the surgeons, in line with a common attitude in the face of a technological innovation, to all possible injuries even if minimal. In fact most of the reported complications are minimal (Table 2) and they probably happen in TPT technique, but the surgeons often neglect them.

Table 2. Panel of complications in LESS

Record	Number of complications	Complications	Partial rate	Total rate
Kuon et al [11]	2/37	bleeding	5,4%	5,4%
Hodgett et al [12]	3/29	pain	2 (6,9%)	10,3%
		urinary incontinence	1 (3,4%)	
Philipp et al [13]	7/29	Wound haematoma	3 (10,3%)	24,1%
		Wound seroma	2 (6,9%)	
		Wound infection	1 (3,4%)	
		Pain	1 (3,4%)	
Curcillo et al [14]	26/297	Minor complications (not listed)	8,7%	8,7%
Edwards et al [15]	7/80	Cystic duct leakage	2 (2,5%)	8,7%
		Accessory duct leakage	2 (2,5%)	
		infection	2 (2,5%)	
		Urinary retention	1 (1,3%)	
Hawasli et al [16]	3/71	Gallbladder perforation	4,2%	4,2%
Roy et al [17]	4/50	spillage of multiple calculi	3 (6,0%)	8,0%
		bleeding	1 (2,0%)	
Roberts et al [8]	3/56	bile leakage	1 (1,8%)	5,4%
		infection	1 (1,8%)	
		Retained common bile duct stone	1 (1,8%)	
Rawlings et al [18]	2/54	Umbilical wound drainage and infection	3,7%	3,7%
Elsey et al [19]	5/238	port site hematomas	1,3%	2,1%
		skin dehiscence at the umbilical site	0,8%	
Romanelli et al [7]	1/22	incarcerated hernia in the fascial incision	4,5%	4,5%
Wen et al [20]	2/50	Wound seroma	4,0%	4,0%

Some of the complications considered in the LESS studies, such as blood lost, are a measure of the learning curve and not the safety and quality of care. We might paradoxically recognize a new technique by measuring the average length of surgery and the amount of blood lost as safe and effective. On the contrary, we have a slight of amount of lesions that can go unrecognized.

Both studies on LESS and TPT do not have a long-term follow-up to assess the impact of the two major complications of the LC: bile duct injuries and hernia at the trocar-site insertion. These also are underestimated for the standard FTT. Particularly the median delay in diagnosis for biliary leak or transection of the bile duct is 1-2 weeks, but for stricture it may be months or years. In the LESS, the umbilical cut is approximately 15-18 mm or 20-30 mm, compared with 10 mm cut in the TPT. From the anatomical point of view, the greater incision in the LESS with the longer operative time could increase the risk of umbilical hernia; however, to date there is still no study on this.

Table 3. Panel of complications in TPT

Record	Number of complications	Complications	Partial rate	Total rate
Agresta et al [21]	10/268	Minor complications (not listed)	--	3,7%
Al-Azawi et al [22]	16/283	abdominal pain	8 (2,8%)	5,7%
		wound infection	4 (1,9%)	
		pleural effusion	2 (0,7%)	
		jaundice	1 (0,4%)	
		port site bleeding	1 (0,4%)	
Tuveri et al [23]	19/1878	bleeding	9 (0,5%)	1%
		bile leakage	3 (0,2%)	
		incisional ernia	3 (0,2%)	
		umbilical fistulas	2 (0,1%)	
		gastric perforation	1 (0,1%)	
		minor common bile duct injury	1 (0,1%)	
Tebala [24]	4/150	bile leakage	2 (1,3%)	2,7%
		haematoma	2 (1,3%)	

Regarding biliary tract lesions, the correct visualization of Calot's triangle is not guaranteed by the technique with single umbilical access, especially if it is performed with only two instruments. The rate of conversion to open is highest in TPT, which could be due to the higher rate of patients with acute cholecystitis or pancreatitis enrolled in studies on TPT (16.1% vs 6.0%). Furthermore, in some study on LESS, acute cholecystitis has been an exclusion criterion, whereas in others it has been a reason to choose the traditional technique from the beginning.

Conclusion

The evaluation of a new technology and/or innovative surgical technique has many problems, related in part to a cultural attitude toward evidence-based surgery. Besides, some factors also bias the best randomized trial with random sampling (Figure 3). Moreover, the success of an intervention is related not only to the surgeon's skills and experience but also to the patient's characteristics (anatomical variants, the subjective perception of pain, etc.).

Diffusion of new techniques in surgery, defined as the total number of surgeons performing the technique, also is related to sociological factors. The demand of new technologies by the patients, the tendency of surgeons to meet this demand, the perception of new as progress, the marketing strategies and especially in the LESS the outlook of a scarless surgery should be the more decisive factors. The cosmetic result seems to be the main difference between LESS and TTT up till now and in the near future it should certainly be the main thrust to the wide use of LESS.

Whatever the quality of innovation, these factors cause its adoption on a large scale, thus making any attempt to objective analysis vain: "It is always too early (for rigorous evaluation) until, unfortunately, it's suddenly too late" (Buxton's law) [10].

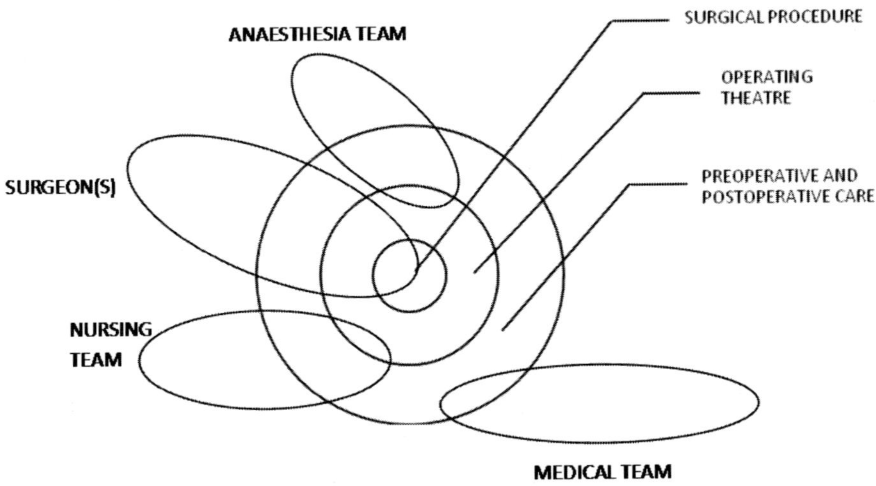

Figure 3. Factors biasing outcome of intervention [modified from [25]].

Table 4. Common challenges and solutions during single-incision laparoscopic surgery (modified from [13])

Challenges	*Solutions*
Clashing of instruments	Use of very-low-profile trocars
Lack of ideal operative ports	Staggering heights and heads of trocars
Interference and deflection of laparoscope's	Use of novel multichannel ports
light source by operating instruments	Use of a laparoscope with a light source
Interference of wires or tubing that connect	on the back of the camera
perpendicularly to instruments (i.e., cautery)	Use of a flexible-tip endoscope
Difficulty with retraction of organs or structures	Use of an extra-long 5-mm angled
Change of surgeon's mindset	laparoscope (50 cm)
Lack of time and patience to learn	Continuous medical education
Use of curved, reticulating, or flexible	
instruments	
	Potential solutions
Additional basic surgical principles	Design of innovative retracting platforms
Maintenance of equivalent operative exposure	Implementation of magnetically anchored
Low threshold for use of additional ports at the	instruments deployed though a single
initial incision site or prompt conversion to	incision
conventional laparoscopy or to open surgery	Design of sigmoid-shaped instruments

In the LESS the outlook of a scarless surgery should be the more decisive factor, despite the presence of critical elements highlighted by the some authors (Table 4). On the other hand rate of complications, although minimal, is higher in LESS and in the only prospective randomized study the more significant finding was a longer operative time for the single-incision technique.

In summary, although LESS cholecystectomy has captured the attention of general surgeons around the world there are few data available from which to make an evidence-based determination as to the real benefits of this technique. Despite the number of publications on LESS cholecystectomy, the vast majority of data available in the literature are from small case series without any comparative data. Studies on LESS show wide heterogeneity with respect to methodological quality and outcome parameters. Many publications report perioperative outcomes only and are largely composed of feasibility studies.

Evidence Based Surgery

As mentioned above, a well-designed comparative studies are desirable to validate the clinical benefits and to ensure that there are no new complications or added costs associated with a new technique. The trials should ensure the presence of few experienced surgeons and the use of same tools, technologies and surgical approach taking into account some fundamental aspects:

- in TTT the incisions are 3 or 5 mm or 1 cm as a maximum in the umbilical site, while in LESS the umbilical incision ranges from 1.5 to 2.5 cm. Against the absence of two scars up to 5 mm, in the LESS the greater umbilical incision might increase the risk of umbilical hernia with the longer operative time;
- according to some authors, the most difficult view of Calot's triangle in the LESS, due to the particular spatial relationship of the instruments, results in a further increase risk of bile ducts injuries, that in standard laparoscopic approach is already twice the open surgery;
- the use of new disposable devices in LESS could lead to higher costs;
- till now there are not complete data on safety and feasibility of both techniques in case of acute cholecystitis, especially for LESS.

References

[1]   Keus F, de Jong JA, Gooszen HG, et al. Laparoscopic versus open cholecystectomy for patients with symptomatic cholecystolithiasis *Cochrane Database Syst Rev.* 2006 Oct 18;(4):CD006231.

[2]   Lau WY, Leow CK, Li AKC History of Endoscopic and Laparoscopic Surgery *World J Surg* 1997; 21, 444 – 453.

[3]   Filipi CJ, Fitzgibbons RJ, Salerno GM Historical review: diagnostic laparoscopy to laparoscopic cholecystectomy and beyond. *Surgical Laparoscopy* 1991, pp. 3–21.

[4]   Sun S, Yang K, Gao M, He X, Tian J, Ma B. Three-Port Versus Four-Port Laparoscopic Cholecystectomy: Meta-Analysis of Randomized Clinical Trials *World J Surg* 2009; 33: 1904-8.

[5]   Reardon PR, Kamelgard JI, Applebaum B, et al. Feasibility of Laparoscopic Cholecystectomy with Miniaturized Instrumentation in 50 Consecutive Cases. *World J Surg* 1999; 23:128-132.

[6] Kumar M, Agrawal CS, Gupta RK. Three-port versus standard four-port laparoscopic cholecystectomy: a randomized controlled clinical trial in a community-based teaching hospital in eastern Nepal. *JSLS* 2007; 11: 358-62.

[7] Romanelli JR, Roshek TB 3rd, Lynn DC, Earle DB Single-port laparoscopic cholecystectomy: initial experience. *Surg Endosc* 2010; 24: 1374-9.

[8] Roberts KE, Solomon D, Duffy AJ, et al Single-incision laparoscopic cholecystectomy: a surgeon's initial experience with 56 consecutive cases and a review of the literature. *J Gastrointest Surg* 2010; 14: 506-10.

[9] Dapri G, Casali L, Dumont H, et al Single-access transumbilical laparoscopic appendectomy and cholecystectomy using new curved reusable instruments:a pilot feasibility study. *Surg Endosc* 2011; 25(4):1325-32.

[10] Barkun JS, Aronson JK, Feldman LS, et al. Evaluation and stages of surgical innovations. *Lancet.* 2009; 374(9695):1089-1096.

[11] Kuon Lee S, You YK, Park JH, et al. Single-port transumbilical laparoscopic cholecystectomy: a preliminary study in 37 patients with gallbladder disease. *J Laparoendosc Adv Surg Tech A.* 2009; 19(4):495-9.

[12] Hodgett SE, Hernandez JM, Morton CA, et al. Laparoendoscopic Single Site (LESS) Cholecystectomy. *J Gastrointest Surg.* 2009; 13:188–92.

[13] Philipp SR, Miedema BW, Thaler K. Single-incision laparoscopic cholecystectomy using conventional instruments: early experience in comparison with the gold standard. *J Am Coll Surg.* 2009; 209(5):632-7.

[14] Curcillo PG 2nd, Wu AS, Podolsky ER, et al. Single-port-access (SPA) cholecystectomy: a multi-institutional report of the first 297 cases. *Surg Endosc.* 2010; 24(8):1854-60.

[15] Edwards C, Bradshaw A, Ahearne P, Dematos P, Humble T, Johnson R, et al Single-incision laparoscopic cholecystectomy is feasible: initial experience with 80 cases. *Surg Endosc* 2010; 24: 2241-7.

[16] Hawasli A, Kandeel A, Meguid A. Single-incision laparoscopic cholecystectomy (SILC): a refined technique. *Am J Surg.* 2010; 199(3): 289-93.

[17] Roy P, De A Transumbilical multiple-port laparoscopic cholecystectomy (TUMP-LC): a prospective analysis of 50 initial patients. *J Laparoendosc Adv Surg Tech A* 2010; 20: 211-7.

[18] Rawlings A, Hodgett SE, Matthews BD, et al Single-incision laparoscopic cholecystectomy: initial experience with critical view of safety dissection and routine intraoperative cholangiography. *J Am Coll Surg.* 2010; 211(1):1-7.

[19] Elsey JK, Feliciano DV. Initial Experience with Single-Incision Laparoscopic Cholecystectomy. *J Am Coll Surg.* 2010; 210(5): 620-4.

[20] Wen KC, Lin KY, Yi Chen, et al. Feasibility of single-port laparoscopic cholecystectomy using a homemade laparoscopic port: a clinical report of 50 cases. *Surg Endosc.* 2011; 25(3):879-82.

[21] Agresta F, Trentin G, Ciardo LF, et al. Laparoscopic cholecystectomy with a three-trocar 5-mm instrument approach. *Chirurgia Italiana.* 2007; 59(3): 371-377.

[22] Al-Azawi D, Houssein N, Rayis AB, et al. Three-port versus four-port laparoscopic cholecystectomy in acute and chronic cholecystitis. *BMC Surgery.* 2007; 13:7-8.

[23] Tuveri M, Tuveri A. Laparoscopic Cholecystectomy: Complications and Conversions With the 3-Trocar Technique. *Surg Laparosc Endosc Percutan Tech.* 2007; 17(5): 380-4.

[24] Tebala GD. Colecistectomia laparoscopica con tecnica a tre trocar e sospensione percutanea della colecisti. *Chirurgia Italiana.* 2008; 60(2): 285-289.

[25] Tsimoyiannis EC, Tsimogiannis KE, Pappas-Gogos G, et al Different pain scores in single transumbilical incision laparoscopic cholecystectomy versus classic laparoscopic cholecystectomy: a randomized controlled trial. *Surg Endosc.* 2010; 24(8):1842-8.

ISBN: 978-1-62257-890-0
© 2013 Nova Science Publishers, Inc.

Chapter X

Single-Incision Laparoscopic Cholecystectomy

Takashi Okuyama, NobumiTagaya and Masatoshi Oya
First Department of Surgery,
Dokkyo Medical University Koshigaya Hospital,
Saitama, Japan

Abstract

Introduction: In general, the term of single-incision laparoscopic cholecystectomy (SILC) has become familiar with the introduction of natural orifice transluminal endoscopic surgery (NOTES) technique. NOTES needs the special surgical instruments, however, SILC can perform by ordinary laparoscopic instruments without any limitations. Therefore, SILC became an attractive surgical procedure from 2007. In fact, we had already started SILC using an abdominal wall-lift method from 1997. However, its outcomes were not acceptable compared with conventional laparoscopic techniques regarding a long operation time, insufficient operative devices and more surgical stress for surgeons. After several novel surgical instruments were introduced into the laparoscopic surgery, SILC was rapidly progressed in many surgical fields. At this time, we are performing SILC using the several new devices consisting of Endo-Grab^{TM}, MIT port^{TM} and pre-bent instruments for the purpose of the elimination of port or instruments, the reduction of clashing between the instruments and laparoscope. We report our technique of SILC and a review of the literature.

Patients and Surgical technique: SILC was performed in 74 patients (40 males, 34 females). The median age was 57 years (range, 30-86 years).The indications for surgery included gallbladder stones in 65 patients (87.7%) and polyps in 9 (12.3%). Under general anesthesia, we made a 2.5-cm skin incision at umbilicus. In pneumoperitoneum method, the incision was applied a wound retractor and a surgical glove or another devices. We used three 5-mm ports technique. In an abdominal wall-lift method, we created using the original abdominal-wall lift with a rigid bar. Two or three 5-mm ports were placed through the same umbilical incision. After retracting the gallbladder upward using an Endo-Grab^{TM}, the cystic duct and artery were divided and identified using pre-bend forceps through the MIT port^{TM} and a laparoscopic coagulating shears (LCS). The cystic artery was dissected by LCS and the cystic duct was also dissected by shears after clipping. The gallbladder was free from the liver bed using LCS. The specimen was retrieved from the umbilical wound.

Results: All procedures were completed without a conversion to open laparotomy. There were no intraoperative complications. The additional ports were required in 3 (4%) cases. The abdominal wall-lift method was changed to pneumoperitoneum in 2 cases (16.7%) out of 10 due to the difficulty of procedure. The Endo-Grab™ eliminated the retraction of the gallbladder by grasping forceps. The mean operative time was 67 min (range, 34-95 min) in the last 20 cases. The MIT port ™ and pre-bend forceps reduced the clashing between the instruments and laparoscope at the intra- and extra-peritoneal cavities. We have to be careful to injure the viscera by the hook locating at the both sides of Endo-Grab™.

Conclusion: SILC is a feasible and safe procedure under the pneumoperitoneum by experienced surgeons. The Endo-Grab™, MIT port™ and pre-bend forceps were very useful in the performance of SILC with the elimination of abdominal instruments and the reduction of clashing between the instruments and laparoscope.

Introduction

Laparoscopic surgery is one of the most significant surgical advances of the twentieth century. Since Eric Muhe performed the first laparoscopic cholecystectomy in 1985, minimally invasive surgery has begun to spread worldwide [1]. This was largely in part due to patient demands for the advantages of laparoscopic surgery, such as less pain, minimal scar, and shorter hospital stay. At present, laparoscopic surgery has become the gold standard for many operative procedures. Thus, the old adage, "the bigger the incision, the bigger the surgeon" has currently changed into "the smaller the incision, the bigger the surgeon."

As a result of the global vision of lessening the size and number of surgical incisions, one major trend has been natural orifice transluminal endoscopic surgery (NOTES). This concept implies that major intra-abdominal surgery might be performed without skin incisions. The natural orifices might provide the entry point for surgical interventions into the peritoneal cavity, thereby avoiding abdominal wall incisions.

Kalloo et al. published the first report of transgastric perineoscopy in a porcine model in 2004, which brought to light the concept of NOTES [2]. Although a substantial number of experimental and clinical NOTES reports appeared in the literature, NOTES was not an easily available alternative for the general laparoscopic surgeon. Many surgeons who searched for something new or an alternative to NOTES re-highlighted single incision laparoscopic surgery (SILS).SILS was first described by Pelosi, who performed a single-puncture laparoscopic appendectomy in 1992 [3]. Navarra et al. performed single-incision laparoscopic cholecystectomy in 1997 using two trocars through one subumbilical incision and three abdominal stay sutures to retract the gallbladder [4].

NOTES needs special surgical instruments and complicated techniques. Compared with NOTES, SILS can be performed using ordinary laparoscopic instruments. Many surgeons currently perform SILS, such as appendectomies [5], Heller myotomy [6], right hemicolectomy [7], sigmoidectomy [8], sleeve gastrectomy [9], and splenectomy [10]. We first performed single-incision laparoscopic cholecystectomy (SILC) using an abdominal-wall lift method in November 1997.

During the past two decades, technology and operative techniques have allowed for surgical procedures to be performed with fewer incisions. We have also improved our method of SILC, and we presently perform this procedure using new devices, consisting of the Endo-Grab[TM] (Virtual ports, Misgav, Israel), a pre-bent instrument (curvedinstrument, Karl Storrz-Endoskope, Tuttlingen, Germany and Adachi Industry Co., Ltd., Gifu, Japan) and a MIT port[TM] (Create Medic Co., Ltd., Yokohama, Japan). The aim of this article is to introduce our techniques of SILC and to compare our results with other reports in the literature.

Patients and Methods

Patients and Indications

From November 1997 to May 1998 (first period)and May 2009 to April 2012 (second period), 74 patients who were referred with benign gallbladder disease and whose diagnoses were routinely verified by ultrasonography, computed tomography, and magnetic resonance cholangiopancreatography (MRCP), underwent SILC in Dokkyo Medical University Koshigaya Hospital, Saitama, Japan and Horie Hospital, Gunma, Japan. For all patients, one author (NT) was part of the operating team, and the operative technique was standardized.

Initially, the exclusion criteria consisted of acute or severe cholecystitis, previous upper abdominal surgery, and body mass index (BMI) greater than 35 kg/m^2, but after several cases and improvement of surgical skills and instruments, there were no exclusion criteria for SILC.

All patients gave their informed consent for SILC; detailed information about the operative strategy of having a single incision in the abdomen with the possibility of additional incisions or conversion to an open procedure, and the difference in cost between SILC and conventional laparoscopic cholecystectomy (CLC) was provided. No patients declined SILC.

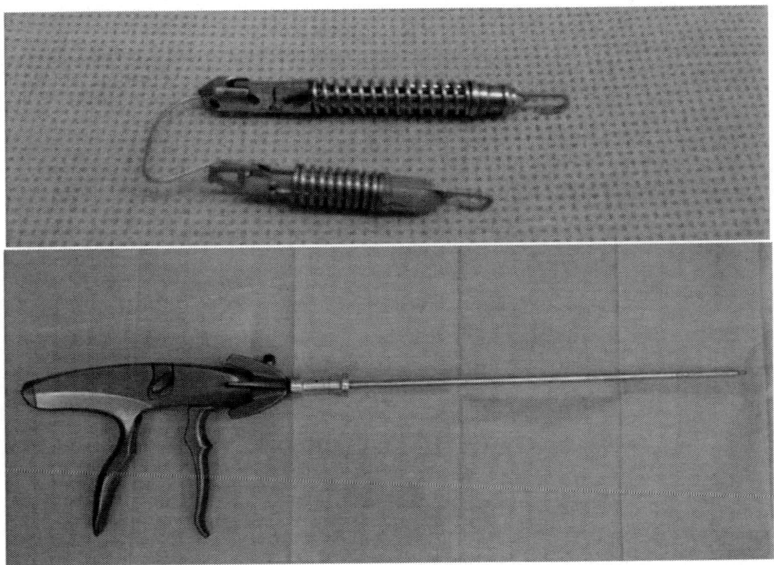

Figure 1. A. The Endo-Grab[TM]. B: The applier of Endo-Grab[TM].

Surgical Techniques

Following routine preoperative care and general anesthesia, patients were placed in the supine position with both upper extremities abducted. The surgeon stood on the left side of the patient unless he or she was left-handed. The assistant stood on the right.

The monitor was put on the right side of the patient's shoulder. A 2.5-cm, transumbilical, vertical incision was made. The linea alba and peritoneum were opened. An Alexis Wound Retractor (Applied Medical Resources Co., Rancho Santa Margarita, CA, USA) and a small surgical glove or another device were used for the single cannel. Once the glove port was in place, a MIT port[TM] and two working 5-mm ports were placed through the fingers of the glove and fixed with ties.

After establishing pneumoperitoneum, the assistant moved to the left side of the patient and manipulated the laparoscope while seated on the chair. In the abdominal-wall lift method, a stainless-steel scaffold with a lifting arm was attached to the operating table. An L-shaped stainless steel bar was inserted into the abdominal cavity through the umbilical wound and connected to the lifting arm with a chain. The right side of the abdominal wall was lifted, and the surgical field was created.

The location of the top of the L-bar must exceed the right costal marginto obtain an adequate operative field. The patient's bed was tilted to a slight reverse Trendelenburg position and 30degrees on the right side.

The camera was placed through the central trocar. A flexible5-mm laparoscope of standard length was used. Other trocars were used for pre-bent instruments, a clip applier, and an electrocautery dissection instrument (laparoscopic coagulating shears: LCS).

The Endo-Grab[TM]applier was inserted through one of the 5-mm ports, and the jaw of the grasper was opened to grasp the gallbladder. The jaw of the positionerlocated on the opposite end of the grasper was then fixed to the anterior abdominal wall. This device could achieve retraction similar to that of CLC.

After retracting the gallbladder upward using the Endo-Grab[TM], the cystic duct and artery were divided and identified using pre-bent forceps and the LCS. Then,a good viewwas obtained, and the cystic duct was clipped with a standard 5-mm clip and dissected using the LCS. The cystic artery was dissected using the LCS.

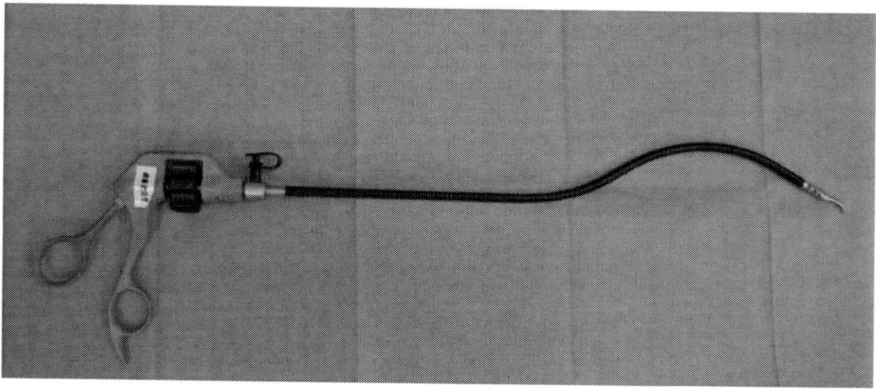

Figure 2. A pre-bend instrument (curved instrument).

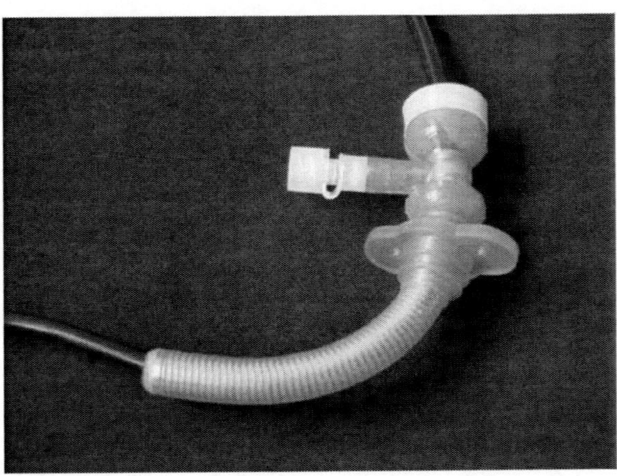

Figure 3. The MIT port[TM].

The gallbladder was then dissected off its bed using the LCS and extracted via the umbilical wound without a disposableplastic bag. Since all patients underwent preoperative MRCP, intra-operative cholangiography was not routinely performed. After ensuring satisfactory hemostasis and evacuation of the pneumoperitoneum, the glove and wound retractor were withdrawn. The fascial incision was closed with 2-0 Vicryl (Ethicon, Johnson and Johnson, New Brunswick, NJ, USA), and the skin was closed using absorbable sutures.

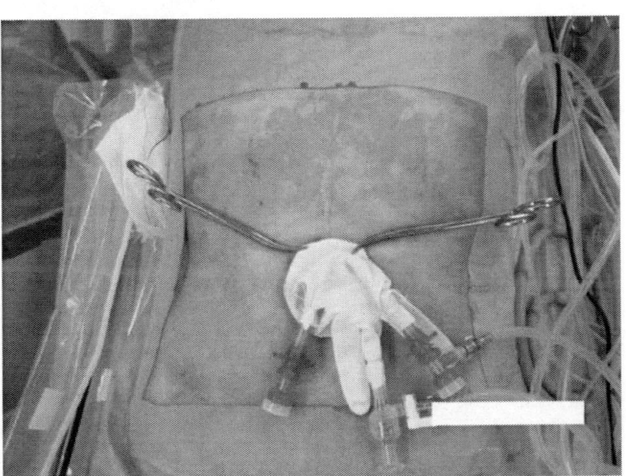

Figure 4. Hand-made single glove-port system.

Clinical Outcomes

Demographic Data

SILC was performed in 74 patients (40 males, 34 females). The median age was 57 years (range, 30-86 years). The indications for surgery included gallbladder stones in 65 patients (87.7%) and polyps in 9 (12.3%). Clinical findings of chronic cholecystitis including atrophic gallbladder and severe adhesions around the gallbladder were found in 9 patients (12.2%).

Two patients (1.4%) had acute cholecystitis after percutaneous transhepatic gallbladder drainage or aspiration. Six patients (8.1%) had previous upper abdominal operative scars after distal gastrectomy, right colectomy,or right nephrectomy. Four patients (5.4%) presented with preoperative bile duct stones, and all underwent endoscopic retrograde cholangiography and stone removal without sphincterotomy.

The operation time in the first period (6 patients) and the second period (68 patients) ranged from 167 to 220 min (median: 192min) and from 34 to 252 min (median: 89 min), respectively. Furthermore, the mean operative time was 67 min (range, 34-95 min) in the last 20 cases. The patients' BMI ranged from 21.8 to 32.4 kg/m^2, with a median of 24.8 kg/m^2. Hospital stay ranged from 2 to 5 days (median: 3 days).

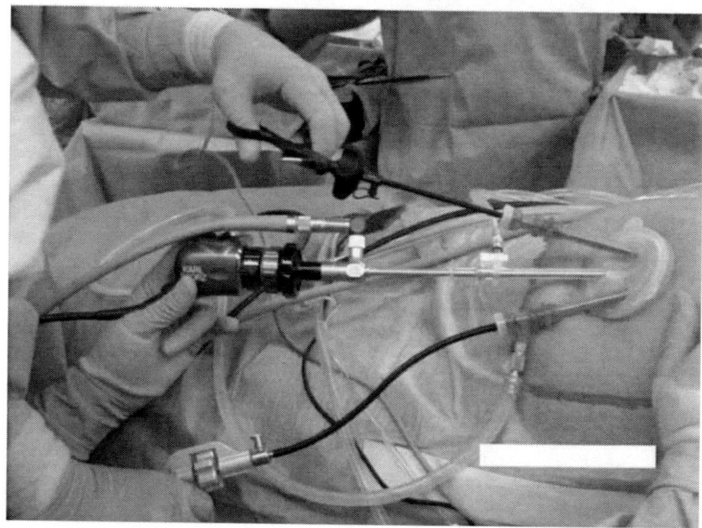

Figure 5. The external setup.

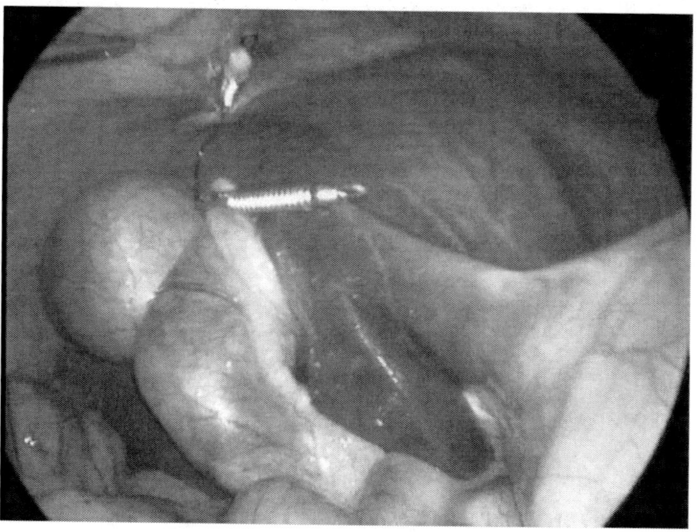

Figure 6. Enough anterior-superior retraction of gallbladder using Endo-Grab^{TM}.

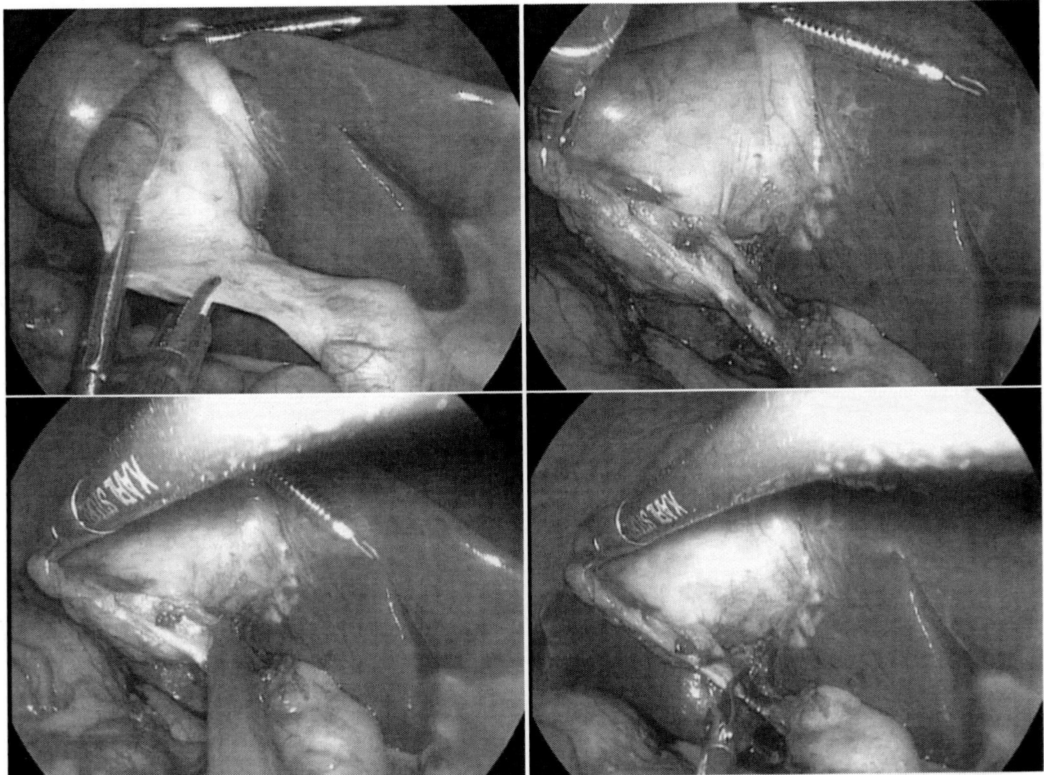

Figure 7. Intra-abdominal procedure. A: The gallbladder ampulla was grasped with a pre-bend forceps and retracted laterally and slightly upward to expose Calot's triangle. B: The cystic duct and cystic artery were verified and skeletonized effectively. C: The cystic artery was dissected using LCS. D: The cystic duct was ligated with two 5-mm clips at a point 5-mm away from the confluence of the cystic duct and the common duct, and another clip was placed as high as possible toward the gallbladder. The cystic duct was dissected using LCS or scissors.

Outcomes and Postoperative Complications

All procedures were performed without conversion to the open approach. There were no major intra- and postoperative complications related to the SILC procedure. Three patients (4.1%) required two or three additional ports to continue the cholecystectomy. The main reason for conversion to multi-port surgery was the difficulty to obtain the critical view of the triangle of Calot. SILC was performed using an abdominal-wall lifting method in 12 patients. Two patients (16.7%) were converted from the abdominal-wall lifting method to pneumoperitoneum due to poor visualization. There were no cases of hernia or infection at the umbilical incision site.

Discussion

CLC, using four abdominal incisions, is the standard operative technique for benign gallbladder disease. The technique of SILC recently emerged as a less invasive alternative to the conventional technique. Several reasons, such as a limited range of motion of the laparoscope and instruments, decreased number of ports, and the close proximity of the working instruments with limited triangulation, make the SILC technique more difficult than CLC. Despite these difficult situations, many surgeons are presently trying this technique using improved instruments and platforms as an alternative to CLC. During the early stage of our experience, we performed SILC using an original rigid bar in an abdominal-wall lift method. Although this method decreases the cardiopulmonary changes compared with the pneumoperitoneum method, visualization was poor,particularly in high-BMI patients [11]. By adapting the pneumoperitoneum method, the operative field has been well maintained throughout the procedure.

Many large healthcare manufacturers have seen this as an emerging market, and new operative hardware is being developed to facilitate the technique. Devices like the SILS port[TM] (Coviden, Norwalk, CT, USA) and Triport[TM] (Advanced Surgical Concepts, Wicklow, Ireland) have made single-site surgery easier and more efficient [12, 13]. Although we initially performed SILC using these novel ports in some cases, we currently prefer to use the glove port that consists of a surgical glove and a wound retractor. This port is not only easy and lessexpensive, but also provides similar manipulation of the instrument compared with other specially designed ports. Additionally, use of a wound retractor may avoid infection of the site incision despite extraction of the gallbladder even without an endo-bag. Although Fransen et al. reported that the wound infection rate was 1% in a review on the complications of SILC, there were no patients with incisional infection in our and other series using the glove port [14-16]. With the glove port, gas leakage at the pipes and cluttering of the instruments were reported [15]. However, the ports were placed through the fingers of the glove and fixed with ties, and air leaks were avoided. Since the external area within which the surgeon's hands are located is much smaller than in conventional laparoscopic surgery, movement of the instruments often results in inadvertent movement of an adjacent instrument, which can make even simple tasks very difficult [17]. This problem will be reduced in time with increasing experience,with increased familiarity with reverse handling of the dissector, and the introduction of new special equipment including multi-lumen ports or trocars with a low profile.

In contrast to CLC, crowding of all instruments within one incision significantly compromises the principle of triangulation, with frequent clashing between the instrument and endoscope. Additionally, visualization during SILC is inevitably obscured to some degree with in-line viewing. When using straight instruments, the laparoscope is aimed along the shaft of the instruments, rendering the tips difficult to visualize. A pre-bent forceps can avoid interference with the other straight instrument or the endoscope and help perform more meticulous dissection of Calot's triangle. The use of this articulating instrument enables local triangulation, enhances dissection capability, and improves operative viewing. Because these instruments could not pass through the usual straight ports, we used a MIT port[TM]that consisted of a flexible tube in a part of endoceliac. A MIT port[TM] makes it possible to pass a pre-bent forceps that can resolve the inherent technical problem arising from the in-line view. Although there is little experience with the use of instrumentsof different lengths, the use of a curved or different length instrument decreases the difficulty of handling and surgeon's stress. Thus, use of variable length and rigid or curved instruments should be re-evaluated to ensure patient safety. Additionally, from our own experience, the ability to manipulate with both hands enables easy and safe dissection of Calot's triangle. In the present series, no patient required conversion to open laparotomy, and only three patients required the addition of one or more ports to complete the procedure.

Several technical methods have been described with regard to gallbladder anchorage and exposure of the Calot's triangle. The two most common methods are gallbladder anchorage with two or three percutaneous sutures, and gallbladder suspension with a grasper [4, 18-20]. We also used a 2-mm instrument for retracting the gallbladder in needlescopic or needle-assistedcholecystectomy [21, 22]. Dominguez et al. described the technique of an extracorporeal magnetic retracting system with magnet forceps attached to the gallbladder [23]. We prefer the Endo-Grab^{TM}for convenience and the reduced number of ports. The Endo-Grab^{TM} is an internally anchored retracting device that can be introduced into the abdomen through a 5-mm port. Additionally, the Endo-Grab^{TM} can be displaced during the operation if it is necessary to displace it. Schlager et al. reported that use of the Endo-Grab^{TM} was safe and provided superior retraction to endoloops [24].

Regarding operation time, the median was 67 min in our last 20 cases. This is similar to other recent reports [25, 26], and these times are acceptable compared with CLC. Naturally, operation times do improve with greater experience, and the expansion of indications for SILC often increases the time. We also believe that the use of pre-bent forceps and the Endo-Grab^{TM} have influenced the operation time. However, we should not gauge the success of SILC by the absolute time for performing the procedure. Safety should always come first and never be sacrificed to do the procedure quickly.

For 3 (4.1%) of the patients, an additional port was placed to aid in the dissection, and for 4 (40%) of the 10 patients, the abdominal-wall lift method was changed to pneumoperitoneum, both due to the difficulty of the procedure.

These changes are not only acceptable but also recommended to maintain safety in aiding the surgeon with the dissection. The most feared complication after laparoscopic cholecystectomy is bile duct injury. Although the incidence of bile duct injury reported in the literature is 1.7% for patients undergoing SILC, there was neither bile duct injury nor other major complications like hemorrhage and subhepatic abscesses in the present series [13]. The dogma is that an incision located on the umbilicus has a higher risk of hernia. In the present study, no postoperative hernias occurred. In other published reports that focused on postoperative incisional hernia in SILC, incisional hernia was rare [14, 27, 28].

Qie et al. concluded that a 2.5-cm trans-umbilical incision provideseasy exposure of every anatomical layer; thus, the layer could be a sutured layer [28]. However, due to the fact that we and other authors had short follow-up periods, we would approach these results with caution.

Conclusion

In selected patients with a low risk of adhesions or technical difficulty, SILC can be an acceptable alternative to CLC. SILC may produce several advantages for the patient compared to CLC, such as less postoperative pain, a better cosmetic result, and a shorter hospital stay. In the present study, there were some drawbacks, such as the small number of patients and selection bias. Nevertheless, SILC was shown to be feasible and safe. Although there are many reports of the safety and positive outcomes of SILC, surgeons should tend toward careful selection of low-risk or healthier patients in need of a cholecystectomy for SILC, in particular when a new technique is used. Based on our experience, a MIT port^{TM}, a pre-bent forceps, and use of the Endo-Grab^{TM} transform SILC, making it safer and more feasible.

This study declares no conflicts of interest.

Reference

[1] Reynold W. The first laparoscopic cholecystectomy. *JSLS* 5: 89-94, 2001.

[2] Kalloo AN, Singh VK, Jagannath SB, Niiyama H, Hill SL, VaughnCA, Magee CA, Kantsevoy SV. Flexible transgastricperitoneoscopy: a novel approach to diagnostic and therapeutic interventions in the peritoneal cavity. *Gastrointest Endosc.* 60: 114-117, 2004.

[3] Pelosi MA, Pelosi MAIII. Laparoscopic appendectomy using a single umbilical puncture (minilaparoscopy). *J. Reprod. Med.* 37: 588-594, 1992.

[4] Navarra G, Pozza E, Occhionorelli S, Carcoforo P, Donini I. One-wound laparoscopic cholecystectomy. *Br. J. Surg.* 84: 695, 1997.

[5] Vidal O, Valentini M, Ginesa C, et al. Laparoscopic single-site surgery appendectomy. *Surg. Endosc.* 24: 686-691, 2010.

[6] Saba SC, Curcillo PG. Single-port access (SPA) surgery: intracorporeal liver retractor for SPA Heller myotomy. *Surg. Endosc.* 22 (Suppl 1): S 285.

[7] Remzi FH, Kirat HT, Kaouk JH, Geisler DP. Single-port laparoscopy in colorectal surgery. *Colorectal. Dis.* 10: 823-826, 2008.

[8] Leroy J, Cahill RA, Peretta S, Marescaux J. Single port sigmoidectomy in an experimental model with survival. *Surg. Innov.* 15: 260-265, 2008.

[9] Saber AA, Elgamal MH, Itawi EA, Rao AJ. Single incision laparoscopic sleeve gastrectomy (SILS): a novel technique. *Obes. Surg.* 18: 1628-1631, 2008.

[10] Targarona EM, Lima MB, Balague C, Trias M. Single-port splenectomy: current update and controversies. *J. Mini Access Surg.* 7: 61-64, 2011.

[11] Gurusamy KS, Samraj K, Davidson BR. Abdominal lift for laparoscopic clolecystectomy. *Cochrane Database Syst. Rev.* (2): CD006574, 2008.

[12] Roberts KE, Solomon D, Duffy AJ, et al. Single-incision laparoscopic cholecystectomy: a surgeon's initial experience with 56 consecutive cases and a review of the literature. *J. Gastrointest. Surg.* 14: 506-510, 2010.

[13] Rao PP, Bhagwat SM, Rane A, Rao PP. The feasibility of single-port laparoscopic cholecystectomy: a pilot study of 20 cases. HPB Oxford 10: 336-340, 2008.

[14] Fransen S, Stassen L, Bouvy N. Single incision laparoscopic cholecystectomy: A review on the complications. *J. Minim. Access Surg.* 8: 1-5, 2012.

[15] Hong TH, You YK, Lee KH. Transumbilical single-port laparoscopic cholecystectomy. *Surg. Endosc.* 23: 1393-1397, 2009.

[16] Barband A, Fakhree MBA, Kakaei F, Daryani A. Single-incision laparoscopic cholecystectomy using glove port in comparison with standard laparoscopic

cholecystectomy SILC using glove port. *Surg. Laparosco. Endosc. Percutan. Tech.* 22: 17-20, 2012.

[17]　Romanelli JR, Earle DB. Single-port laparoscopic surgery: an overview. *Surg. Endosc.* 23: 1419-1427, 2009.

[18]　Philipp SR, Miedema BW, Thaler K. Single-incision laparoscopic cholecystectomy using conventional instruments: early experience in comparison with the gold standard. *J. Am. Coll Surg.* 209: 623-637, 2009.

[19]　Chow A, Purkayastha S, Aziz O, et al. Single-incision laparoscopic surgery for cholecystectomy: an evolving technique. *Surg. Endosc.* 24: 709-714, 2010.

[20]　Hirano Y, Watanabe T, Uchida T, Yoshida S, Tawaraya K, Kato H, Hosokawa O. Single-incision laparoscopic cholecystectomy: Single institution experience and literature review. *World J. Gastroenterol.* 16: 270-274, 2010.

[21]　Tagaya N, Rokkaku K, Kubota K. Needlescopic cholecystectomy versus needlescope assisted laparoscopic cholecystectomy. *Surg. Laparosc. Endosc. Percutan. Tech.* 17: 375-379, 2007.

[22]　Tagaya N, Kubota K. Reevaluation of needlescopic surgery. *Surg. Endosc.* 26: 137-143, 2012.

[23]　Dominguez G, Durand L, De Rosa J, Danguise E, Arozamena C, Ferraina PA. Retraction and triangulation with neodymium magnetic forceps for single-port laparocopic cholecystectomy. *Surg. Endosc.* 23: 1660-1666, 2009.

[24]　Schlager A, Khalailth A, Shussman N, Elazary R, Keidar A, Pikarsky AJ, Shibolt O, Horgan S, Talamini M, Zamir G, Rivkind AI, Mintz Y. Providing more through less: current methods of retraction in SIMIS and NOTES cholecystectomy. *Surg. Endosc.* 24: 1542-1546, 2010.

[25]　Hawasli A, Kandeel A, Meguid A. Single-incision laparoscopic cholecystectomy (SILC) : a refined technique. *Am. J. Surg.* 199: 289-293, 2010.

[26]　Raakow R, Jacob DA. Single-incision cholecystectomy in about 200 patients. *Minim. Invasive Surg.* 2011: 915735.

[27]　Curcillo II PG, Wu AS, Podolsky ER, Graybeal CG, Katkhouda N, Saenz A, Dunham R, Fendley S, Neff M, Copper C, Bessler M, Gumbs AA, Norton M, Iannelli A, Mason R, Moazzez A, Cohen L, Mouhhlas A, Poor A. Single-port-access (SPATM) cholecystectomy: a multiple-institutional report of the first 297 cases. *Surg. Endosc.* 24: 1854-60, 2010.

[28]　Qie Z, Sun Y, Pu Ying, Jiang T, Cao J, Wu W. Learning curve of transumbilical single incision laparoscopic cholecystectomy (SILS): A preliminary study of 80 selected patients with benign gallbladder diseases. *World J. Surg.* 35: 2092-2101, 2011.

ISBN: 978-1-62257-890-0
© 2013 Nova Science Publishers, Inc.

Chapter XI

Single Incision Cholecystectomy: Moving towards Less Invasive Approaches While Maintaining Patient Safety

***Camille D. Blackledge and Melissa S. Phillips**[*]*
University of Tennessee Graduate School of Medicine, Knoxville,
Tennessee, US

Abstract

Laparoscopic cholecystectomy has been accepted by the surgical community as the "standard of care" for the treatment of biliary disease. When compared to open cholecystectomy, laparoscopic approaches do carry a higher complication rate for biliary injury but offer many beneficial advantages in reduced postoperative pain and shorter recovery times. With the introduction of single incision approaches to cholecystectomy, it is important that the surgical community maintain similar operative standards as these new techniques are introduced into clinical practice. This article will focus on the outcomes and complications of laparoscopic cholecystectomy as well as ways to reduce these potential injuries. The role for intraoperative cholangiography will also be addressed. It will also analyze the available data regarding single incision cholecystectomy with regards to advantages and potential complications from this new and evolving operative technique.

The first cholecystectomy was performed by Dr. Carl Langenbuch in 1882 [1] and, since that time, surgical therapy for the treatment of gallbladder diseases has become the mainstay of treatment. Open cholecystectomy offers a reliable, safe therapy with a low complication profile. When laparoscopic cholecystectomy was first reported by Dr. Eric Mühe in 1985 [2], the concept of minimally invasive approaches in the treatment of gallbladder disease was

---

[*] Corresponding Author/Contact Information: Melissa S. Phillips, MD. University Surgeons Associates, PC, 1930 Alcoa Highway, Suite 240, Knoxville, TN 37920. (865) 305-9620; Phillips.Melissa@gmail.com

initially met with hesitation. When compared to open cholecystectomy, LC has been associated with improved cosmesis, shorter hospital stay, and faster return to normal activities [3] but these positive outcomes are offset by an increased rate of biliary complications [4]. Over the past 25 years, however, laparoscopic cholecystectomy (LC) has established itself as the "gold standard" for the treatment of cholelithiasis, acute and chronic cholecystitis, and biliary dyskinesia.

As surgeons have gained more experience with laparoscopic equipment and technique, there has been an increased interest in even more minimally invasive approaches, including the idea of natural orifice surgery and single incision approaches. It was postulated that single incision laparoscopic cholecystectomy (SILC) could offer better cosmetic outcome as well as less postoperative pain [5] when compared to the traditional four port approach. These efforts led to the first single incision laparoscopic cholecystectomy described by Navarro et al in 1997 [6] in a population of 30 patients. This technique is gaining popularity with both patients and surgeons, but the literature to support the benefits of this approach remains in its infancy. At the time of this chapter, there have been thirteen randomized controlled trials comparing SILC and LC [7-19] published in the literature. As it true with the introduction of any new surgical technique, SILC must meet the standards that the surgical community holds for the safety and efficacy of LC while adding benefit above the accepted "gold standard."

Open cholecystectomy was the primary surgical options for almost a century. It offered a low complication profile and a low rate of biliary injury, averaging 0.2-0.3% [20-22]. When laparoscopic techniques for cholecystectomy where introduced, the surgical community was forced to evaluate this new operative approach with regards to outcomes and complications. Many large studies [20, 23-25] have shown LC to have less post operative pain, shorter recovery periods, faster return to work, and shorter hospital stays. The trade off for these benefits was seen initially as a higher rate of biliary complications. This was reported initially as high as 0.9% but has decreased with the learning curve of this new technique, now commonly accepted at 0.6% [26]. In 1992, the National Institute of Health published a consensus [27] of multidisciplinary experts regarding surgical treatment for biliary disease. This consensus summarized the literature, without a large randomized controlled trial comparing open and laparoscopic techniques, and established LC as the "gold standard" as it reduced pain and disability after cholecystectomy. The increase in the risk of biliary complications remains an accepted risk for the advantages offered by the laparoscopic approach in the eyes of most surgeons today.

With the exception of the incision, the technical aspects of the SILC are similar to those of a conventional LC. The traditional laparoscopic cholecystectomy is described as a four port technique with the camera port is placed at the umbilicus with the other three working ports in a subcostal position. This configuration allows for triangulation of working instruments and thus adequate visualization during dissection. Most commonly for SILC, a single skin incision is placed at the umbilicus and either a specialized single incision port device (available from multiple commercial vendors) or multiple standard laparoscopic trocars (three 5 mm ports or one 10 mm port and two 5 mm ports) are inserted through separate fascial incisions within the umbilical skin incision.

The working instruments are placed inside the abdomen, and the gallbladder hilum is dissected using the surgeon's instrument of choice. The cystic duct and artery are carefully dissected in order to adequately expose the triangle of Calot. Visualization of the "critical view of safety" (CVS) [28] should be a requirement for all multi- or single port cholecystectomies as this decreases the possibility of anatomic misidentification and, thus, injury to the common bile duct. If an intraoperative cholangiogram (IOC) is performed, it is completed at this time. After identification of biliary anatomy, gallstones, or other biliary pathology, the cystic duct and artery are ligated and cut using laparoscopic scissors. The gallbladder is dissected from the liver bed using either sharp dissection, electrocautery, or an ultrasonic scalpel. The gallbladder is removed through the 10 mm port site or through the single incision port site. The fascia and skin are closed at the discretion of the surgeon with the authors of this text preferring an interrupted, absorbable suture on fascia and an absorbable, subcuticular suture at the skin.

One concern regarding the use of SILC is the lack of triangulation and, thus, inadequate visualization of the CVS. In the original technique described by Navarra [6], three sutures were placed through the top of the fundus, neck, and infundibulum to provide exposure of the triangle of Calot. Others [5] have described the use of a single, transabdominal suture through the dome of the gallbladder to provide the equivalent retraction of the missing instrument. In addition to the placement of sutures which increase the risk for bile leakage during the procedure, the use of a flexible tip laparoscope, instruments with different lengths, and/or instruments with articulating tips have been described [29] with the hope of improving visualization.

In a study of 54 patients, Rawlings et al [30] demonstrated the feasibility in obtaining the CVS and maintaining the basic principles of dissection during SILC. In that report, 92% of patients also underwent successful intraoperative cholangiography using a needle puncture technique. As this new approach for cholecystectomy is introduced, it is essential that surgeons maintain their current standards for identification of biliary anatomy and do not compromise on the safety of this operation.

One challenge is how to teach this new technique to practicing surgeons. When laparoscopic cholecystectomy was determined to be the standard of care, the NIH consensus panel [27] also clarified that surgeons should be properly trained and credentialed in this technique before introduction into practice. Training surgeons in the techniques of SILC has also raised similar questions. Muller et al [31] advocate the avoidance of the traditional Halstedian model, but rather the use of a formal team-based proficiency training. The authors consider the precision and technical skills needed to manage interactions between instruments, which are controlled by different operating team members, beyond a level that can be learned under an apprentice model. Khandelwal et al [32] have developed a defined training algorithm for single incision laparoscopy including both inanimate and animal-based simulation modules, a supervised clinical introduction, and review of early outcomes with plans for improvement of the training process.

When looking at SILC specifically, the learning curve reported for proficiency in the literature covers a broad range, from 5-20 cases [33, 34]. In these, proficiency is defined as normalization of the operative time to that equivalent to standard LC. Others [35] have defined proficiency not only in terms of operative time but have also included the point of proficiency to have no increased rate of additional trocar placements or conversion to open surgery. In a prospective study of 150 patients, this study separated patient outcomes into groups of 25 patients, demonstrating similar conversion and complication rates above the initial 25 cases. Additionally, the authors showed a significant decrease in operative time after the completion of 75 SILC cases.

The steep learning curve associated with SILC is mainly due to technical limitations. The restricted working area creates several obstacles that a surgeon must overcome to complete the procedure including collision of instruments, inadequate triangulation, a compromised field of view, and inadequate exposure/retraction [36, 37]. Laparoscopic instruments share an access point, and this confinement of the fascial entry can cause external and internal collision between instruments and the laparoscope. This "sword fighting" is due to the instruments being in-line as opposed to triangulated. The obstacles of colliding instruments can be overcome by the use of internal retraction, shorter ports, and different length instruments as well as angled, or articulating instruments. Angled or flexible-tip laparoscopes can provide a better field of view. The instruments chosen for retraction can potentially limit the ease with which the critical view can be obtained. Intra-abdominal retractors have the advantage of changing angles of exposure as compared to static extraperitoneal suture placement. Strategic placement of retracting sutures or instruments can aid in providing adequate exposure when intra-abdominal options are costly or unavailable. Again, it is essential that the surgeon be willing to place an additional trocar or convert to a standard laparoscopic approach is he or she cannot get adequate exposure for safe visualization of the anatomy.

As expected, when introducing a new technology, patient selection can make a significant difference on the outcomes. Only two [14, 16] of the 13 published randomized controlled trials have allowed inclusion of patients with a diagnosis of cholecystitis. When looking at body mass index, some authors [9, 16, 17] have limited patient enrollment to SILC to those less than 30 kg/m^2, while others [11, 12] have had less stringent enrollment, allowing BMI up to 45 kg/m^2. Other relative contraindications for SILC include previous open intra-abdominal surgery, pancreatitis, cholangitis, choledocholithiasis, a high ASA score, and suspicion for gallbladder cancer [36-38]. As surgeons gain experience with SILC, the inclusion criteria is expanding to include patients with more complex biliary disease and previously perceived contraindications may no longer be applicable.

Complications of SILC are similar to those of laparoscopic surgery as well as complications related to laparoscopic cholecystectomy and are reported in the literature to be around 5% [39]. Complications related to laparoscopy include intra-abdominal injuries secondary to trocar placement, deep venous thrombosis, need for placement of additional ports, conversion to open celiotomy, trocar site hernia formation, and postoperative wound infection. More serious complications related to cholecystectomy include common bile duct injury with either stricture or leak formation, retained common bile duct stones, injury to or bleeding from hepatic artery and/or portal vein, and inability to adequately visualize proper anatomy.

The largest meta-analysis [40] of the above mentioned 13 randomized controlled trials, containing 892 patients from 12 individual trials, showed no difference in length of hospitalization, postoperative pain, postoperative complication rate, and conversion rate. There was a significant increase in operative length and patient satisfaction scores associated with SILC. These findings were also confirmed by a study by Markar et al [38] who also found no differences in postoperative pain, length of hospital stay, or post-operative complications. Some of the individual randomized trials, however, have shown a statistical difference in complication rates between SILC and LC. Garg et al [41] reported an increase in the rates of seroma formation with 17% in SILC and 0% in LC while we [11] reported an increase in wound complications with 10% in SILC compared to 3% in LC. In continued follow up from that published data, our group has also found a difference in hernia formation with an increase in SILC at 8% when compared to LC at 1% [unpublished data].

When addressing the possible complication profile of SILC, some authors [42, 43] have advocated caution with the widespread introduction of this technique given an increase in biliary complication rate when compared to historic controls. Many of the SILC cases have had strict inclusion criteria, excluding acute cholecystitis which is a known factor for biliary leak [44]. Because the outcomes are currently reported for this more ideal population, one must consider the possibility that a selection bias is masking an increased complication rate when this technique is applied to the general population.

Routine versus selective intraoperative cholangiography (IOC) continues to be a controversial discussion in regards to laparoscopic cholecystectomy. Due the increase in bile duct injury with the use of laparoscopic cholecystectomy, the argument has been made that the use of intraoperative cholangiography can decrease the number of injuries by allowing identification of biliary anatomy. Advantages of IOC include confirmation of biliary anatomy, identification of stones, and identification of common bile duct injury. Disadvantages of IOC include increased operative time, exposure to radiation, additional costs, and false positives resulting in unnecessary procedures. Typically, indications for selective IOC includes, but is not limited to elevated liver enzymes, jaundice, preoperative evidence of common bile duct dilation, choledocholithiasis, or abnormal intraoperative anatomy [45].

A study by Debru et al [46] supported the use of IOC in identifying common bile duct injuries, however, it did not demonstrate a decrease in common bile duct injury (CBDI). In this prospective study of 3145 patients, use of routine cholangiography identified intraoperative CBDI at a rate of 0.16%, similar to the historic controls cited above. When identified and repaired intraoperatively, CBDI repair may have the advantage of less inflammation and contamination and, thus, may be a less complex undertaking than delayed repair. Other retrospective studies support the use of cholangiography in decreasing the incidence of common bile duct injuries. Waage et al [47] showed a 34% decrease in the risk of common bile duct injury with the use of IOC. Flum et al [48], in a study of over 1.5 million cholecystectomies, reported a decrease in CBDI from 0.58% without IOC to 0.39% with IOC and this difference persisted even after adjustment for both patient and surgeon specific factors. In this group of 40210 physicians, only 21.5% performed routine IOC, defined as >75% of cases. This study further demonstrated a decrease in CBDI with increased use of IOC by surgeons. A meta-analysis [49] of prospective, randomized trials comparing the use of IOC in laparoscopic cholecystectomy failed to demonstrate a statistically significant decrease in the rate of common bile duct injury with the use of IOC, but was limited by a small study population of only 1715 patients with two cases of CBDI. Although not supported by a large, prospective randomized controlled trial, the authors feel that the retrospective evidence [50] available supports the use of routine intraoperative cholangiography, which is our standard practice. Literature supports the use of intraoperative cholangiography in SILC, when deemed appropriate by the operating surgeon [37, 43]. Whether using selective or routine IOC, surgeons should still maintain basic principles of dissection and obtain the critical view of safety to define intra-abdominal anatomy.

The currently accepted gold standard of laparoscopic cholecystectomy sets a high bar for the surgical treatment of gallbladder disease. When compared to open cholecystectomy, the standard laparoscopic approach offers a short recovery period, short length of stay, improved cosmesis, and a low complication profile. Because of these high standards for comparison, the introduction of a new surgical technique, specifically SILC, the standards of safety and technical proficiency must be maintained. Single incision laparoscopic cholecystectomy has been proven to be technically feasible for the treatment of uncomplicated gallbladder disease. Further studies are needed to demonstrate the universal applicability of SILC in a more complex patient population. With regards to long term follow-up, there is still limited data available. As wide spread introduction with regards to the learning curve of this new approach occurs, surgeons must continue to follow closely the surgical outcomes. It is essential that, with the introduction of a new technique including SILC, surgeons maintain established the surgical principles of dissection and obtaining the critical view of safety as the foundation for a safe cholecystectomy. There should be no compromise on safety, including the use of cholangiography, following introduction of a new approach. Training modules and courses regarding single incision technique will be an important step in the wide-spread introduction of SILC to assure that surgeons are familiar and well

References

[1] Sparkman, R.S., 100th anniversary of the first cholecystectomy. *Arch Surg,* 1982. *117*(12): p. 1525.

[2] Reynolds, W., Jr., The first laparoscopic cholecystectomy. *JSLS,* 2001. *5*(1): p. 89-94.

[3] Nagle A, S.N., Laparoscopic cholecystectomy and choledocholithotomy. *Blumgart's surgery of the liver,* 5th ed. Jarnagin WR, Blumgart LH. Eds. 5th ed. Elsevier. Philadelphia., 2012. *Ch34*: p. 511-531.

[4] Targarona, E.M., et al., How, when, and why bile duct injury occurs. A comparison between open and laparoscopic cholecystectomy. *Surg Endosc,* 1998. *12*(4): p. 322-6.

[5] Elsey, J.K. and D.V. Feliciano, Initial experience with single-incision laparoscopic cholecystectomy. *J Am Coll Surg. 210*(5): p. 620-4, 624-6.

[6] Navarra, G., et al., One-wound laparoscopic cholecystectomy. *Br J Surg,* 1997. *84*(5): p. 695.

[7] Asakuma, M., et al., Impact of single-port cholecystectomy on postoperative pain. *Br J Surg. 98*(7): p. 991-5.

[8] Lai, E.C., et al., Prospective randomized comparative study of single incision laparoscopic cholecystectomy versus conventional four-port laparoscopic cholecystectomy. *Am J Surg. 202*(3): p. 254-8.

[9] Tsimoyiannis, E.C., et al., Different pain scores in single transumbilical incision laparoscopic cholecystectomy versus classic laparoscopic cholecystectomy: a randomized controlled trial. *Surg Endosc. 24*(8): p. 1842-8.

[10] Marks, J., et al., Prospective randomized controlled trial of traditional laparoscopic cholecystectomy versus single-incision laparoscopic cholecystectomy: report of preliminary data. *Am J Surg. 201*(3): p. 369-72; discussion 372-3.

[11] Phillips, M.S., et al., Intermediate results of a prospective randomized controlled trial of traditional four-port laparoscopic cholecystectomy versus single-incision laparoscopic cholecystectomy. *Surg Endosc. 26*(5): p. 1296-303.

[12]   Sinan, H., et al., Single-incision laparoscopic cholecystectomy versus laparoscopic cholecystectomy: a prospective randomized study. *Surg Laparosc Endosc Percutan Tech.* 22(1): p. 12-6.

[13]   Lee, P.C., et al., Randomized clinical trial of single-incision laparoscopic cholecystectomy versus minilaparoscopic cholecystectomy. *Br J Surg.* 97(7): p. 1007-12.

[14]   Bucher, P., et al., Randomized clinical trial of laparoendoscopic single-site versus conventional laparoscopic cholecystectomy. *Br J Surg.* 98(12): p. 1695-702.

[15]   Lirici, M.M., et al., Laparo-endoscopic single site cholecystectomy versus standard laparoscopic cholecystectomy: results of a pilot randomized trial. *Am J Surg.* 202(1): p. 45-52.

[16]   Cao, Z.G., et al., Randomized clinical trial of single-incision versus conventional laparoscopic cholecystectomy: short-term operative outcomes. *Surg Laparosc Endosc Percutan Tech.* 21(5): p. 311-3.

[17]   Aprea, G., et al., Laparoendoscopic single site (LESS) versus classic video-laparoscopic cholecystectomy: a randomized prospective study. *J Surg Res.* 166(2): p. e109-12.

[18]   Zheng, M., M. Qin, and H. Zhao, Laparoendoscopic single-site cholecystectomy: a randomized controlled study. *Minim Invasive Ther Allied Technol.* 21(2): p. 113-7.

[19]   Ma, J., et al., Randomized controlled trial comparing single-port laparoscopic cholecystectomy and four-port laparoscopic cholecystectomy. *Ann Surg.* 254(1): p. 22-7.

[20]   A prospective analysis of 1518 laparoscopic cholecystectomies. The Southern Surgeons Club. *N Engl J Med*, 1991. 324(16): p. 1073-8.

[21]   Giger, U., et al., Bile duct injury and use of cholangiography during laparoscopic cholecystectomy. *Br J Surg.* 98(3): p. 391-6.

[22]   Nuzzo, G., et al., Bile duct injury during laparoscopic cholecystectomy: results of an Italian national survey on 56 591 cholecystectomies. *Arch Surg*, 2005. 140(10): p. 986-92.

[23]   Soper, N.J., et al., Laparoscopic cholecystectomy. The new 'gold standard'? *Arch Surg*, 1992. 127(8): p. 917-21; discussion 921-3.

[24]   Cuschieri, A., et al., The European experience with laparoscopic cholecystectomy. *Am J Surg*, 1991. 161(3): p. 385-7.

[25]   Schirmer, B.D., et al., Laparoscopic cholecystectomy. Treatment of choice for symptomatic cholelithiasis. *Ann Surg*, 1991. 213(6): p. 665-76; discussion 677.

[26]   Diamantis, T., et al., Bile duct injuries associated with laparoscopic and open cholecystectomy: an 11-year experience in one institute. *Surg Today*, 2005. 35(10): p. 841-5.

[27]   Gallstones and laparoscopic cholecystectomy. *NIH Consens Statement*, 1992. 10(3): p. 1-28.

[28]   Strasberg, S.M., Avoidance of biliary injury during laparoscopic cholecystectomy. *J. Hepatobiliary Pancreat Surg*, 2002. 9(5): p. 543-7.

[29]   Gumbs, A.A., et al., Totally transumbilical laparoscopic cholecystectomy. *J. Gastrointest Surg*, 2009. 13(3): p. 533-4.

[30] Rawlings, A., et al., Single-incision laparoscopic cholecystectomy: initial experience with critical view of safety dissection and routine intraoperative cholangiography. *J. Am. Coll Surg. 211*(1): p. 1-7.

[31] Muller, E.M., et al., Training for laparoendoscopic single-site surgery (LESS). *Int J Surg. 8*(1): p. 64-8.

[32] Khandelwal, S., et al., Single-incision laparoscopy: training, techniques, and safe introduction to clinical practice. *J Laparoendosc Adv Surg Tech* A. *21*(8): p. 687-93.

[33] Kravetz, A.J., et al., The learning curve with single-port cholecystectomy. *JSLS*, 2009. *13*(3): p. 332-6.

[34] Qiu, Z., et al., Learning curve of transumbilical single incision laparoscopic cholecystectomy (SILS): a preliminary study of 80 selected patients with benign gallbladder diseases. *World J Surg. 35*(9): p. 2092-101.

[35] Hernandez, J., et al., The learning curve of laparoendoscopic single-site (LESS) cholecystectomy: definable, short, and safe. J Am Coll Surg. *211*(5): p. 652-7.

[36] Shussman, N., et al., Single-incision laparoscopic cholecystectomy: lessons learned for success. *Surg Endosc. 25*(2): p. 404-7.

[37] Rivas, H., E. Varela, and D. Scott, Single-incision laparoscopic cholecystectomy: initial evaluation of a large series of patients. *Surg Endosc. 24*(6): p. 1403-12.

[38] Markar, S.R., et al., Single-incision laparoscopic surgery (SILS) vs. conventional multiport cholecystectomy: systematic review and meta-analysis. *Surg Endosc. 26*(5): p. 1205-13.

[39] Roberts, K.E., et al., Single-incision laparoscopic cholecystectomy: a surgeon's initial experience with 56 consecutive cases and a review of the literature. *J Gastrointest Surg. 14*(3): p. 506-10.

[40] Pisanu, A., et al., Meta-analysis of Prospective Randomized Studies Comparing Single-Incision Laparoscopic Cholecystectomy (SILC) and Conventional Multiport Laparoscopic Cholecystectomy (CMLC). *J Gastrointest Surg.*

[41] Garg, P., et al., A Prospective Controlled Trial Comparing Single-incision and Conventional Laparoscopic Cholecystectomy: Caution Before Damage Control. *Surg Laparosc Endosc Percutan Tech. 22*(3): p. 220-5.

[42] Joseph, M., et al., Single incision laparoscopic cholecystectomy is associated with a higher bile duct injury rate: a review and a word of caution. *Ann Surg. 256*(1): p. 1-6.

[43] Fransen, S., L. Stassen, and N. Bouvy, Single incision laparoscopic cholecystectomy: A review on the complications. *J Minim Access Surg. 8*(1): p. 1-5.

[44] Antonopoulos, C., et al., Bile leaks after cholecystectomy: the significance of patient selection. *Surg Laparosc Endosc Percutan Tech,* 2009. *19*(5): p. 379-83.

[45] Nickkholgh, A., S. Soltaniyekta, and H. Kalbasi, Routine versus selective intraoperative cholangiography during laparoscopic cholecystectomy: a survey of 2,130 patients undergoing laparoscopic cholecystectomy. *Surg Endosc,* 2006. *20*(6): p. 868-74.

[46] Debru, E., et al., Does routine intraoperative cholangiography prevent bile duct transection? *Surg Endosc,* 2005. *19*(4): p. 589-93.

[47] Waage, A. and M. Nilsson, Iatrogenic bile duct injury: a population-based study of 152 776 cholecystectomies in the Swedish Inpatient Registry. *Arch Surg,* 2006. *141*(12): p. 1207-13.

[48] Flum, D.R., et al., Intraoperative cholangiography and risk of common bile duct injury during cholecystectomy. *JAMA*, 2003. *289*(13): p. 1639-44.

[49] Ford, J.A., et al., Systematic review of intraoperative cholangiography in cholecystectomy. *Br J Surg*. 99(2): p. 160-7.

[50] Buddingh, K.T., et al., Intraoperative assessment of biliary anatomy for prevention of bile duct injury: a review of current and future patient safety interventions. *Surg Endosc*. 25(8): p. 2449-61.

ISBN: 978-1-62257-890-0
© 2013 Nova Science Publishers, Inc.

Chapter XII

Laparoscopic Single Site Cholecystectomy: Preparation, Procedure, and Outcomes

Angel M. Rodriguez[1] and Andrew A. Gumbs[2]
[1]Department of Surgery, Mercy Catholic Medical Center,
Philadelphia, PA, US
[2]Department of Surgical Oncology,
Summit Medical Group, Berkeley Heights, NJ, US

Abstract

Several case series have been published demonstrating the feasibility of single site laparoscopic cholecystectomy in both the adult and pediatric population with satisfactory results. The advantage of the procedure, as compared to traditional multi-port laparoscopic cholecystectomy, is to achieve better cosmesis and decrease post-operative pain. Several reports have addressed the outcomes and complication rates, reporting the safety and feasibility of the procedure. This chapter describes preoperative preparation, instrumentation and details of the procedure. Also, it discusses the outcomes and complication rates of laparoscopic single site cholecystectomy as compared to multi-port laparoscopic cholecystectomy. Being cosmetically superior with comparable outcomes to multi-port laparoscopic cholecystectomy, the single site approach can be easily performed with standard laparoscopic instruments and techniques.

Introduction

The first cholecystectomy was performed in 1882 [1] and more than a hundred years later, in 1985, Muhe performed the first laparoscopic cholecystectomy [2]. However, it was not until 1992, when a consensus was reached making the laparoscopic approach the treatment of choice for benign gallbladder disease [3]. Nowadays, laparoscopic cholecystectomy has become the "gold standard treatment" for gallbladder disease, even for the treatment of malignancy [4].

Table 1. Reported mean BMI in published series

Study	Mean BMI
Cuesta [6]	23
Chow [7]	26.5
Dominguez [8]	28
Hernandez [9]	29
Hong [10]	25.2
Kirschniak [11]	27.8
Kravetz [12]	30.2
Kuon Lee [13]	22.3
Rivas [14]	29.8
Roberts [15]	30.2
Romanelli [16]	32.7
Schlager [17]	27
Tacchino [18]	30
Brody [19]	29.2
Ersin [20]	26.5

Single site laparoscopic cholecystectomy was first described by Navarra, et al. in 1995 with a series of 30 patients [5]. Since then several case series have been published demonstrating the feasibility of the procedure in both the adult and pediatric population. The proposed advantages of the procedure, as compared to traditional multi-port laparoscopic cholecystectomy, have been to achieve better cosmesis, decrease post-operative pain and obtain a faster recovery. So far, several reports have addressed outcomes and complication rates, reporting the safety and feasibility of the procedure, especially in well-selected patients.

The aim of this chapter is to describe preoperative preparation, the instrumentation, and procedure, as well as the outcomes and complication rates of laparoscopic single site cholecystectomy as compared to traditional multi-port laparoscopic cholecystectomy.

Preparation

Like any laparoscopic procedure, patient selection is the single most important factor in preparation for this procedure. Single site laparoscopic cholecystectomy has been performed for several gallbladder diseases. These include, but are not limited to: symptomatic cholelithiasis, gallbladder polyps, biliary dyskinesia, biliary pancreatitis, acute and chronic cholecystitis. In order to maintain the feasibility and safety of the procedure, many advocate excluding patients with a BMI$> 35m^2/kg$, history of pancreatitis, large gallstones, previous upper abdominal surgery, pregnancy and an ASA score of III/IV. We advocate that in the early surgeon's experience the inclusion criteria should simply be limited to patients without complicated biliary disease who would be suitable candidates for a laparoscopic cholecystectomy at an ambulatory surgical center.

The surgeon and his/her team should be highly experienced with the four port traditional laparoscopic cholecystectomy either using the American or the French technique [21,22]. The surgeon should also be familiar with the different instruments, ports, and camera systems available at his/her institution in order to prepare for the procedure. Training in simulators and/or animal models is highly recommended. Also, assisting and/or being supervised until surpassing the learning curve is encouraged, recognizing that surgeon's experience is the most significant factor associated with an adverse outcome in a laparoscopic cholecystectomy [23]. There is short learning curve for this procedure, which is believed to be about 20 cases and may be considered an estimate for safe adoption of the procedure in clinical practice [17].

Table 2. Exclusion criteria in reported series of single site laparoscopic cholecystectomies

Study	Exclusion critera
Bresadola [24]	Acute cholecystitis
Cuesta [9]	Acute cholecystitis
Rao [25]	Acute cholecystitis, history of pancreatitis
Binenbaum [26]	Acute and chronic cholecystitis
Dominguez [11]	Acute cholecystitis, pregnancy, implanted pacemaker
Dunning [27]	Acute cholecystitis, large gallstones
Hong [13]	Acute cholecystitis, complicated cholecystolithiasis, cirrhosis, peritonitis, previous upper abdominal surgery, severe obesity, high-risk for anesthesia
Kirschniak [14]	Acute cholecystitis, cholestasis
Kuon Lee [16]	Previous upper abdominal surgery, acute cholecystitis, suspicion of malignancy
Petrotos [28]	Acute cholecystitis
Roberts [18]	Pregnancy, ASA score III and IV
Schlager [20]	BMI 35 m2/kg, acute cholecystitis, elevated liver enzymes, ASA III and IV
Erbella [29]	Acute cholecystitis, biliary pancreatitis
Ersin [23]	Acute cholecystitis

Procedure

Single site laparoscopic cholecystectomy achieves better cosmesis, may decrease post-operative pain, and can lead to a faster recovery. The approach requires a 2 cm umbilical incision with multiple trocar insertions through a single incision site, and this has shown to be feasible even in obese patients. The initial cases in literature identified multiple problems, and thus required different modifications of technique and instrumentation. By entering all of the instruments through a single site, there is loss of triangulation and clashing of the instruments. But, using modified instruments with roticulating properties and angulated shafts, and ports with flat profiles, have allowed free play of the instruments despite their proximity to each other. Also, it is difficult for both the surgeon and assistant to work in the same area and the camera cable can interfere with the movement of the instruments. For this reason camera holders and/or flexible cameras have been used to make the procedure more comfortable. A broad variety of methods have been used to describe the approach to perform a single site laparoscopic cholecystectomy. Type and size of trocars as well as instruments and optics vary tremendously in the reported literature. All have one thing in common: they follow the same principles as a laparoscopic cholecystectomy in terms of safety and adequate gallbladder retraction to unmistakably expose Calot's triangle. The two most common differences in technique include gallbladder anchorage with percutaneous sutures or looped wire vs. using a roticulating or conventional grasper to suspend the gallbladder.

To perform a single site laparoscopic cholecystectomy we recommend following the steps described in the video publication *Totally Transumbilical Laparoscopic Cholecystectomy* [38].

Table 3. Number, size and type of trocars used in single site laparoscopic cholecystectomies

Study	No of trocars	Size and type of trocars
Navarra [5]	2	10 mm, 10 mm
Bresadola [24]	2	10 mm, 5 mm
Piskun [30]	2	5 mm, 5 mm
Cuesta [9]	2	5 mm, 5 mm
Rao [25]	1	Mutiport system (10 mm, 5 mm or 5 mm, 5 mm, 5 mm)
Binenbaum [26]	2	12 mm, 5 mm
Bucher [31]	1	12 mm
Chow [10]	2-3	12 mm, 5 mm, 5 mm
Dominguez [11]	1	12 mm
Dunning [27]	2	5 mm, 5 mm
Hernandez [12]	2	5 mm, 5 mm
Hong [13]	1	12 mm and 2 pipes through a surgical glove
Kirschniak [14]	3	5 mm, 5 mm, 5 mm
Kravetz [15]	1	Multiport system (12 mm, 5 mm, 5 mm)
Kuon Lee [16]	3	5 mm, 5 mm, 5 mm
Langwieler [32]	1	12 mm, 5 mm, 5 mm
Petrotos [28]	3	5 mm, 5 mm, 5 mm
Philipp [33]	2-3	NR
Rivas [17]	1-3	Multiport system or 5 mm
Roberts [18]	1 or 3	Multiport system or 5 mm, 5 mm, 5 mm
Romanelli [19]	1-3	Multiport system or 12 mm, 5 mm, 5 mm or 12 mm
Schlager [20]	1-3	15 mm or 5 mm, 5 mm, 5 mm
Tacchino [21]	3	NR
Vidal [34]	3	12 mm, 5 mm, 5 mm
Zhu [35]	3	5 mm, 3 mm, 3 mm
Brody [22]	3	5 mm, 5 mm, 5 mm
Curcillo [36]	3	5 mm, 5 mm, 5 mm
Erbella [29]	2	5 mm, 5 mm
Ersin [23]	3	5 mm, 5 mm, 5 mm
Gumbs [37]	4	Multiport system or 5 mm, 5 mm, 5 mm, 5 mm

NR Not reported.

Table 4. Instruments and optics used in single site laparoscopic cholecystectomies

Study	Instruments	Optics
Navarra [5]	Conventional	10 mm 0° or 30° Laparoscope
Bresadola [24]	Conventional	10 mm 30° Laparoscope
Piskun [30]	Conventional	5 mm 0° or 30° Laparoscope
Cuesta [9]	Conventional	5 mm 30° Laparoscope
Rao [25]	Roticulating	5 mm 30° Laparoscope
Binenbaum [26]	Roticulating	Laparoscope, gastroscope
Bucher [36]	Conventional	10 mm 0° Laparoscope with a 6 mm channel
Chow [10]	Roticulating	5 mm 30° Laparoscope
Dominguez [11]	Conventional	11 mm 0° Laparoscope with a 6 mm channel
Dunning [27]	Conventional	5 mm 0° and 5 mm 30° Laparoscope
Hernandez [12]	Roticulating	NR
Hong [13]	Conventional	5 mm 30° Laparoscope
Kirschniak [14]	Conventional	5 mm 30° Laparoscope
Kravetz [15]	Roticulating	5 mm 30° Laparoscope
Kuon Lee [16]	Roticulating	5 mm Laparoscope
Langwieler [32]	Conventional	5 mm 30° Laparoscope
Petrotos [28]	Roticulating	5 mm 30° Laparoscope
Philipp [33]	Conventional	5 mm Angulated or flexible-tip laparoscope
Rivas [17]	Conventional/roticulating	5 mm 30° Laparoscope or flexible endoscope
Roberts [18]	Roticulating	NR
Romanelli [19]	Roticulating	NR
Schlager [20]	Roticulating	Gastroscope or 5 mm 30° Laparoscope
Tacchino [21]	Roticulating	5 mm 30° Laparoscope
Vidal [34]	Roticulating	5 mm or 10 mm 30° Laparoscope
Zhu [35]	Conventional	5 mm 30° Laparoscope
Brody [22]	Conventional	5 mm 45° Laparoscope
Curcillo [37]	Conventional/roticulating	5 mm 30° Laparoscope
Erbella [29]	Roticulating	5 mm 0° Laparoscope
Ersin [23]	Roticulating	5 mm 30° Laparoscope
Gumbs [40]	Roticulating	Roticulating 5 mm Laparoscope

NR Not reported.

Following routine preoperative work up and anesthesia, the patient is placed in a supine position with both upper extremities abducted. Depending on the surgeon's comfort he or she stands on the left side of the patient vs. between the legs if using the French technique. Then, a 2 cm incision is made through the umbilicus and the fascia is exposed. Pneumoperitoneum is obtained and three separate 5 mm trocars are placed in separate fascial sites within the incision. The use of three separate fascial insertion points could create a problem with a gas leak. To avoid this, trocars should be placed more than 2mm apart. A gelport can also be used as described in *Laparoendoscopic Single-Site Cholecystectomy: Using a Gelport Device* [40]. In this approach a wound protector is placed after the fascia is opened. Then, three 5 mm trocars (one with a balloon tip for insufflation) are placed in the gelport. The working trocars are placed in a semilunar fashion at the inferior aspect of the gelport before mounting it onto the wound protector. An additional 4th trocar can also be placed at the superior aspect of the gelport.

A 5 mm deflecting/articulating laparoscope is used with a robotically controlled camera holder to improve visualization and surgeon's comfort. At least one roticulating instrument is used to avoid clashing of the instruments and/or blocking the view during the surgery.

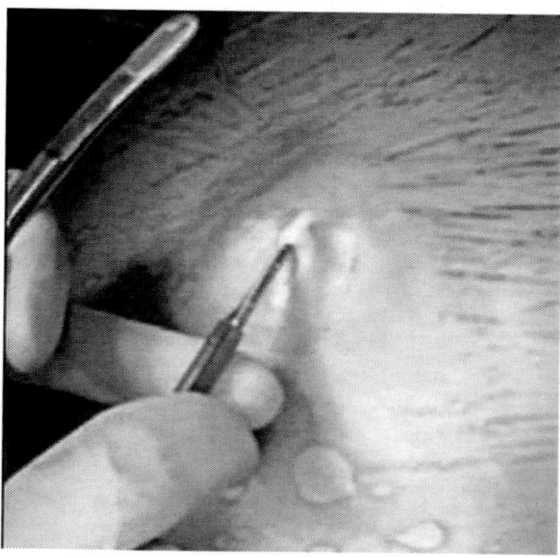

Figure 1. Umbilical skin incision.

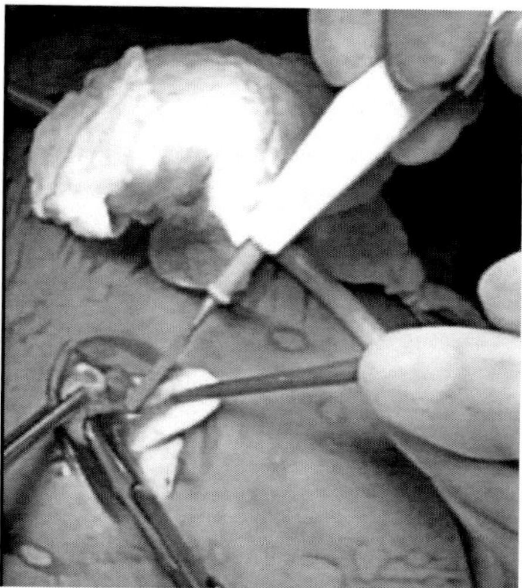

Figure 2. Dissection to expose umbilical area fascia.

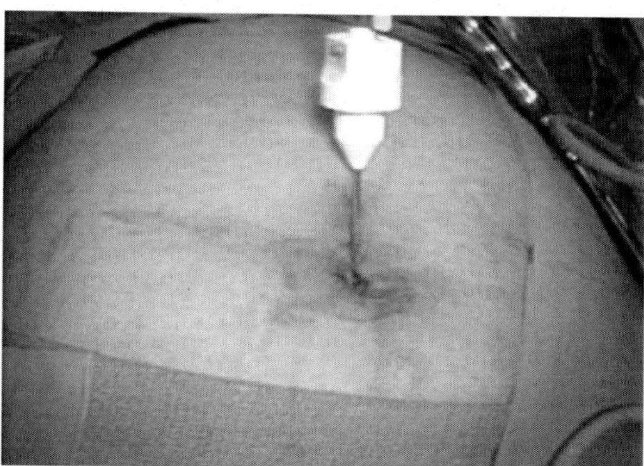

Figure 3. Insufflation of intrabdominal cavity.

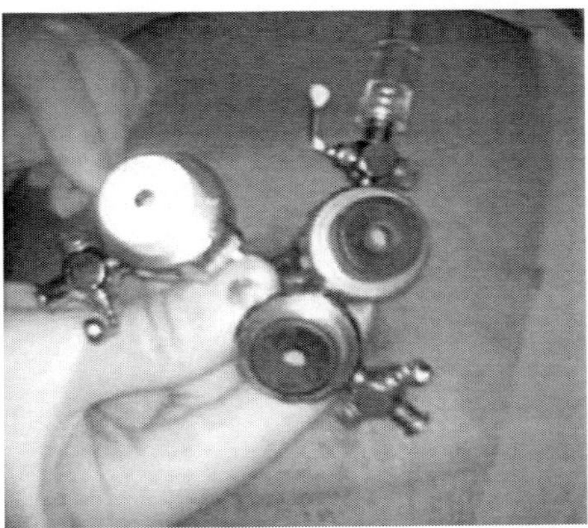

Figure 4. Insertion and positioning of trocars directly through umbilical fascia.

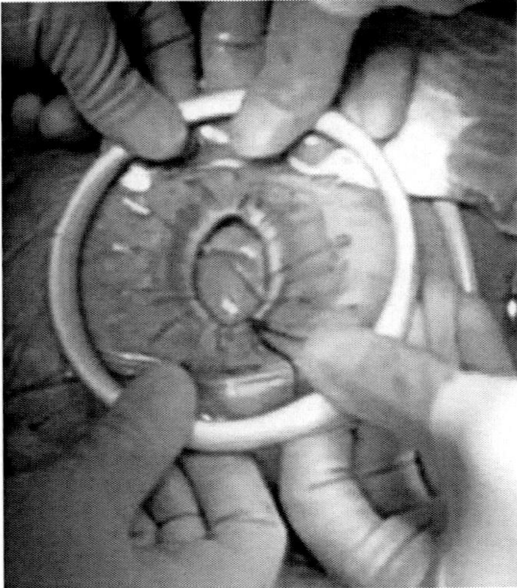

Figure 5. Wound protector placement after the umbilical fascia is opened.

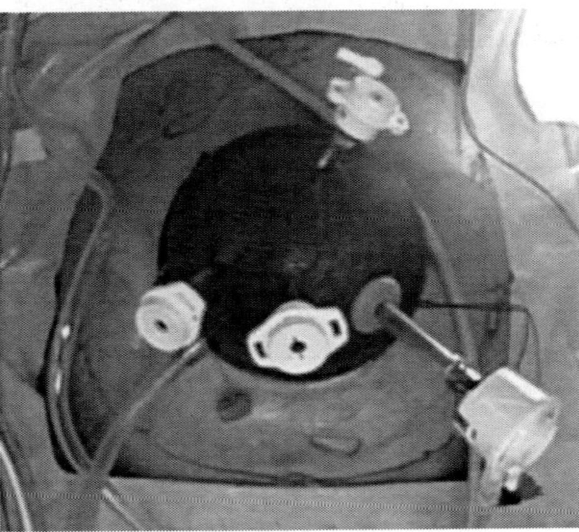

Figure 6. Placement of trocars in the gelport (Gelpoint, Applied Medical, Rancho Santa Magarita, CA). Three trocars are placed in a semilunar fashion inferiorly and an additional trocar is placed superiorly. Left inferior trocar with balloon tip is used for insufflation.

Angel M. Rodriguez and Andrew A. Gumbs

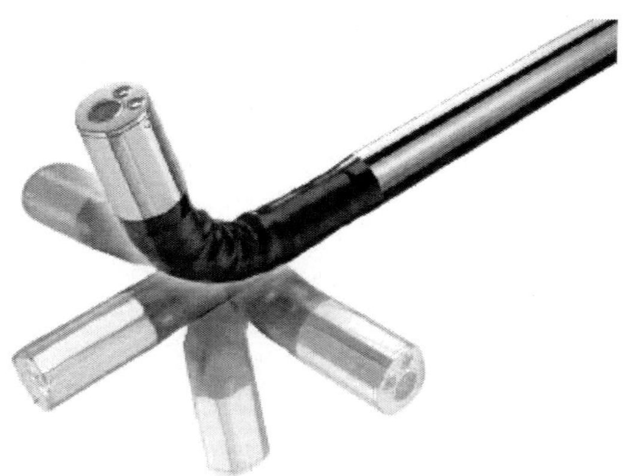

Figure 7. Five-millimeter deflectable tip video laparoscope (Olympus, Orangeburg, NY, USA).

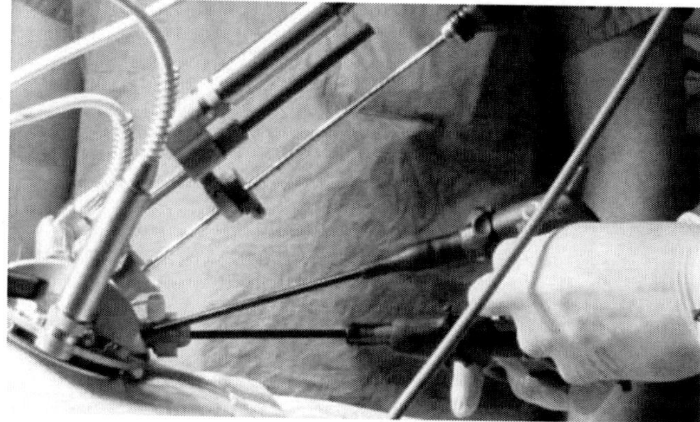

Figure 8. Camera holder system.

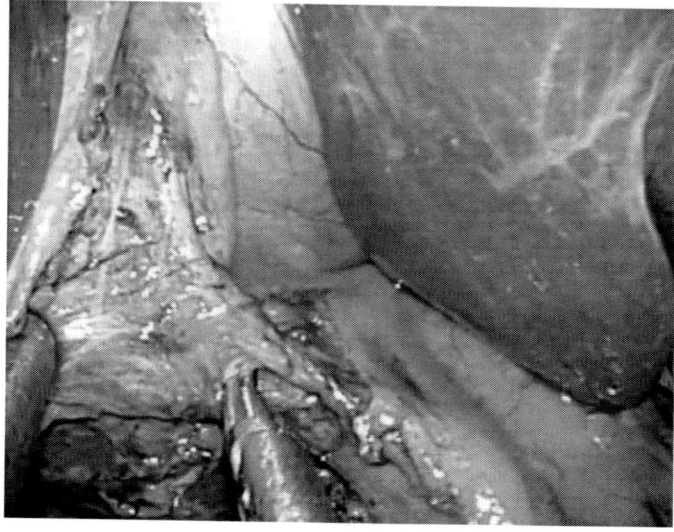

Figure 9. Laparoscopic dissection of cystic artery and duct.

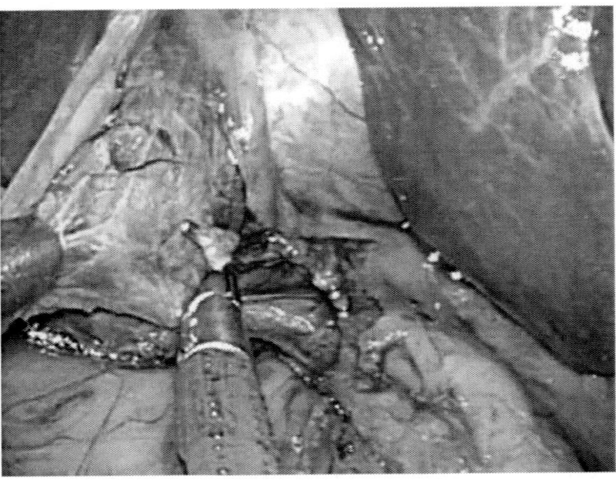

Figure 10. Laparoscopic dissection of cystic duct after clipping and transection of cystic artery.

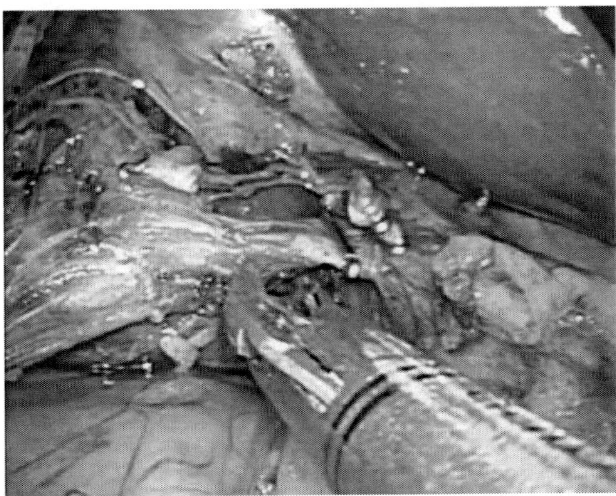

Figure 11. Clipping of cystic duct.

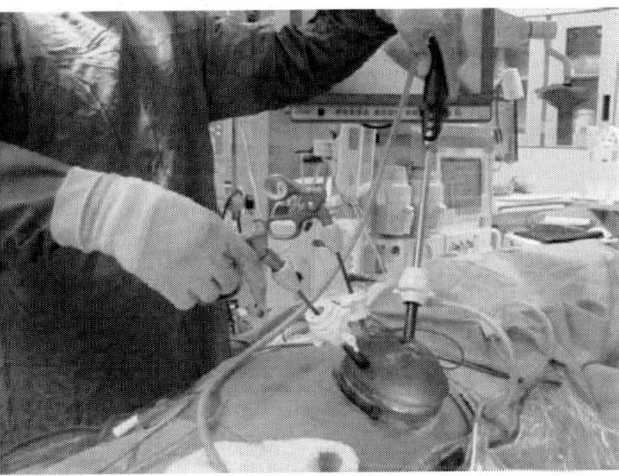

Figure 12. Triangulation using a gelport device. (Single-Incision Laparoscopic Takedown of a Hartmann's Colostomy [39]).

After the table has been positioned in reverse Trendelenburg with mild rotation to the patient's left side, the gallbladder is identified and retracted cephalad and laterally. The gallbladder should be grasped in a "sweet spot" that allows both adequate visualization of the Calot's triangle and retraction of the cystic duct off the common bile duct. If retraction is difficult with only one instrument, percutaneuos or internally fixated sutures can be used to help obtain an adequate view. A second instrument is then used to dissect and complete the procedure in a similar manner as a standard laparoscopic cholecystectomy, first dissecting the cystic duct and cystic artery, followed by clipping and transection of these structures. The gallbladder can be then dissected of the liver bed using electrocautery and placed in a specimen retrieval bag.

Even though intra-operative cholangiograms are not routinely done for every cholecystectomy, it is feasible to perform it with this technique if necessary. A cholangiogram catheter may be placed using one of the trocars within the umbilical incision or a separate right upper quadrant wound can be added without the need of a separate trocar.

Fascial incisions can be then interconnected or one of the trocars can be exchanged to a 12mm port to allow for the use and retrieval of the bag. Finally, the fascial and skin openings are closed with absorbable sutures.

Outcomes

When single site laparoscopic cholecystectomy was first described, the mean operative time was 123 min. and the mean length of stay was 1.8 days [5]. The original technique used three extracorporeal sutures and two working 10 mm ports. Once the procedure gained popularity, 5 mm and 3 mm ports were then adopted and roticulating and deflecting laparoscopes were employed to lessen the need of extracorporeal sutures and improve the exposure.

This technique significantly achieves better cosmesis and patient satisfaction by decreasing the wound length and hiding it in the umbilical region. It also possibly decreases post-operative pain, need for post-operative analgesia, length of stay, and lead to a faster recovery. Decreasing the number of ports during a multi-port cholecystectomy from 4 to 3 has significantly shown to decrease use of analgesics, length of stay, and number of days to return to normal daily activities [40]. However, with several scattered studies it has been difficult to prove these benefits when comparing single-site vs. multi-port laparoscopic cholecystectomy.

In a recent systematic review by Antoniou, et al. over 1100 single site laparoscopic cholecystectomies have been reported in the literature demonstrating the safety and feasibility of the procedure [41]. In this retrospective review success rate was found to be 90.7%, where the most common reason for technical failure was inadequate exposure of Calot's triangle due to inflammation, adhesions, or insufficient gallbladder retraction. The cumulative intra-operative complication rate was 2.7% with gallbladder perforation/bile spillage being the most common complication (2.2%) followed by hemorrhage (0.3%) and bile duct injury (0.1%). Postoperative complications included: wound infection and hematoma (2.1%), bile leak (0.4%) and choledocholithiasis (0.3%). The cumulative complication rate was 3.4%. Type of instrumentation did not affect success rate, operative time or morbidity. A mean age of <45 years, was reported to have significant (p=0.04) lower complication rate, whereas there was no difference in success rate and morbidity with regards to sex distribution and mean BMI. Cumulative mean operative time of 70 min and cumulative hospital stay of 1.4 days were also observed.

Several retrospective studies have been published reporting the safety of the single site laparoscopic cholecystectomy with no difference in complication rate and similar length of stay as compared to traditional multi-port laparoscopic cholecystectomy [12,34,42,43,44,45,46,47]. However, these studies have several limitations including selection bias with less ill patients in the single site group and/or randomly selected with no matched multi-port patients.

Table 5. Intraoperative and postoperative complication rates in single site laparoscopic cholecystectomies

Study	Intraoperative complication (%)	Postoperative complication (%)
Navarra [5]	0	0
Bresadola [24]	0	0
Piskun [30]	0	0
Cuesta [9]	10	0
Rao [25]	0	0
Binenbaum [26]	0	0
Bucher [31]	0	0
Chow [10]	0	7.1
Dominguez [11]	5	2.5
Dunning [27]	0	0
Hernandez [12]	1	1
Hong [13]	2.7	0
Kirschniak [14]	0	5.3
Kravetz [15]	0	0
Kuon Lee [16]	32.4	0
Langwieler [32]	0	0
Petrotos [28]	20	0
Philipp [33]	0	20.1
Rivas [17]	0	1
Roberts [18]	0	5.4
Romanelli [19]	0	4.5
Schlager [20]	0	5
Tacchino [21]	0	16.7
Vidal [34]	0	0
Zhu [35]	1	0
Brody [22]	1.7	1.7
Curcillo [36]	2.4	6.7
Erbella [29]	1	0
Ersin [23]	0	0
Gumbs [40]	5	5

Table 6. Mean operative time and mean hospital stay in single site laparoscopic cholecystectomies

Study	Mean operative time (min)	Mean hospital stay (days)
Navarra [5]	123	1.8
Bresadola [24]	94	NR
Piskun [30]	NR	1
Cuesta [9]	70	<1
Rao [25]	40	1
Binenbaum [26]	149.5	<1
Bucher [31]	52 (median)	<1 (median)
Chow [10]	142.9	<1
Dominguez [11]	93	NR
Hernandez [12]	72	1
Hong [13]	79	1.6
Kirschniak [14]	67.1	4.4
Kravetz [15]	73.1	1.2
Kuon Lee [16]	83.6	2.7
Petrotos [28]	85 (median)	1
Philipp [33]	85 (median)	0 (median)
Rivas [17]	50.8	NR
Roberts [18]	80	0.3
Romanelli [19]	80.8	NR
Schlager [20]	136	NR
Vidal [34]	62	<1
Zhu [35]	62	2
Brody [22]	92.6	1.2
Curcillo [36]	71	1.5
Erbella [29]	30	1
Ersin [23]	94	1
Gumbs [40]	81	<1

NR Not reported.

To eliminate selection bias, several randomized controlled trials have been performed in which patients underwent either single site or multi-port cholecystectomy. In a recent systematic review and meta-analysis of these controlled studies, seven were selected to evaluate postoperative complications, postoperative pain, operative time and length of stay of single site laparoscopic cholecystectomy as compared to multi-port cholecystectomy [48]. There were 20 (10.3%) complications in the single site group and 16 (8.9%) complications in the multi-port group with no statistical difference between the groups (p=0.81). There was also no difference in postoperative pain (p=0.42, 6-24h after surgery) or length of stay (p=0.25). Operative time was significantly longer in the single site group compared to the multi-port group (weighted mean difference = 2.13, p=0.0001), with many advocating lower operative times as experience increased.

Laparoscopic single site cholecystectomy is safe and feasible in most cases of uncomplicated gallbladder disease, rarely requiring additional ports. When performing the procedure in complicated and/or high risk patients one should have a low threshold for additional ports and/or conversion to a traditional four-port cholecystectomy to maintain the safety of the procedure. Intra-operative cholangiogram can be easily implemented as necessary by using one of the ports in the umbilical incision or using a separate stab wound in the right upper quadrant.

Being cosmetically superior with only few simple modifications, this technique offers an alternative to NOTES being a more reasonable step for today's surgeon not requiring opening hollow organs and avoiding complications related to visceral closure. It can be easily performed with standard laparoscopic instruments and requires only the techniques that are necessary for a multi-port laparoscopic cholecystectomy.

The procedure is rapidly gaining attraction among patients and surgeons, and is very likely that it will be in demand the same way that multi-port laparoscopic cholecystectomy was a few decades ago.

References

[1] vanGulik TM. Langenbuch's cholecystectomy, once a remarkably controversial operation. *Neth J Surg.* 1986;38:13841.

[2] Reynolds W. The first laparoscopic cholecystectomy. *JSLS.* 2001;5:89 –94.

[3] National Institutes of Health, Consensus Development Conference. Gallstones and laparoscopic cholecystectomy. *NIH Consens Statement.* 1992;10:1–28.

[4] Gumbs AA, Rodriguez Rivera AM, Matteotti R and Hoffmam JP: Cancer of the hepato-biliary system, gallbladder and extrahepatic ducts. *Minimally Invasive Surgical Oncology – State of the art cancer management.* 2011;1(6), 297-308.

[5] Navarra G, Pozza E, Occhionorelli S, Carcoforo P, Donini I. One-wound laparoscopic cholecystectomy. *Br J Surg.* 1997;84:695.

[6] Cuesta MA, Berends F, Veenhof AA. The "invisible cholecystectomy": a transumbilical laparoscopic operation without a scar. *Surg Endosc.* 2008;22:1211–1213.

[7] Chow A, Purkayastha S, Paraskeva P. Appendicectomy and cholecystectomy using single-incision laparoscopic surgery (SILS): the first UK experience. *Surg Innov.* 2009;16:211–217.

[8] Dominguez G, Durand L, De Rosa J, Danguise E, Arozamena C, Ferraina PA. Retraction and triangulation with neodymium magnetic forceps for single-port laparoscopic cholecystectomy. *Surg Endosc.* 2009;23:1660–1666.

[9] Hernandez JM, Morton CA, Ross S, Albrink M, Rosemurgy AS. Laparoendoscopic single site cholecystectomy: the first 100 patients. *Am Surg.* 2009;75:681–685.

[10] Hong TH, You YK, Lee KH. Transumbilical single-port laparoscopic cholecystectomy—scarless cholecystectomy. *Surg Endosc.* 2009;23:1393–1397.

[11] Kirschniak A, Bollmann S, Pointner R, Granderath FA. Transumbilical single-incision laparoscopic cholecystectomy:preliminary experiences. *Surg Laparosc Endosc Percutan Tech.* 2009;19:436–438.

[12] Kravetz AJ, Iddings D, Basson MD, Kia MA. The learning curve with single-port cholecystectomy. *JSLS.* 2009;13:332–336.

[13] Kuon Lee S, You YK, Park JH, Kim HJ, Lee KK, Kim DG. Single-port transumbilical laparoscopic cholecystectomy: a preliminary study in 37 patients with gallbladder disease. *J Laparoendosc Adv Surg Tech A.* 2009;19:495–499.

[14] Rivas H, Varela E, Scott D. Single-incision laparoscopic cholecystectomy: initial evaluation of a large series of patients. *Surg Endosc.* 2009;24(6):1403-1412.

[15] Roberts KE, Solomon D, Duffy AJ, Bell RL. Single-incision laparoscopic cholecystectomy: a surgeon's initial experience with 56 consecutive cases and a review of the literature. *J Gastrointest Surg.* 2009;14(3):506-510.

[16] Romanelli JR, Roshek TB 3rd, Lynn DC, Earle DB. Single-port laparoscopic cholecystectomy: initial experience. *Surg Endosc.* 2009;24(6):1374-1379.

[17] Schlager A, Khalaileh A, Shussman N, Elazary R, Keidar A, Pikarsky AJ, Ben-Shushan A, Shibolet O, Horgan S, Talamini M, Zamir G, Rivkind AI, Mintz Y. Providing more through less: current methods of retraction in SIMIS and NOTES cholecystectomy. *Surg Endosc.* 2009;24(7):1542-1546.

[18] Tacchino R, Greco F, Matera D. Single-incision laparoscopic cholecystectomy: surgery without a visible scar. *Surg Endosc.* 2009;23:896–899.

[19] Brody F, Vaziri K, Kasza J, Edwards C. Single incision laparoscopic cholecystectomy. *J Am Coll Surg.* 2010;210(2):e9-e13.

[20] Ersin S, Firat O, Sozbilen M. Single-incision laparoscopic cholecystectomy: is it more than a challenge? *Surg Endosc.* 2010;24:68–71.

[21] Cuschieri A, Dubois F, Mouiel J, Mouret P, et at. The European experience with laparoscopic cholecystectomy. *Ann J Surg.* 1991;161:385-7.

[22] Begos DG, Modlin IM. LC: from gimmick to gold standard. *J Clin Gast.* 1994;19(4):325-30.

[23] Moore MJ, Bennett CL. The learning curve for laparoscopic cholecystectomy. The Southern Surgeons Club. *Am J Surg.* 1995;170:55-59.

[24] Bresadola F, Pasqualucci A, Donini A, Chiarandini P, Anania G, Terrosu G, Sistu MA, Pasetto A. Elective transumbilical compared with standard laparoscopic cholecystectomy. *Eur J Surg.* 1999;165:29–34.

[25] Rao PP, Bhagwat SM, Rane A, Rao PP. The feasibility of single port laparoscopic cholecystectomy: a pilot study of 20 cases. *HPB.* 2008;10:336–340.

[26] Binenbaum SJ, Teixeira JA, Forrester GJ, Harvey EJ, Afthinos J, Kim GJ, Koshy N, McGinty J, Belsley SJ, Todd GJ. Single-incision laparoscopic cholecystectomy using a flexible endoscope. *Arch Surg.* 2009;144:734–738.

[27] Dunning K, Kohli H. Transumbilical laparoscopic cholecystectomy: a novel technique. *Arch Surg.* 2009;144:957–960.

[28] Petrotos AC, Molinelli BM. Single-incision multiport laparoendoscopic (SIMPLE) surgery: early evaluation of SIMPLE cholecystectomy in a community setting. *Surg Endosc.* 2009;23(11):2631-2634.

[29] Erbella J Jr, Bunch GM. Single-incision laparoscopic cholecystectomy: the first 100 outpatients. *Surg Endosc.* 2010;24(8):1958-1961.

[30] Piskun J, Rajpal S. Transumbilical laparoscopic cholecystectomy utilizes no incisions outside the umbilicus. *J Laparoendosc Adv Surg Tech.* 1999;9:361–364.

[31] Bucher P, Pugin F, Buchs N, Ostermann S, Charara F, Morel P. Single port access laparoscopic cholecystectomy (with video). *World J Surg.* 2009;33:1015–1019

[32] Langwieler TE, Nimmesgern T, Back M. Singleport access in laparoscopic cholecystectomy. *Surg Endosc.* 2009;23:1138–1141.

[33] Philipp SR, Miedema BW, Thaler K. Single-incision laparoscopic cholecystectomy using conventional instruments: early experience in comparison with the gold standard. *J Am Coll Surg.* 2009;209:632–637.

[34] Vidal O, Valentini M, Espert JJ, Ginesta C, Jimeno J, Martinez A, Benarroch G, Garcia-Valdecasas JC. Laparoendoscopic single-site cholecystectomy: a safe and reproducible alternative. *J Laparoendosc Adv Surg Tech A.* 2009;19:599–602.

[35] Zhu JF, Hu H, Ma YZ, Xu MZ. Totally transumbilical endoscopic cholecystectomy without visible abdominal scar using improved instruments. *Surg Endosc.* 2009;23:1781–1784.

[36] Curcillo PG II, Wu AS, Podolsky ER, Graybeal C, Katkhouda N, Saenz A, Dunham R, Fendley S, Neff M, Copper C, Bessler M, Gumbs AA, Norton M, Iannelli A, Mason R, Moazzez A, Cohen L, Mouhlas A, Poor A. Single-port-access (SPA(TM)) cholecystectomy: a multi-institutional report of the first 297 cases. *Surg Endosc.* 2010;24(8):1854-60.

[37] Gumbs AA, Rassi ZE, Chouilliard EK. Laparoendoscopic single-site cholecystectomy: using a gelport device. *Surg Laparosc Endosc Percutan Tech.* 2011;21(6):e306-7.

[38] Gumbs AA, Milone L, Sinha P and Bessler M. Totally Transumbilical Laparoscopic Cholecystectomy. *J Gastrointest Surg.* 2009;13:533-534.

[39] Tsai T, Siripurapu V, Gumbs AA. Single-Incision Laparoscopic Takedown of a Hartmann's Colostomy. *J Laparoendosc Adv Surg Tech Part B Videoscopy.* 2011;21.

[40] Osborne D, Boe B, Rosemurgy AS, Zervos EE. Twenty-millimiter laparoscopic cholecystectomy: fewer ports results in less pain, shorter hospitalization, and faster recovery. *Am Surg.* 2005;71:298-302.

[41] Antoniou SA, Pointner R and Granderath FA. Single-incision laparoscopic cholecystectomy: a systematic review. *Surg Endosc.* 2011;25:367–377.

[42] Hodgett ST, Hernandez JM, Morton CA, Ross SB, Albrink M, Rosemurgy AS. Laparoendoscopic single site (LESS) cholecystectomy. *J Gastrointest Surg.* 2009;13:188–192.

[43] Khambaty F, Brody F, Vaziri K, Edwards C. Laparoscopic versus single-incision cholecystectomy. *World J Surg.* 2011;35(5):967–972.

[44] Chang SK, Tay CW, Bicol RA, Lee YY, Madhavan K. A case–control study of single-incision versus standard laparoscopic cholecystectomy. *World J Surg.* 2011: 35(2):289–293.

[45] Prasad A, Mukherjee KA, Kaul S, Kaur M. Postoperative pain after cholecystectomy: conventional laparoscopy versus single-incision laparoscopic surgery. *J Minim Access Surg.* 2010;7(1):24–27.

[46] Fronza JS, Linn JG, Nagle AP, Soper NJ. A single institution's experience with single incision cholecystectomy compared to standard laparoscopic cholecystectomy. *Surgery.* 2010;148(4):731–734.

[47] Tsimoyiannis EC, Tsimogiannis KE, Pappas-Gogos G, Farantos C, Benetatos N, Mavridou P, Manataki A. Different pain scores in single transumbilical incision laparoscopic cholecystectomy versus classic laparoscopic cholecystectomy: a randomized controlled trial. *Surg Endosc.* 2010;24(8):1842–1848.

[48] Markar SR, Karthikesalingam A, Thrumurthy, et al. Single-incision laparoscopic surgery (SILS) vs. conventional multiport cholecystectomy: systematic review and meta-analysis. *Surg Endosc.* 2012;26:1205-1213.

Index

J

L